D0780519

Managing Health

Nancy M. Kane
Nancy C. Turnbull

Managing Health
An International Perspective

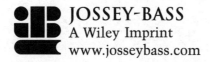

JOSSEY-BASS
A Wiley Imprint
www.josseybass.com

Copyright © 2003 by Nancy M. Kane and Nancy C. Turnbull. All rights reserved.

Published by Jossey-Bass
A Wiley Imprint
989 Market Street, San Francisco, CA 94103-1741   www.josseybass.com

No part of this publication may be reproduced, stored in a retrieval system, or transmitted in any form or by any means, electronic, mechanical, photocopying, recording, scanning, or otherwise, except as permitted under Section 107 or 108 of the 1976 United States Copyright Act, without either the prior written permission of the Publisher, or authorization through payment of the appropriate per-copy fee to the Copyright Clearance Center, Inc., 222 Rosewood Drive, Danvers, MA 01923, 978-750-8400, fax 978-750-4470, or on the web at www.copyright.com. Requests to the Publisher for permission should be addressed to the Permissions Department, John Wiley & Sons, Inc., 111 River Street, Hoboken, NJ 07030, 201-748-6011, fax 201-748-6008, e-mail: permcoordinator@wiley.com.

Jossey-Bass books and products are available through most bookstores. To contact Jossey-Bass directly call our Customer Care Department within the U.S. at 800-956-7739, outside the U.S. at 317-572-3986 or fax 317-572-4002.

Jossey-Bass also publishes its books in a variety of electronic formats. Some content that appears in print may not be available in electronic books.

Library of Congress Cataloging-in-Publication Data

Kane, Nancy M.
    Managing health : an international perspective / Nancy M. Kane and
    Nancy C. Turnbull.— 1st ed.
        p. ; cm.
    Includes bibliographical references and index.
    ISBN 0-7879-6899-4 (alk. paper)
    1. Health services administration—Case studies. 2. Public health administration—Case studies. 3. Managed care plans (Medical care)—Case studies. 4. Health facilities—Administration—Case studies.
    [DNLM: 1. Managed Care Programs—economics. 2. Cross-Cultural Comparison. 3. Organizational Case Studies. 4. Quality of Health Care. W 130.1 K16m 2003]
        I. Turnbull, Nancy C. II. Title.
    RA971.K325 2003
    362.1'068—dc21
                                                            2003006248

Printed in the United States of America
FIRST EDITION
HB Printing   10 9 8 7 6 5 4 3 2 1

~~~ Contents

——— Tables, Figures, and Exhibits

TABLES

FIGURES

EXHIBITS

This book is dedicated to our families, who put up with our extended absences in faraway places with grace and good humor.

~~~ Acknowledgments

We especially wish to thank Tim Donohue, who arranged many interviews, trips, and conferences, sponsors, and publishers. Without Tim, this book would not have been possible. Special recognition as well goes to Mary Jane Nappi, whose cheerful voice and professionalism kept us calm and moving in the right direction no matter where in the world we were.

The financial and intellectual support of Astra Zeneca and the former Astra USA were essential to our work on this book. Special thanks to Bradley Fleahman and Nancy Featherstone, whose vision and willingness to take a chance made a big difference.

Debts of gratitude are also owed to all those who sponsored and facilitated our cases and epilogues, including Carlos Felipe of Astra-Zeneca Brazil, Jie Chen and Ying Yao Chen of Shanghai Medical University, Sabine Richard of the German sickness fund BKK, David Colin-Thome of Castlefields Health Center and the British National Health Service, Andrzej Rys of Jagiellonian University and the Polish Ministry of Health, Paul Campbell of Harvard University School of Public Health, George Isham and Maureen Peterson of HealthPartners, William Hoffman and Charles Gayney of the United Auto Workers, Gene Clayton of Westinghouse, Roberta Herman of Harvard Pilgrim Health Care, John Ludden, Susan Moore, Kate K. Willrich, and Diane Flanders of the Massachusetts Division of Medical Assistance.

We are also indebted to the dozens of individuals who agreed to be interviewed for the cases presented in each chapter. The interviews were made possible by the professional services of translators in China, Poland, Germany, and Brazil, several of whom also provided personal stories and impromptu tours that greatly enriched our cultural appreciation of these countries.

For their assistance in writing cases and teaching notes, we appreciate the professional assistance provided by Kirin Verma and Ingrid

Nembhard. Thanks to Margot Kane for her able assistance with references and tables.

Thank you to Andrew Pasternack and Seth Schwartz of Jossey-Bass, who displayed incredible patience and were always ready to help. We also thank Hilary Powers, whose careful editing improved our writing and educated us about some of the finer points of the English language.

⁓ The Authors

Nancy M. Kane is a professor of management at the Harvard School of Public Health. She teaches in executive and master's degree programs in the areas of accounting, financial analysis, and competitive strategy. Her research interests include measuring hospital financial performance, quantifying community benefits and the value of tax exemption, and global applications of managed care concepts.

Kane earned her master's and doctoral degrees in business administration from Harvard Business School.

Nancy C. Turnbull is a lecturer in health policy at the Harvard School of Public Health. She teaches in executive and master's degree programs in the areas of managed care policy and provider payment systems. Her research interests include regulation of health insurers, access to health insurance, and global applications of managed care concepts.

Turnbull earned her MBA from the Wharton School of the University of Pennsylvania.

Managing Health

CHAPTER ONE

The Practicalities of Managing Cost, Care, and Health

Teaching Cases from Six Countries

—◦◦◦—

he eleven teaching cases in this book are intended to provide students of health care systems with an international perspective on tools and mechanisms commonly employed to make health care affordable and high quality, and on the practicalities of using those tools in a range of international health settings. Our major purpose is to focus on the challenges of implementation in order to encourage a deeper understanding of variations among health systems, and to stimulate debate on what works, what does not work, and why.

In the United States, many of these mechanisms fall under the rubric of *managed care,* while other countries use terms such as *general practitioner fundholding, primary care trusts, practice networks, indicative budgets, gatekeepers,* and *list of essential drugs.* Regardless of terminology, all these mechanisms are used to accomplish the same goals: to contain costs at affordable levels, improve quality and access, and advance the health of populations—enrollees, communities, or whole countries.

The advent of the new millennium witnessed the continuation of a prolonged backlash against managed care in the United States,

1

evident in both public policy and popular culture. This backlash has, to varying degrees, constrained the ability, and sometimes the willingness, of managed care plans and many purchasers in the United States to use certain managed care techniques as vigorously as in the past. However, many of the tools and techniques of managed care—selecting provider networks, establishing drug formularies, negotiating prices between purchasers and providers, adopting provider payment methods that share financial accountability with providers, implementing disease management programs, providing health education and disease prevention programs—are in use in countries around the world. Even the managed care backlash has not eliminated the presence or the need for managed care in the United States; in fact, managed care mechanisms may be needed more now than ever before as the U.S. population ages and develops more chronic conditions needing long-term management. Modern-day epidemics of obesity, substance abuse, and depression require behavioral, social, and educational interventions that can be coordinated with medical solutions and targeted to at-risk populations. By looking at how several countries approach these challenges, we believe the United States might come up with more effective solutions for its own problems.

TREND TOWARD DECENTRALIZED FINANCING AND COMPETITIVE PROVIDER SYSTEMS

The adoption of managed care mechanisms to control costs and to improve care and health goes hand in hand with the trend toward decentralization of health financing, splitting the roles of purchaser and provider, and efforts to increase responsiveness of health systems to consumer demands. In countries where all providers are government-owned or employed and government is the sole source of financing, it is difficult to implement an arm's-length price negotiation between purchaser and providers, or a network selection process that leaves out some providers. In such systems, an internal budgetary process controls prices and utilization of services, and government policy determines what services are provided and who is covered under the government financing scheme.

However, many countries are abandoning centralized, government-financed, government-owned health delivery systems, and instead seeking ways to make providers both independent and more accountable for the cost and quality of their services. Some countries are also allowing private sector or quasi-governmental insurance plans to supplement or replace the central government as a financing agent. These decentralized financing agents may try to harness competition among providers (for contracts or for patients) as a lever for encouraging responsive behavior by providers. The competition may be driven primarily by demands of purchasers (which may be governments or private insurers) or by consumers of health services, depending on the extent and nature of consumer choice possible in a particular health delivery system.

Managing Cost, Managing Care, Managing Health

Part of the backlash to managed care in the United States is related to the gap between what advocates of managed care promised and what managed care has actually delivered to date. These promises are viewed categorically in this book as managing *cost*, managing *care*, and managing *health*. As our cases illustrate, an overemphasis on managing cost, or alternatively, an underemphasis on managing care or health, contributes to hostility toward managed care and skepticism about its potential to improve health system performance. Sometimes the competitive conditions that facilitate the successful management of costs are counterproductive to the cooperative environment necessary to successfully manage care and health.

Managing cost involves three general undertakings, which are facilitated by the use of competitive forces among payers and providers:

- *Managing insurance risk:* This involves activities such as benefit design (what services will be covered), underwriting policies (who will be covered and under what terms and conditions), product pricing, and marketing strategy.
- *Managing provider and supplier prices:* This is accomplished by developing networks of providers, negotiating for price discounts or rebates (often in exchange for promises of increased numbers of patients), and adopting drug formularies or preferred drug lists based on price discounts.
- *Managing utilization of services:* This is accomplished by the use of techniques such as prior authorization of services, concurrent review, provider financial incentives, and consumer cost sharing.

Managing care involves cooperation between purchasers and providers, along with coordination or integration of efforts to deliver health services more effectively. Although competition might create incentives for better management of care, it can also interfere with efforts at cooperation and integration. Managing *care* involves activities such as the following:

- Developing and implementing community-wide practice guidelines or protocols for prevention or treatment of specific conditions, and the monitoring and evaluation of outcomes
- Care pathways, usually for management of acute care episodes
- Case management, to coordinate the care of patients with high-cost conditions to improve continuity and quality across multiple care settings
- Disease management across the continuum of care, potentially shifting resources from institutional to community-based sites, inpatient to ambulatory sites, and acute to long-term sites

Managing health is a third dimension of managed care, and the hardest to achieve, particularly in highly competitive and decentralized delivery systems. It involves such activities as these:

- Population-based interventions, including risk assessment, outreach, interventions (counseling, education, and behavioral and environmental modifications), monitoring, evaluation, and follow-up
- Pooling or shifting of resources among health, social services, housing, education, transportation, and other sectors to address the causes of poor health

The Practicalities of Managing Cost, Care, and Health

The relative success that any country experiences in implementing and using the tools of managed care is greatly affected by six features of its health care system:

- Level of system funding
- Structure of the provider market
- Proportion of population covered by health insurance

• Information and communication systems infrastructure
• Consumer expectations
• Sociopolitical values

LEVEL OF FUNDING. Countries with relatively low overall levels of health system funding generally have less political will and ability to invest in the administrative and managerial infrastructure needed to manage cost, care, or health. Managing care requires diverting financial resources from direct provision of services to more active management of those services: patient registration; provider contracting; collecting, processing, and disseminating information; designing and implementing interventions; and monitoring and follow-up activities.

The six countries in our cases represent a wide range in terms of the percentage of gross domestic product (GDP) absorbed by health expenditures, from China (3–4 percent), Poland and England (6–7 percent), and Brazil (8 percent) to Germany (10–11 percent) and the United States (13–14 percent). The resistance to investing in administrative infrastructure is understandably highest in the countries with the lowest levels of health spending. Some sample quotes from our cases illustrate the nature of the challenge:

"But there would be tensions if we devoted more of our resources to administrative costs and managing care instead of providing medical services."
—*Shanghai Medical Insurance Bureau official,
from Chapter Two*

The PCGs [primary care groups that would manage care] are a classic English administrative concept—no staff, no budgets, and no power. They are at an early stage of development, spending more time bickering about fees for management services than clinical initiatives. But the GPs [general practitioners] do not see the value in what the health authority does. We ran seminars to try to educate doctors about what we do but they did not come. They don't understand or value administration and bureaucracy.
—*A National Health Service officer in England,
from Chapter Twelve*

In Brazil, where almost 8 percent of GDP is spent on health care, observers disagree as to whether the system is underfunded or just poorly managed.

In the late 1990s, the World Bank Operations Evaluation Department conducted a study of the Brazilian health system that identified four problems in the health sector:

- Severe underfinancing of the public system, resulting in regional inequalities and a perceived decline in quality
- Weak incentives for cost-effectiveness and quality
- Tension between decentralization and maintaining the quality of care
- Overemphasis on curative services. . . .

But many officials reject the idea that lack of money is the major issue in the SUS [the Brazilian public health system]. "We have other sectors in Brazil without lots of money and they work quite well," said one federal official. "The problem in Brazil with health care is not the level of the spending but the quality of the spending. There is lots of corruption, waste, and mismanagement in the health system."

—*From Chapter Four*

Clearly, a major challenge to managing care is balancing the desire for a more professionally managed health system with the realities of political, managerial, and budgetary feasibility. Lower levels of health spending are associated with greater reluctance to invest in the managerial infrastructure needed to manage care.

PROVIDER MARKET STRUCTURE. The structure of provider markets, as well as consumer perceptions of provider services (particularly those of physicians), is influential in the design and relative success of managed care mechanisms. A provider market dominated by multi-specialty physician group practices with strong medical leadership enhances the potential of managed care to achieve its goals. Both availability of and consumer respect for primary care practitioners exert a significant influence as well.

Our cases provide examples of markets with very different provider structures. For instance, in our Twin Cities case (Chapter Nine), the ability to establish evidence-based protocols covering a large percentage of medical care for the entire metropolitan area was greatly enhanced by a physician market structure dominated by very large medical group practices.

The mission of ICSI [a physician-managed organization that designs evidence-based medical protocols and monitors compliance community-wide] is to "champion the cause of health care quality and to accelerate improvement in the value of the health care we deliver." ICSI provides health care improvement services to seventeen participating medical groups affiliated with HealthPartners [a local managed care plan]. Most of the groups are multi-specialty practices and range in size from fourteen practitioners to more than a thousand physicians. The combined medical groups represent nearly twenty-five hundred doctors. All but two of the large medical groups in the Twin Cities metropolitan area are members of ICSI. HealthPartners and BHCAG [another health insurer] accept membership in ICSI as meeting their requirements for continual improvement processes and accept ICSI guidelines.

—From Chapter Nine

Besides being amenable to community-wide protocols, large multi-specialty group practices facilitate standardization of internally developed disease management programs:

"The structure and culture of the health centers [large multi-specialty group practices] make it much easier in most ways to do disease management," observed one clinician. "The doctors are all in one place, so you can do centralized education, and the chiefs can require people to attend. The asthma nurses are on site, so they get to know the nurses and the case managers, and it becomes second nature to refer patients to the program. . . . And although the doctors have no financial incentive to be innovative, because they are salaried, there is peer pressure and a culture of excellence. All in all, it's easy in the health center to get people to do the right thing in terms of asthma care."

—From Chapter Seven

In contrast, a physician market structure dominated by solo and small, single-specialty group practices makes managing care much more difficult:

"Disease management makes sense for managed care plans, because they care for large populations of members. But physicians don't think of themselves as caring for populations—they care for individual patients. Physicians get excited about improving the quality of care, but you have to approach them with a patient-centered not population-centered approach. And the program has got to make life easier for the doctors. Adhering to practice guidelines may be easy in settings where there are computerized practice guidelines and reminders for physicians. But we are very low-tech in my practice—and it would take a huge investment to develop the necessary infrastructure. I don't hear any of the HMOs willing to help us with that investment. Instead, a lot of the information we get from them is outdated, or incomplete and not very helpful."

—*A primary care physician in a four-person practice,*
contracting with Harvard Pilgrim and other
health plans, from Chapter Seven

The challenge for the English National Health System, which is seeking to create a "primary-care-driven system," will be to change what has been a tradition of solo-practice GPs into "care managers" across a broad spectrum of health services. A sample quote from our case illustrates the problem:

"Most GPs did not go into medicine to have to worry about how to make decisions about spending limited amounts of money. . . . GPs are very insular about things—they face toward their patients, not the system as a whole. Personal medical services and public health are not the same. GPs are not experts in public health. GPs are not good at meeting public health and population health needs—they are experts at anatomy and physiology and individual ill health. They don't have the skills or outlook to think about public health—they run small businesses."

—*A National Health Service official, from Chapter Twelve*

Some health systems simply do not have primary care capacity. They tend to have many specialists, few primary care practitioners, and inadequate methods of communicating among providers of care. In Brazil, for example, the government has begun to foster a small but growing primary practice sector:

"General practice is not high status and is badly paid, so most physicians specialize. But the government is finding out that GPs are cheaper so we are undertaking efforts to promote the development of GPs."

—*Government official in Brazil's Ministry of Health,*
from Chapter Four

A similar problem has affected Poland's ability to manage care:

Overspecialization of physicians is also a problem in Poland, with a ratio of specialists to primary care providers of 3:1. "Primary care is very low stature and poorly paid," said one official. "Patients want to see specialists." Although primary care doctors are supposed to operate as gatekeepers to specialty care, they are regularly bypassed by patients who go directly to specialists, whom they perceive to be better trained and have better resources. Even when patients do initially see a primary care doctor, most primary care visits end in a referral to a specialist.

—*From Chapter Five*

Germany has one of the least conducive provider market structures for managing care:

Strict financial and structural divisions separate the different sectors of the German health system, and German providers have little history of cooperation or coordination of care. In particular, there is a strict separation between ambulatory physicians, who are private contractors and practice mainly in solo or two-person offices, and hospital-based physicians, who are salaried employees of the hospitals. . . . This separation . . . has resulted in serious problems of coordination and quality, including lack of communication among physicians and widespread duplication of tests by hospital doctors.

—*From Chapter Six*

PROPORTION OF POPULATION COVERED BY HEALTH INSURANCE. The insurance or financing systems that provide the greatest opportunities to manage care and health are those that are either universal in nature or have mature and dominant private health insurers (that is, insurers that have a monopoly or oligopoly), because enrollees are likely to be with them for a length of time that merits long-term investment in health outcomes. On the opposite end of the scale, the insurance systems least conducive to care management or health improvement are those in which large proportions of the population are uninsured and paying for care out-of-pocket.

Our cases provide examples from a range of financing arrangements: from England with its single payer and universal coverage structure, Germany with universal coverage financed through a large number of private sickness funds, and Brazil with 80 percent of the population insured by the central government financing scheme, to the highly fragmented, competitive, and noncomprehensive financing scheme in the United States and the highly fragmented, noncompetitive, and noncomprehensive financing systems in Poland and China.

The latter systems are among the least conducive to effective managed care mechanisms, for reasons that are obvious. Fragmented financing systems create multiple, often conflicting incentives for providers—and often for payers as well—regarding the cost and quality of care. Noncomprehensive systems produce many uninsured people who come into the system only when they are sick. In Poland and China, the governments historically had strong public health orientations, which enabled both countries to achieve major improvements in basic health outcomes (such as reducing infant mortality and increasing childhood immunization) in decades past. However, now both countries are facing a growing prevalence of major chronic disease burdens and high-cost medical problems that public health measures alone have been unable to address. Both countries now have fragmented insurance systems that fail to cover large segments of their populations and that focus coverage primarily on the acute care sector while not covering many preventive services, community-based care, and prescription drugs.

Excerpts from cases that present countries at either end of the health insurance spectrum illustrate the practicalities faced by the types of insurance markets or health financing schemes they represent.

> The government's goals for the new NHS [National Health Service] are quite simple:
> - To improve the health of the population as a whole
> - To improve the health of the worst-off in society and to narrow the health gap
> - To modernize the health and social care system
>
> —*From Chapter Twelve*

England's ambitious health reforms of the late 1990s include creating a primary care–driven health system that is locally controlled and responsive to the health and social service needs of the entire community.

In contrast, in the late 1990s, the wealthiest province in China, Shanghai, was able to reform only a part of its health financing scheme, the employer-based health system, representing roughly 45 percent of the population in the province. (Nearly 12 percent of the population was uninsured, and the others were covered under a variety of different insurance systems.) Shanghai's approach to reform was to pool portions of the hospitalization funds of all insured employees to equalize the cost across employer groups. However, the reforms were limited to pooling only the funds for inpatient and selected outpatient procedures. According to a local health ministry official,

> "We considered an insurance program for all care, . . . But Shanghai is too large, too diverse, and has too many retirees to adopt a comprehensive approach. . . . Our goals were to reduce the rate of increase in inpatient hospital costs, lower the medical costs of the employers, make the use of hospital services more equitable, and impose more supervision on the hospitals."
>
> —*From Chapter Two*

With health spending accounting for only 3 percent of GDP, China has limited ability to manage care or health of its population, and the fragmentation of coverage and limited services covered further reduce the scope of reform that it can hope to undertake.

In more generously financed but still fragmented financing systems, such as those in the United States, faith in managed care organizations to go beyond simply managing cost is not very strong among many parties:

> "We believe strongly in the need to focus on changing the organization and delivery of care," said one UAW [United Auto Workers union] official. "But employers have a false idea that competition will lead to efficiencies in the delivery system; there's no evidence of that. HMOs sell cost containment, but then they skim good risks, cost-shift, squeeze the providers, and increase administrative costs. HMOs and competition are not changing the system. . . . The appropriate way to focus on delivery system issues is not competition but cooperation and collaboration among all stakeholders."
>
> —*From Chapter Ten*

Even greater criticism can be made about the fragmented *public* financing system in the United States, particularly in the case of

low-income, chronically ill elderly people who are covered by both
Medicare (a federal program covering primarily acute care and hospitalization) and Medicaid (a combined state and federal program
covering long-term institutional care for elders):

> "Frankly, the current system could not really be much worse. The fed-
> eral government spends more on Medicare because it doesn't control
> long-term care; nursing homes push their elderly patients unneces-
> sarily into hospitals and other acute care providers to try to shift costs
> to Medicare. Meanwhile Medicaid doesn't control the acute medical
> care system for elders, which often practices in a way that leads to
> higher use of the long-term care services covered by Medicaid services.
> No one is in charge of the patients—doctors don't know their patients
> have gone into nursing homes and home care case managers don't
> know people have gone to the hospital. Care is incredibly fragmented
> and uncoordinated. The patients get bounced around with lousy
> results—high rates of preventable hospitalizations, unnecessary nurs-
> ing home admissions and higher costs for everyone."
> —*An advocate for the elderly, as quoted in Chapter Eight*

However, in some local U.S. markets that have a few dominant
insurers and a relatively stable insurance market, health insurers are
able to develop systems to manage care and improve the health of
communities. The Twin Cities case (Chapter Nine) describes the
efforts of one dominant insurer to improve the health of the community as well as that of its own enrollees, sometimes by cooperating
with other area insurers (ensuring community-wide evidence-based
standards of practice, educating providers to recognize and deal with
domestic violence, teaching new parents to read to their babies and
young children). However, these efforts were vulnerable to competitive pressures and employer concerns:

> Many employers seem skeptical about the involvement of health plans
> in community health activities. "There's a split among businesses
> about these issues," reported one employer representative. "Some of
> them think business needs to be accountable to the community. But
> this is not a core business for the employers and many are very
> frustrated with the health plans. They do not want the plans focused
> on public health. They want them to focus on taking care of sick
> people and show good performance doing that. . . . They don't want
> business to have a public health agenda—that's government's role. The

obligation of business is to keep its health insurance premiums down to be accountable to stockholders."

—From Chapter Nine

INFORMATION AND COMMUNICATION INFRASTRUCTURE. An essential ingredient to managing care is timely, accurate, and detailed medical utilization, cost, and outcome data, spanning the continuum of care, that can be transformed into useful information for managing care and health. The information infrastructure is a challenge in all health systems, regardless of how generously they are funded.

In underfunded developing countries, obtaining very basic patient and cost information is highly labor-intensive:

> Lack of data is a significant obstacle to program design. The health stations have some patient medical and cost information, but only in paper files. . . . Jinshanwei Hospital has medical records for patients, but no computerized medical records system, although some administrative functions are computerized (accounting, admissions, and discharge). It appears impossible to obtain detailed information on hospital utilization or costs without doing sampling of medical records or surveys (for example, keeping a daily log of medications dispensed by the hospital pharmacy to identify the most frequently prescribed drugs). The Shanghai Medical Insurance Bureau has two years of inpatient claims data on insureds in Jinshanwei, but the claims forms contain limited information (patient ID number, age, gender, diagnosis at admission, length of stay, charges by type of service). The claims data are available in a computerized format.
>
> *—From Chapter Two*

In Poland, decentralization of the financing system to regional "sickness funds" became a nightmare for practicing physicians seeking to register patients and obtain their capitation payments because of the lack of basic information systems and poor communication systems (including not enough phone lines):

> "We have had difficulty getting our patients registered with the practice so we can receive the capitation from the insurance fund. . . . We are spending a tremendous amount of physician time at night and on the weekends entering data into the computer to create a list of our patients for the fund. We tried to hire a data entry person to put the information into the computer but it would have cost us the equivalent of two

physicians' salaries. . . . We don't know which hospitals and which specialists have contracts with the insurance fund, so we're not sure where to refer. The health insurance fund is not providing any information and no one answers the phones. So we have to take half days away from our practice to go to the fund to try to meet with people and get our questions answered. . . . Based on our experience so far, we have great concerns about the competency of the funds to perform many of their new functions."

—Primary care physician in Krakow, from Chapter Five

At the opposite extreme, however, is the United States, where one corporate benefit manager exclaimed, "We are drowning in data and starving for information." This case continues:

"We have lots of data," said one staff member. "In fact, in a way we have too much data. The quality of the data is good but we don't know how to use it. And the people who work for our data vendor are data crunchers, not analysts or producers of information." . . . But corporate staff remain frustrated that vendors request the data for administrative purposes and have not been interested or excited in using the data warehouse as a resource for identifying opportunities for clinical or programmatic interventions. "So we are just left with interesting data and useless information."

—From Chapter Three

Even at the health plan level in the United States, data and information problems abound, hampering efforts to manage even the simplest diseases:

Getting timely information is also a problem because of the lag in the availability of outpatient data for the Medical Groups and the network. "In Harvard Vanguard [a medical group] we have every outpatient visit in the system within forty-eight hours. It takes three to four months to get complete claims data from the network." Another problem is inaccurate diagnostic coding. For example, a recent study by NCQA found that using claims data to identify asthmatics resulted in many false positives on the East Coast compared to other parts of the country, because many cases coded as asthma turn out to be something else, like pneumonia or chronic obstructive pulmonary disease (COPD).

—From Chapter Seven

Finally, there is the problem best illustrated by the German health system, where information is gathered but kept confidential for both political and privacy reasons:

> The data available to [the insurers] . . . are also limited. Although [the insurers] have detailed data on hospital and drug expenditures, because they pay providers directly for those services, the [insurers] do not have access to data on utilization and costs for office-based physicians, who are paid by the [physician associations]. . . . Although the [insurers] are interested in working with the [physician associations] to establish a more comprehensive and coordinated information system, . . . serious nationwide concerns about protecting the confidentiality of patient information have led to strong resistance to permitting centralized organizations to create large comprehensive databases. Physician organizations have also been able to exploit the public's fear about privacy to resist providing their associations or [insurers] with more information on their practices.
>
> —*From Chapter Six*

CONSUMER EXPECTATIONS. Consumer willingness to accept limits on choice, particularly choices among specialists, drugs, and hospitals, has a major impact on the potential effectiveness of managed care. Systems that require consumer choice to be influenced by financial responsibility are more conducive to managed care, all else being equal. Our cases provide examples of countries where consumers have quite different expectations about health care, choice of provider, and consumer financial responsibility.

From the perspective of consumer expectations, Germany is the country in our cases that is least conducive to managed care:

> Germans are permitted unrestricted freedom of choice of provider. Sickness funds are required by law to provide standard [very comprehensive] benefits with little variation. . . . Cost-sharing is minimal. . . . Copayments cannot exceed 2 percent of income in any year, and many groups are exempt from copayments. . . . Sickness funds are financed through salary-based payroll deductions [at fixed regional or national levels].
>
> —*From Chapter Six*

Whereas these consumer rights in Germany are guaranteed by extensive federal law, in the United States, a few groups have similar consumer protections built into their health insurance. One such group is the unionized auto workers in Michigan:

> The UAW–Big Three workers have one of the most extensive health insurance programs of any U.S. industry. . . . Members are eligible for medical, dental, and vision benefits. Most UAW members can choose from a range of options. . . . Regardless of the options selected, UAW members make no contribution to premiums; the entire cost of the UAW health program is borne by the automakers. . . .
>
> "Opposing cost-sharing is as high a priority as we have, ahead of wage increases," said one union official. "It is an article of faith for our members. The membership has to ratify any agreement and would view cost-sharing as a violation of the faith. It would never be implemented without a strike."
>
> *—From Chapter Ten*

Unlike the UAW members, most insured consumers in the United States make significant contributions to the cost of their health insurance, both through premium contributions and copayments for services. Consumer cost-sharing has grown dramatically over the last ten years, and was a major force fueling the expansion of managed care enrollment to over 90 percent of the under-sixty-five privately insured, employer-based market. One of the attractive features of managed care plans for most consumers was more limited cost-sharing than in unmanaged plans. In general, consumers were financially motivated to accept some restrictions on their choice of provider in return for these lower out-of-pocket costs (although the more successful managed care plans in terms of enrollment generally had the least restrictive networks and the least effective controls on cost or care management).

In contrast to the United States or Germany, in England, where highly restricted choice and a strong primary care gatekeeping system have been a part of the National Health System since its inception, many consumers embraced the notion of managed care as represented by "GP Fundholding." GP fundholders were primary care physicians who received budgets to purchase a broader scope of services than those they provided directly for their panel of patients. The GP fundholder scheme described in Chapter Eleven (the first of two dealing with England), in which general practitioners sought to create "preferred provider networks" for their panels of patients, was widely viewed as giving patients better access to care than non-fundholder patients could obtain. In fact, acknowledgment of that effect contributed to the demise of GP fundholding:

> Many advocates of reform, including many family physicians, believed that fundholding provided an opportunity to raise standards of clinical practice and improve quality of care. . . . [However, opponents argued (among other things)] that the initiative would create a two-tier system of care in which the patients of non-fundholding GPs would have less access to care.
>
> —*From Chapter Eleven*

One might expect consumers in countries where access to care is severely limited by individual financial responsibility (Poland, China, even Brazil to some extent) to be particularly open to managed care as a way to keep health care accessible and affordable. However, in some cases, at least among the insured portions of the population (for instance, in China), consumers do not readily accept limits on provider choice.

> "We need to have a gatekeeper," said a physician at the community health center in Jinshanwei. "People are going directly to the hospital who could be treated at the health center or at a health station. This is inefficient and a waste of resources." . . .
> "In Shanghai selectively contracting with hospitals is something that could work potentially, but it would be very difficult culturally and politically."
>
> —*Official from the Shanghai Medical University, from Chapter Two*

SOCIOPOLITICAL VALUES. Strongly held social values about equity and efficiency, which ultimately are expressed through the political system in most countries, affect the successful implementation of managed care programs. In England, when the managed care program of GP fundholding was used to improve quality of care and access for a set of enrollees, these results were viewed as creating an "unequal" system of care. This flaw was ultimately fatal for the GP fundholding scheme, despite its perceived successes in improving the responsiveness and quality of hospital and specialist care for fundholder patients. As Chapter Twelve notes, the GP fundholder scheme, originated by the

Conservative Party, was ultimately dismissed by the Labour Party as a "divisive internal market system of the 1990s . . . an approach which was intended to make the NHS more efficient but ended up fragmenting decision-making and distorting incentives to such an extent that unfairness and bureaucracy became its defining features."

The creation of competing health systems that vied for patient business by managing care or cost was widely viewed in both Germany and China as undermining "solidarity"—that is, the principle that all people should have equal access to the same level of services (although in China's case this meant only those who were insured). In Germany, the basis for competition among health insurers could not include restrictive provider networks or consumer cost-sharing because of concerns that these managed care mechanisms might create a two-tier or multiple-tier health system. Although since 1996 Germans have increased freedom to choose among sickness funds, the funds have been given very little room to compete in terms of benefit design, product pricing, consumer cost-sharing, and provider contracting. Chapter Six quotes one government official as describing the federal approach to managed care in these terms: "We are experimenting with managed care for a limited time. . . . But there is no competitive or managed care strategy, just room for some managed care and competitive elements."

In contrast, in the United States, a societal belief in individual responsibility is far more prevalent than the notion of solidarity. One by-product is a high societal tolerance for inequities in access to affordable, high-quality health care. These values may have contributed to a greater emphasis in our country on the use of managed care tools to reduce cost rather than to improve quality of care or health outcomes. The U.S. faith in competitive markets also fosters cost competition but creates obstacles to the cooperation needed within a geographic area to implement uniform care management or health intervention and education programs.

SUMMARY

The cases presented in this book provide students, health care managers, and policymakers with an opportunity to understand some of the unique features of the health systems of six countries from a range of hemispheres and continents. These countries are very different in terms of the resources they have devoted to health care, and also in the decisions and choices they have made about how to structure, finance, and manage their health care systems. Yet despite these differences, the countries in our cases face many similar challenges as they seek to make health care affordable, accessible, and high-quality, and to improve the health of their populations. Our cases illustrate, in particular, the common managerial problems and themes that arise in the efforts of each country to use managed care techniques within its own unique health system to craft solutions to its own particular problems. Despite the universal absence of easy solutions in any country, we can learn a great deal from what has worked well and not so well in each country. Ironically, these lessons may be particularly relevant for the United States, where—despite the predominance of managed care—the ability of managed care approaches to improve system performance and health has been severely limited by other aspects of our health care financing and delivery system. This book is dedicated to encouraging better understanding and more discussion, in the United States and elsewhere, of the problems and implementation issues involved in improving health and health care, with the goal of inspiring more effective health policies and reform in the future.

PART ONE

Managing Cost

CHAPTER TWO

Managed Care in Shanghai
Another Long March or a Great Leap Forward?

I n February 1998, the temperature in the conference
room at Shanghai Medical University (SMU) was chilly—at least for
U.S. visitors accustomed to central heating—but the discussion was
lively as Jie Chen and her colleagues discussed their ideas about how
managed care might be used to deal with some of the problems in the
health care system in Shanghai. "We may be able to use a managed
care pilot to achieve a number of goals in the targeted area," said Chen.
"These include reducing costs, improving access, improving quality
of care, improving provider efficiency, strengthening referral systems,
and redirecting resources to prevention. A pilot would be an important program in and of itself. But if it were successful, it could also be
the catalyst to facilitate a broader program of health reform in China.
Managed care could help us rationalize resource use and provide more
appropriate care to more of our people."

This case was originally written by the authors in 1998. Funding was provided
by Astra USA. The authors thank Dr. Jie Chen and her colleagues at Shanghai
Medical University for their interest and assistance in preparing the case.

The SMU group had targeted Jinshanwei, a suburb about forty miles southwest of Shanghai, as a promising site for a managed care pilot. Chen and her staff had been working on the project in collaboration with the largest employer in Jinshanwei, Shanghai Petrochemical Company, as well as with officials from the provider community and state insurance system. The group was also receiving technical assistance from Kaiser Permanente, a health plan in northern California. So far, the group had completed some preliminary planning and data analysis. It was now ready to develop a specific project design and approach.

BACKGROUND

China is the largest country in the world, with a population of 1.2 billion in a geographic area about the size of the United States. Approximately 80 percent of the population live in rural areas and 20 percent in urban areas.

Since the Communist Party assumed power in 1949, China has made tremendous strides at improving the health of its population with limited resources. These improvements were achieved by a combination of actions including improvements in socioeconomic conditions, an emphasis on prevention (with massive immunization campaigns, improved nutrition, sanitation, water quality, and attacks on specific diseases and carriers) and promoting access to primary care, especially in rural areas. As a result, China has seen significant drops in infant mortality from 200/1,000 births in 1949 to 31/1,000 in 1995, and increases in life expectancy from thirty-five years in 1949 to seventy years in 1995. Since 1970, infectious disease rates have plummeted—from 7,061/100,000 to 176/100,000 in 1995. In rural areas, 400 million people now have piped water, and primary health care plans are in place in 1,538 of China's 2,404 counties.

For the first thirty years after the Revolution, China had a centrally directed economy, including its health care system. In 1979, the country began a program of economic reform, moving from central direction and planning to the use of market forces, creating a new system often characterized as a "socialist market economy." A major purpose of this shift was to emphasize economic growth and end disruption and stagnation in industry and agriculture. Economic growth has accelerated since 1979, along with a significant increase in foreign investment in China. Average income levels have risen significantly, although the distribution of income has broadened as well. In the last decade, China has developed an urban middle class of independent businesspersons, private sector lawyers, and employees of joint-venture companies. At the same time, many workers are being laid off from state-owned factories that have been too inefficient to compete in the global marketplace. Even among those with jobs, income disparities are growing; for instance, in Beijing in 1997, a typical urban manager of a private company made $8,000/year, while a worker in the company averaged only $1,000/year (Rosenthal, 1998).

As part of this overall economic shift, there were fundamental changes in the ways health care was organized and financed. One intent of the changes was to limit the proportion of health care spending financed by the government. Since 1980 the proportion of total health care expenditures financed by the government has declined from 30 percent to 20 percent. Half of government spending is for direct medical services; the other half goes to prevention, public health, medical education, and research. The other 80 percent of health care expenditure is financed almost equally by a combination of out-of-pocket payments by patients and payments by employment-based health insurance programs. As of 1997, China spent approximately 3.8 percent of its GDP on health care, up from 2.9 percent in 1985. In the past two decades, health care spending by government and nongovernment sources has risen faster than the overall Chinese GDP.

The Health Insurance System

China has no national health insurance program. Where a person lives and works are the major determinants of whether the person has health insurance, and, if insured, the type and scope of coverage. Patients either pay for services out of pocket or are covered by one of two major insurance systems.

The Government Insurance System *(gonfei yiliao)* covers all government employees and retirees, college students and teachers, and certain military personnel. Dependents are also generally covered. Approximately 29 million people have coverage through this system.

The Labor Insurance system *(laodong baoxian)* is provided by state enterprises as a requirement and is voluntary for other employers. Dependents may or may not be covered, depending on the employer. Approximately 144 million people have labor insurance. In most parts of China, labor insurance is operated largely on an employer self-funded basis. Under the policies of the socialist market economy, many state-owned enterprises are failing or closing. In 1997 in Shanghai, where state-owned enterprise employed 2.96 million, 168,000 lost their jobs in state-owned enterprises; in the same year, only 17,900 new jobs were created in the private sector ("Shanghai's Folks Obese . . . ," 1998).

There are significant regional variations in the proportion of people who have insurance coverage. Urban workers are much more likely than rural workers to be covered, as are people who live in higher-income provinces. As much as half of the urban population has no health insurance, and 85 percent of the rural population is uninsured.

The benefits provided by the insurance programs vary among regions and employers. In general, coverage is more comprehensive for inpatient services, and benefits are oriented to curative care, although there are some disease prevention benefits.

Cost-sharing is an important component of the insurance systems. The level of cost-sharing varies widely among employers. The cost-sharing levels for the government insurance system are determined by the provincial governments. In general, coinsurance for inpatient care is around 8 percent and is 10–20 percent for outpatient care. Co-insurance is higher for dependents than for workers. Workers in wealthier provinces generally have lower cost-sharing because of the greater ability of the provinces to absorb health care costs. Shanghai is the wealthiest province in China and has one of the lowest coinsurance levels, 10 percent, compared to 40 percent in poorer provinces. In recent years, differences in company financial performance have affected the comprehensiveness of health insurance coverage offered by employers. In addition, the economic reforms have increased income differences among regions and created a relatively more mobile population, which has made health insurance coverage more insecure for many people.

Traditional insurance programs function as third-party payers separate from providers, and generally play no role other than financing services. For example, they make no attempt to influence referrals or level of care. Although some insurance plans require insureds to use contracting hospitals, there appear to be few, if any, sanctions on patients who do not comply with these requirements.

Medical Insurance Reform in Shanghai

Beginning in 1995, Shanghai undertook a major reform of the medical insurance system in the city and surrounding areas. The reform essentially combined the inpatient coverage component of the government and labor insurance programs, and replaced the separate employer-based insurance system with a single medical insurance program that now covers workers in state-owned, collectively owned, and privately owned companies, self-employed individuals, and all government workers. The new plan, run by the Shanghai Medical Insurance Bureau, a public agency, now covers almost 6 million people. The remainder of the population of Shanghai is covered under separately administered schemes for primary and middle school students (2 million), rural health cooperatives (4 million), and uninsured individuals (1.6 million). The Bureau has also recently set up a special medical relief fund to cover laid-off and unemployed workers.

Any employer in Shanghai that provides insurance to its workers must participate in the program, called "Shanghai Urban Enterprise Employee's Hospitalization Insurance." (The plan will be referred to as Shanghai Medical Insurance or SMI.) SMI originally provided coverage only for inpatient services. "We considered an insurance program for all care, similar to the pilot programs in the Zhenjiang and Jiujiang regions that began in 1994," said an official at the Bureau. "But Shanghai is too large, too diverse, and has too many retirees to adopt a comprehensive approach. So we took a more limited approach . . . consistent with our principles of wanting to have a program that is prudent, vigorous, and safe . . . and our strategy of overall planning, properly exercising in steps, progressively promoting, and continually improving." SMI's coverage was expanded in May 1997 to include certain outpatient services, including emergency room care, chemotherapy, radiotherapy, and dialysis for patients with severe kidney disease. "We are exploring how to expand social insurance to cover other services, including home care and health education," said the official. "Maybe we will extend the program in the future."

Outpatient care for the elderly is an increasing factor as an increasing proportion of urban elderly do not live with their children or grandchildren. According to the *China Daily News* ("Aging Society," 1998), in Beijing, less than 50 percent of elderly people live with their children.

The SMI program has significant cost-sharing. There is a deductible for inpatient and emergency care, which varies by type of hospital, as well as 15 percent coinsurance. The deductible and coinsurance must be "reasonably shared" between the employer and employee. On the outpatient side, the coinsurance is 30 percent, which must also be shared reasonably between employer and employee. (See Table 2.1 for a summary of the benefit structure.)

1. Inpatient Services
   a. Deductible per admission
      • Primary hospital: RMB 1,500
      • Secondary hospital: RMB 2,000
      • Tertiary hospital: RMB 2,500
   b. Cost-sharing for inpatient care after deductible
      • 85 percent paid by SMI
      • 15 percent paid by employer and employee
2. Emergency care
   • 85 percent paid by SMI
   • 15 percent reasonably shared by employer and employee
3. Covered Outpatient services
   • 70 percent paid by SMI
   • 30 percent reasonably shared by employer and employee

Table 2.1.   Cost-Sharing in Shanghai Medical Insurance Program.
Source: Shanghai Medical Insurance Bureau. Unpublished data provided to authors during interview with officials in February, 1998.
Note: 1 RMB (yuan) = roughly US$0.12, that is, 8.27 RMB to the U.S. dollar (summer 1998 exchange rate).

Other cost-containment mechanisms used by the program include retrospective review of medical records for "medical necessity." Roughly once a month a claim is denied on such grounds. However, standards for the determination of medical necessity have not yet been developed.

Technically, the SMI program provides coverage only at contracting hospitals. But, as an official of the Bureau explained, "At the moment, we contract with all hospitals—that is safer for everyone. But the hospitals must obey the principles and play by the rules." The Bureau has implemented a number of quality assurance activities. When it detects problems, it issues a warning to the hospital to change its behavior, with a threat of not paying for services in the future or seeking a refund for services already provided.

The SMI program is financed by a uniform premium rate, set as a percentage of wages, paid by employers to the Bureau. The premium rate in 1997 was 6.5 percent, of which 4.5 percent went to finance inpatient services, and 2 percent was used to cover emergency and outpatient care. In 1998, the premium rate increased to 7.5 percent. SMI's administrative costs are paid by the government and not charged back to the employers through the premium.

Officials from the Bureau believe the program has been very successful at achieving its goals. "First, we have covered 98 percent of eligible individuals and we are collecting 97 percent of premium," said one official. "Second, we have made good progress in achieving the objectives of the reform. Our goals were to reduce the rate of increase in inpatient hospital costs, lower the medical costs of the employers, make the use of hospital services more equitable, and impose more supervision on the hospitals. We have positive results in all these areas." In support of this conclusion, the officials provided the following data for the period July 1, 1996, to June 30, 1997:

- Total inpatient costs and average cost per admission for individuals covered by SMI increased 12 percent, compared to a target of 15 percent.
- Medical costs of the employers rose 9 percent, compared to an average annual increase of 23 percent in the prior three years.
- The hospitalization rate for the lowest-income workers increased from 3.3 percent to 4.8 percent, while the rate for the highest-income workers declined from 6.0 percent to 5.6 percent.
- The plan is covering a much higher proportion of high-cost bills (28 percent of bills of less than RMB 3,000 compared to 80 percent of bills above RMB 100,000).

The Health Care Delivery System

China's delivery system is often described as being "three-tiered." This model, which was established in the late 1950s, differs somewhat in rural and urban areas. In urban areas, the three tiers are as follows:

- Local providers, including township health stations and community health centers that provide basic medical care
- District providers, including community hospitals providing secondary care, disease control centers, centers for women and children, and disease prevention and health education and training services
- City hospitals, which provide tertiary care

Preparation of medical personnel at the various levels entails anywhere from three to six months of training after middle school (for health

Measure	1985	1990	1994	Percentage Change 1985–1994
Number of hospitals	59,614	62,454	67,857	+14
Number of beds (million)	2.23	2.62	2.83	+21
Hospital occupancy (percent)	83	81	69	−17
Average length of stay (days)	15.8	15.9	15.0	−5
Number of doctors (million)	1.41	1.76	1.88	+33
Number of outpatient and emergency visits (trillion)	1.14	1.27	1.14	0

Table 2.2.   Selected Measures of Medical Resources and Utilization: 1984–1994.

Source: Shanghai Medical University. Unpublished data provided to authors during interviews with officials in February 1998.

station doctors) to three years of postsecondary medical education (for community health centers and hospital physicians) and four to five years' postsecondary medical education for physicians in the tertiary centers (Hsiao, 1995).

During the 1980s, China made massive investments in health care facilities, personnel, and technology. There are now 123 medical and pharmacy universities producing sixty-one thousand graduates a year. Health care resources increased dramatically. Overall hospital utilization did not keep pace with the increasing inpatient capacity, and hospital occupancy declined, as shown in Table 2.2. There are, however, significant regional variations in the distribution and use of medical resources. For example, hospital occupancy tends to be much higher in city hospitals than in community facilities.

Provider Payment and Pricing

Health insurers and patients pay providers on a fee-for-service basis. Prices are set by the government and have major effects on the amount and type of care that is provided.

HOSPITALS.   Prior to the economic reforms of the late 1970s, hospitals received most of their operating and capital funds from the government. As part of the reforms, hospitals were required to cover most of their nonstaff, noncapital costs from fee-for-service charges, either from patients or insurance. Government now funds only basic personnel costs and new capital expenditures—only about one-quarter of total hospital costs. In recent years, government spending has grown less quickly than total expenditures, and health facilities have become increasingly dependent on fee-for-service revenues.

PHYSICIANS. In the early 1980s, the Chinese government began to allow "diversity of provision" in health care, including permitting physicians to have private practices. But less than 5 percent of doctors are in private practice. Most physicians work in community-based or hospital settings. Physicians are paid by a combination of salary and bonus. The salary component is financed in part by the government and in part by the hospital. A physician's salary is based on rank and number of years' experience. The bonus payment is linked to specialty, productivity, and the amount of revenue the physician generates. Up to 50 percent of a doctor's income may be accounted for by the bonus. Total compensation for the average physician in China is approximately two or three times the average urban wage of $1,000.

PRICING. The Chinese government sets the prices providers can charge. In a deliberate attempt to make basic medical care affordable, it keeps the prices of most services low. Pricing policy and principles are established by the state finance bureau and adjusted at the provincial level. The fees for services that were in use in the late 1950s, when fees were first set (doctor visits, inpatient care, surgery) are generally set below costs (in part because at that time there were no accurate cost data), and even with attempts to update prices in 1985, most fees are still considerably below costs. Older price guidelines do not exist for new technologies, and many of these services are priced above costs (such as CT scans, lab services, dialysis, ultrasound, coronary care). Hospitals negotiate fees for new technologies with local health and price bureaus, typically on the basis of the likely average cost of the service and assumptions regarding volume. This process creates an incentive for hospitals to project moderate levels of use, and then use the service more intensively to generate more revenue. Another result is that hospitals acquire and use any technology that is priced above cost, regardless of whether it is obsolete or of questionable effectiveness. (Examples of such technologies are myopia correction machines and the use of hyperbaric oxygen chambers to treat a wide range of conditions, including stroke and cancer.)

Hospitals and other providers are allowed to mark up the price of drugs by 10–18 percent over the wholesale price for which they acquire them. The markup for traditional Chinese medicine (TCM) averages 20–25 percent. The markups are intended to cover the costs of storage and distribution. Drugs are a major profit source for health care providers, and almost every health facility in China, including the outpatient clinics, has a pharmacy that sells Western and TCM drugs, including prescription and over-the-counter medicines. China manufactures most of its drugs at low cost, and drugs are widely available. The types of drugs available at outpatient facilities have expanded greatly since the economic reforms. Marketing of drugs is active in China, and drug companies pay bonuses to physicians who use new and expensive drugs. Many drugs are advertised directly to consumers through TV, newspaper, and magazine advertisements.

Drugs account for half of total health care expenditures in China. The average annual increase in drug costs consistently exceeds 10 percent. Drug utilization is very high: on average, 2.3 drugs are prescribed per outpatient visit. Inappropriate utilization is common. For example, it is estimated that between one-third and one-half of prescriptions written include an antibiotic, and many are for injectables.

The insurance programs have established formularies. Only drugs on the formulary are covered; insureds must pay out of pocket for nonformulary drugs. The formulary used by the Shanghai Labor and Government Insurance programs contains approximately fourteen hundred drugs, including many over-the-counter drugs like ibuprofen and Tylenol. In general the list is quite broad, with many therapeutic classes included, although the choice of drug within class is often quite limited. The formulary list also includes medications used in the inpatient setting (such as IV solutions and additives, and anesthetics). One of the notable omissions in the Shanghai formulary is drugs used in treatment of HIV/AIDS. (China reports low HIV prevalence, although the real prevalence level is believed by many experts to be much higher.)

It is widely agreed that the payment system creates strong incentives for providers to overuse overpriced services, in part to subsidize the cost of underpriced ones. A number of studies have found high levels of inappropriate use for a number of services (such as CT scans and coronary care). The pricing of services has also created incentives for providers to acquire certain types of technologies and services. (For example, there are sixty-seven CT scanners in Shanghai.) It is common for hospitals to have outpatient infusion rooms that treat minor complaints with IV medication, so that a patient with a cold or fever might receive IV fluids with some added antibiotics. Another incentive for overutilization is the bonuses providers receive based on how much revenue they generate for the hospital (largely through ordering prescriptions and high-cost technologies).

Rising Costs

Total health care expenditures in China have increased rapidly in recent years, at an average annual rate of approximately 13–14 percent in real terms. (See Figures 2.1 and 2.2.) The costs of the two major insurance systems have also increased rapidly in recent years. For example, in the last few years, the average annual increase in spending by the government insurance plan has been nearly 13 percent. Expenditures by the Labor Insurance Program have increased from 5.5 percent of wages to nearly 10 percent.

The rate of growth of health care spending in China has been fueled by a number of factors, including changing patterns of disease, with an increased incidence of chronic illness; an increased number of people with insurance; the health care financing and pricing systems, which have created strong incentives to provide services on which profits can be earned; and an aging population. By the end of the twentieth century, China will have one of the world's highest

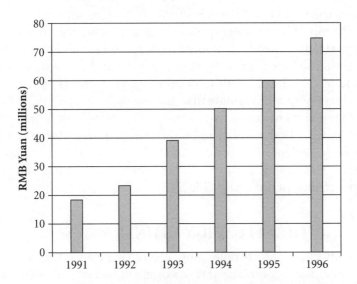

Figure 2.1.   Total Health Expenditures.

Source: Shanghai Medical University. Unpublished data provided to authors during interviews with officials in February 1998.

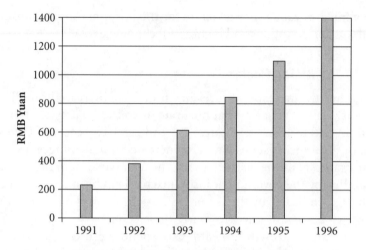

Figure 2.2.   Health Care Cost per Capita.
Source: Shanghai Medical University. Unpublished data provided
to authors during interviews with officials in February 1998.

proportions of elderly people. In Shanghai, the proportion of people
over the age of sixty is projected to be almost 20 percent in 2000, up
from 16 percent in 1995; the percentage of residents over eighty will
increase from 10 percent to 13 percent in this same five-year period.

The mix of health care expenditures has also changed, with a larger
proportion of spending devoted to hospital care and drugs and a
declining share of spending going to basic and preventive health
spending. The use of health services by insured people is much greater
and increasing more rapidly than the use by uninsured individuals.
The level and growth of cost-sharing has created significant access
problems for both insured and uninsured people, and there is considerable evidence that the cost of medical care has become both a
barrier to access and a source of serious financial hardship, and often
impoverishment, for many Chinese.

THE SITUATION IN JINSHANWEI

Jinshanwei, about forty miles southwest of Shanghai, is China's major
petrochemical region. The area was originally developed in 1972 and
is now dominated by two huge enterprises: Shanghai Petrochemical
Company (SPC) and Shanghai Jinshan Industrial Company (SJIC).
SPC is owned by China Petrochemicals, a publicly traded company

since 1993. SPC is primarily engaged in the processing of crude oil into a broad range of synthetic fibers, resins, plastics, intermediate petrochemicals, and petroleum products. SJIC does engineering contracting, design, construction, machine manufacturing, and a range of other activities, including real estate development.

Jinshanwei has a population of approximately 120,000, with a surrounding rural population of 300,000. SPC employs approximately 52,000 people, representing 107,000 covered lives. The area is relatively young, with an average age of thirty-two. Only 10 percent of the population is over the age of sixty. The population is also predominantly male (the ratio of males to females is 157:100). With low birth and death rates, Jinshanwei has a stable population that is growing slightly.

Since its inception, SPC played the role of builder and financier for the district's health, education, housing, and other social support systems. Until 1997, all workers employed by these social services were employees of SPC and covered by SPC's own labor insurance program. However, as part of China's long-term economic reforms, SPC has been reorganized, shedding its paternalistic role (although retaining substantial residual financial responsibilities) of owning and operating housing units, schools, hospitals, and other social services. Social service workers have become employees of the district government, and are now covered by government, rather than labor, insurance.

Like other employers, SPC was self-insured before the implementation of the SMI program. Its cost escalated rapidly throughout the 1990s, at rates that generally mirrored the increases for other employers in Shanghai. (See Table 2.3.)

Year	Total Medical Care Spending (RMB million)	Percentage Increase Over Prior Year	Per Capita Spending	Percentage Increase Over Prior Year
1991	17.9	—	265	—
1992	23.8	34	390	46
1993	38.5	62	645	65
1994	51.2	33	870	26
1995	60.5	18	1,094	26
1996	74.6	23	1,412	29

Table 2.3.   Medical Spending by Shanghai Petrochemical Company 1991–1996 (Excluding SPC Subsidies to Jin Shan Hospital).
Source: Shanghai Petrochemical Company. Unpublished data provided to authors during interviews with officials in February 1998.

Initially, SPC reacted to rising costs by increasing cost-sharing somewhat, but the changes had little effect. In 1996, SPC tried giving its workers a small sum of money each month, which they could keep or use to defray the cost of coinsurance. "At first there was a reduction in utilization," said the official. "But before long the workers said, 'ah, it is only ten yuan,' and it had no real effect." SPC is now thinking of limiting its liability for outpatient services by giving its employees a fixed sum each year for outpatient care, rather than providing a self-funded insurance plan for these services. "But we are concerned that this will lead people to defer care and will cost us more in the long run as we have to pay for things that are preventable or become more serious because of not being treated."

According to company officials, the implementation of the SMI plan has not helped SPC. "We are paying even more for medical care now than we were before the health insurance program started. Our costs have increased an average of 20 percent every year since the plan started. Health care costs are becoming a competitive issue for us—not within China but with other countries." The medical insurance system has many problems, including the provider payment mechanism. We would like to take our workers out of the insurance pool and try another model." One source claimed that only 50 percent of the premium paid by SPC into SMI came back into Jinshanwei as claims payments for SPC employees and dependents.

Chen and her colleagues believe that Jinshanwei has a number of attributes that make it a good site for a managed care pilot. She explained:

> Jinshanwei is an isolated area geographically, which is a very unusual situation in China and would give us a captive population and group of providers. In Shanghai selectively contracting with hospitals is something that could work potentially, but it would be very difficult culturally and politically. But here there is only one hospital. . . . The area also has a younger population, with relatively high incomes. Health indicators are good and meet national standards. And the pattern of disease is similar to other areas. Finally, the area has lots of health resources. These conditions present good opportunities for improvement and have the potential to produce results that could be replicated in other areas of China.

Tables 2.4 and 2.5 present some data collected by the SMU team on disease prevalence and causes of death in the region.

Condition	Prevalence/1,000: 1991	Prevalence/1,000: 1996
Hypertension	15	25
Mental illness and substance abuse	5	7
Cardiovascular	3	3
Tumors	2.5	2.5
Tuberculosis	2.0	1.0

Table 2.4.   Chronic Disease Prevalence in Jinshanwei: 1991 and 1996.

Source: Shanghai Medical University. Unpublished data provided to authors during interviews with officials in February 1998.

Cause of Death	Percentage of All Hospital Deaths: 1996	Death Rate/ 100,000 Population: 1991	Death Rate/ 100,000 Population: 1996
Cancer	39	70	90
Circulatory disease	25	35	65
Respiratory disease	10	25	25
Trauma	7	0	20
Digestive disorders	6	N/A	N/A

Table 2.5.   Causes of Death and Death Rates in the Petrochemical District: 1991 and 1996.

Source: Shanghai Medical University. Unpublished data provided to authors during interviews with officials in February 1998.

Medical Resources in Jinshanwei

Jinshanwei has forty-six medical facilities, including a tertiary hospital; forty-two health stations (fourteen located in SPC factories that provide care only to SPC workers); one public health anti-epidemic station; one community health center; and one mental health clinic (with 150 beds). There are a total of 1,813 medical personnel, including 564 doctors, 429 nurses; and 184 medical technicians. Table 2.6 describes the relative richness of health resources in Jinshanwei compared to Shanghai County as a whole.

Units/1,000 Population:	Jinshanwei	Shanghai County
Professional staff	12.3	8.51
Physicians	6.75	4.13
Registered nurses	4.97	2.77
Beds	6.3	5.5

Table 2.6.   Relative Health Resources.

Source: Shanghai Medical University. Unpublished data provided to authors during interviews with officials in February 1998.

Health Stations

As in other urban areas, the health stations in Jinshanwei provide primary and preventive care. According to the staff at one health station in Jinshanwei, the most common problems treated at the station are the common cold and chronic ailments such as hypertension and ulcers. At this health station, which served a population of employees working in a plastics factory owned by SPC, the top five diseases causing absenteeism at the factory were hepatitis, tumors (smoking was very popular), cardiac conditions, gastroenteritis, and fever (variety of reasons).

Workers are assigned to health stations based on residence and employment. The stations serving SPC workers are given a budget (by SPC) within which they are expected to cover all worker and dependent copayments and deductibles for use of hospital and other ambulatory services, including drugs. The health stations are supposed to act as a gatekeeper for certain services, including hospital care, but they report seeing a significant shift of care from the stations to the hospital as patients seek more advanced types of care directly from hospitals. Table 2.7 contains some descriptive data for the plastics factory health station in Jinshanwei.

The station expenses in 1996–1997 totaled RMB 3.3 million, broken down into direct salaries and bonuses (13 percent), direct prescription of drugs (27 percent), other direct supplies (4 percent), and payments

Assigned Population	2,700 workers, 350 retirees, 1,000 dependents
Staff	25 workers, including 14 station doctors, 2 nurses, and 4 clinical assistants
Number of visits (annual)	33,000 (roughly 8.1 visits per person)
Number of prescriptions written (annual)	34,000 (roughly 8.4 scripts per person)
Lab tests	600
Other diagnostic tests	840
ER visits to Jin Shan Hospital	801 (197.8/1,000 enrollees)
Inpatient admissions to Jin Shan Hospital	181 (44.7/1,000 enrollees)
Inpatient admissions to other Shanghai hospitals	41 (10.1/1,000 enrollees)

Table 2.7.   SPC Plastics Factory Health Station in Jinshanwei: Selected Data for 1997.

Source: Shanghai Petrochemical Company. Unpublished data provided to authors during interviews with officials in February 1998.

to outside vendors such as hospitals and other health stations for prescribed drugs (22 percent), worker copayments for inpatient (7 percent) and outpatient (18 percent) services, dependent copayments for all outside services (5 percent), and health exams given to workers (4 percent). Roughly 24 percent of outside vendor payments were for workers who had retired.

Community Health Center

The community health center's role has traditionally been the "public health" arm of the medical system. In Jinshanwei, the community health center had four units:

- *Preventive:* Within this function, clinicians visit schools and neighborhoods to provide preventive health services and home care visits for asthma, COPD, and other chronic respiratory ailments.

- *Outpatient Elderly Care:* Community center clinicians visit hypertensive patients in the elderly housing units to take blood pressure and prescribe and deliver medicines. The center manages hypertensives at three levels of care, the most intensive of which involves daily home visits.

- *Maternal and Child Care:* Pregnant women are assigned to community health centers based on proximity to work or home. This unit supervises maternal care for assignees; its staff also work in the community to prevent anemia, rickets, and dental disease in children ages one through six.

- *Internal Medicine:* The center also offers a primary care unit that provides internal medicine and TCM services to patients.

Despite little change in the service or patient mix of the center for the last five years, community health center leaders are concerned about a steady drop in volume since 1995. "Shanghai Petrochemical Company used to control our center but now control has been transferred to the district," explained a physician at a community health center, who continued:

> SPC no longer wants its workers to come here for care because it is cheaper for them to go to the company-run health stations. And the Labor Insurance System lets patients go directly to the hospital without

a referral. In the last two years, the number of visits here has dropped by more than 30 percent. Because of this decline, we are very overstaffed. We have one hundred staff providing an average of 108 visits per day (excluding home care and community education programs). We also have very strong clinical programs, like our asthma management program, but no patients. Labor Insurance has not helped us because we have no inpatient beds. The county is pressuring us to find alternative sources of revenue, perhaps by opening a dental care center or converting to private ownership.

Jin Shan Hospital

The district's one hospital is Jin Shan Hospital, a 570-bed facility that was historically managed and financially supported jointly by SPC and SJIC. It receives more than 90 percent of hospital admissions of Jinshanwei residents. The hospital, which is affiliated with Shanghai Medical University, was originally built in 1975 and upgraded in 1990. It offers a broad range of services including internal medicine, surgery, obstetrics, pediatrics, anesthesia, TCM, ENT, ophthalmology, occupational health, oral surgery, dermatology, rehabilitation, cardiology, pulmonology, and gastroenterology. Among its ancillary services are laboratory, pathology, pharmacy, nuclear medicine, physical therapy, laser, ultrasound, EKG, EEG, pulmonary function, and endoscopy. The hospital has a variety of high-tech equipment, including a CT scanner and a high-pressure oxygen chamber. "The oxygen chamber is one of our busiest services," said the medical director of the hospital, pointing to a roomful of patients waiting for their appointments. "We use it to treat all types of conditions, such as bone diseases, deafness, and vascular conditions."

Before 1997, SPC was the source of unlimited financial subsidies for the hospital's operating deficits and capital needs. But in May 1997, the district government assumed responsibility for services that had previously been financed by SPC, including schools, transportation, and the hospital. SPC now negotiates an annual operating subsidy payment to the hospital. In 1996, SPC's subsidy was RMB 16 million, roughly 15 percent of the hospital's operating cost. SPC also makes a capital contribution to the hospital, also established through negotiation.

In 1997, the hospital's occupancy level was 80 percent. Average length of stay was approximately eighteen days, down from twenty-two days in the early 1990s. This is probably influenced by an eighteen-day limit on inpatient stays instituted by the new SMI. If a patient needs to stay longer, an appeal to SMI must be made. Hospital officials were concerned that appeals would give the hospital a reputation for poor quality. Instead, patients needing more days were frequently discharged and readmitted (triggering a new deductible, roughly RMB 2,500 ($302) at Jin Shan Hospital). Table 2.8 provides data collected by Shanghai Medical University on the major admission diagnoses at Jin Shan Hospital in 1997. Table 2.9 shows data on the top reasons for hospital admission of the population in Jinshanwei, regardless of where the admissions occurred, and Table 2.10 provides summary income statement information for Jin Shan Hospital.

Disease	Number of Admissions	Percentage of Total Admissions
1. Pneumonia	544	7.0
2. Broken bone	393	5.1
3. Head injury	389	5.0
4. Inflamed gallbladder	261	3.4
5. Benign tumor	247	3.2
6. Disease of female fertility organs	241	3.1
7. Appendicitis	235	3.0
8. Cancer	218	2.8
9. Other heart disease	197	2.5
10. Perinatal care (including neonate disease)	180	2.3
Total: TOP 10	4,525	37

Table 2.8.   Top Ten Diseases at Admission, Jin Shan Hospital: 1997.
Source: Jin Shan Hospital and Shanghai Medical University. Unpublished data provided to authors during interviews with officials in February 1998.

Disease	Percentage of Total Admissions
Gastrointestinal and digestive	17
Respiratory disease	14
Trauma or poisoning	14
Circulatory conditions	10
Tumor, including cancer	8

Table 2.9.   Hospital Admissions by Disease Category: Top Five Conditions in 1997, All Hospitalizations for Jinshanwei Population (Regardless of Where Admitted).
Source: Shanghai Medical University. Unpublished data provided to authors during interviews with officials in February 1998.

	1995	1996
Revenues:		
Inpatient	25,159,254	27,707,888
Outpatient	28,923,951	45,283,952
Total revenues	54,083,205	72,991,840
Expenses:		
Wages	8,948,970	10,766,053
Bonuses	3,557,441	1,259,652
Drugs:		
Western	20,990,846	22,982,664
TCM	3,122,862	4,479,944
Equipment purchase	0	2,626,881
Lab supplies	365,663	894,193
Other expenses	1,421,644	2,418,749
Total expenses	38,407,425	45,428,135

Table 2.10.   Revenues and Expenses, Jin Shan Hospital (in RMB).

Source: Jin Shan Hospital. Unpublished data provided to authors during interviews with officials in February 1998.

THE MANAGED CARE PILOT PROGRAM IN JINSHANWEI

Chen and her colleagues at Shanghai Medical University have been working with key parties in Jinshanwei for several months to explore ideas for a managed care pilot. Many participants are enthusiastic about the potential of a managed care approach; they see many areas where managed care techniques could have a positive effect. "We need to have a gatekeeper," said a physician at the community health center in Jinshanwei. "People are going directly to the hospital who could be treated at the health center or at a health station. This is inefficient and a waste of resources." Others echoed the concern about inefficient use of resources. "The health stations are overstaffed and underused," said one observer. "Provider supply has been determined based on the size of the population, not need or use. And it's hard for health stations to compete when the hospitals have a much broader range of services, a wider range of drugs, more high-technology equipment and, frankly, often higher quality even for basic services."

The need to reduce hospital utilization was discussed as a major opportunity. As mentioned earlier, lengths of stay are long. Many patients have lengthy preoperative stays and there is very little discharge planning. "There is too much hospital use, at least in part because of the payment mechanism," said a member of Chen's team at Shanghai Medical University. "We have a saying, 'It used to be hard to be admitted to a hospital, now it's hard to get out. . . . Hospitals have no incentive to be more efficient. If a hospital runs a deficit, it is made up by the government. Hospital administrators have limited ability to change staffing patterns or take other actions to become efficient. There is tremendous waste and excess capacity in many hospitals, including Jin Shan." A walk through the hospital at 3 P.M. one weekday found very little activity in many outpatient areas, except at the pharmacy and hyperbaric oxygen machine.

Studies have found that length of stay is considerably longer for insured patients than for those who are uninsured. There is also evidence that insurance status affects the use of other resources. For instance, insured patients receive many more drugs than uninsured patients, with no evidence of improved outcomes. Controlling drug use is seen as a key goal of any managed care pilot program. "If we can control the use and cost of drugs, we can free up a tremendous amount of resources for other uses," said a member of the Shanghai Medical University team. "If we move to capitation, there would be incentives to do more prevention, patient education, and demand management." One of his colleagues added, "Managed care and capitated payment could help us rationalize our resource use. It would also make future planning better. At the moment, China makes future investment decisions based on historical utilization rates, which are distorted by the insurance, pricing, and payment systems."

Others hope that managed care can lead to more coordinated and integrated care. One clinician said, "Our recent efforts have focused on cost control and waste. We need better integration of social supports and medical services. If managed care helped with that, it would be useful."

However, not everyone involved in the Jinshanwei project is an enthusiast about managed care. "We do not know if managed care has potential," said an official at the Shanghai Medical Insurance Bureau. "We just do not know and we have not considered it. . . . But there would be tensions if we devoted more of our resources to administrative costs and managing care instead of providing medical services." A representative of a labor group echoed this concern, then added, "Also, an HMO plan may reduce quality, as we read has happened in the United States. . . . Who would oversee the managed care plan?"

Others expressed concerns about the goals of the project. "We must be careful whose interests we are serving," said one participant. "The goal of Shanghai Petrochemical Company is to reduce its costs. But we must also consider the hospital. It cannot lose too much money or its ability to serve will be threatened." An official at the Bureau added, "The major motivation for the project seems to be SPC's concern about its premium contribution going up. But that's the reason for insurance, to share costs broadly. . . . A managed care pilot might undermine the government insurance system. We need a uniform mechanism to share costs broadly and to facilitate movement from one job to another."

The project team had identified at least three possible approaches to a pilot program:

- An HMO, providing comprehensive inpatient and outpatient services. This approach would require the support and active participation of the Shanghai Medical Insurance Bureau.
- An outpatient-only program, which would avoid the need to integrate the pilot and the SMI plan.
- A much more limited and focused managed care plan, targeted at a few diseases and conditions, perhaps using a disease management approach.

Lack of data is a significant obstacle to program design. The health stations have some patient medical and cost information, but only in paper files. As part of its technical assistance, Kaiser Permanente has been collecting data from a sample of health stations on costs, utilization, referral patterns, and staffing ratios. Jin Shan Hospital has medical records for patients, but no computerized medical records system, although some administrative functions are computerized (accounting, admissions, and discharge). It appears impossible to obtain detailed information on hospital utilization or costs without doing sampling of medical records or surveys (for example, keeping a daily log of medications dispensed by the hospital pharmacy to identify the most frequently prescribed drugs). The Shanghai Medical Insurance Bureau has two years of inpatient claims data on insureds in Jinshanwei, but the claims forms contain limited information (patient ID number, age, sex, diagnosis at admission, length of stay, charges by type of service). The claims data are available in a computerized format.

The participants in the project are ambitious and optimistic, but also aware that the pilot must be appropriate to the specific situation and conditions in the area. "Medical development is related to economic development," said one team member. "China is still an underdeveloped country—our medical benefits are very good for our stage of development. Our social policy issue is how to get the biggest benefit for the available money—there are many trade-offs that must be made. If managed care can help with these decisions, it would be very helpful." Chen was particularly aware that the design of the pilot was both an economic and a political endeavor. "The medical care system is complex," she said. "We need to figure out a role for the different parties. The design of the program is very important if it is to get broad support and be successful."

~~~ Epilogue: Managed Care in Shanghai, November 2002

Based on information provided to the authors by Dr. Ying Yao Chen, Shanghai Medical University

Although the Kaiser Permanente consultants submitted a feasibility analysis to Shanghai Medical University detailing how much money could be saved under different managed care scenarios in Jinshanwei, no one pursued the idea further. Efforts to introduce managed care in urban areas of China continue in the form of grants to do feasibility studies and set up pilot programs. But nothing has been proposed on a large scale by the provinces or by the federal government.

Instead, Shanghai province has continued to reform the medical insurance system. At the time of the case, the Shanghai Medical Insurance Bureau had pooled into a single insurance plan all employer-based inpatient coverage, which covered 4.95 million employees and retirees. The premium started at 4.5 percent of payroll, and was raised to 6.5 percent in 1997 when some emergency and selected outpatient services were included for employees. In July 1999 outpatient coverage was extended to retirees, and the premium rose to 8.5 percent of payroll.

On January 1, 2001, Shanghai Medical Insurance Bureau introduced a new medical insurance scheme, called New SMIS. It is composed of a Basic Medical Insurance (BMI), and an Additional Medical

Insurance (AMI). The premium was raised to 12 percent of payroll for BMI (the employee pays 2 percent of payroll and the employer 10 percent) and an additional 2 percent of payroll for AMI (paid by the employer only). New SMIS benefits cover ambulatory, emergency, and inpatient care, with deductibles, copayments, and coinsurance based on the age of enrollees. New SMIS covers 6.5 million enrollees, including 2 million retirees, 3.5 million employees, and 1 million government workers.

The New SMIS splits the BMI into two accounts, the "sickness fund" and the "individual account." The sickness fund covers inpatient, emergency resulting in admission, and major outpatient (dialysis, chemotherapy, radiotherapy) services, while the individual account covers other outpatient and emergency services, and can be drawn upon to cover copayment and coinsurance up to the limit of the amount set aside in the individual account (roughly 40 percent of the BMI premium). Once a patient has gone over the ceiling in the BMI accounts, the AMI covers the additional inpatient and outpatient costs.

While the financing system changed, the payment system to hospitals remained fee-for-service, and the Shanghai Medical Insurance Bureau continues its retrospective review of hospital bills.

The major policy focus of the Shanghai Medical Insurance Bureau is on pharmaceutical policy, classification of hospitals, and managing the medical insurance plan. There is little policy interest in managed care.

References

"Aging Society." *China Daily News,* Feb. 16, 1998.

Hsiao, W. C. "The Chinese Health Care System: Lessons for Other Nations." *Social Science and Medicine,* 1995, *41*(8), 1047–1055.

Rosenthal, E. "China's Middle Class Savors Its New Wealth." *New York Times,* June 19, 1998, Section A, p.1

"Shanghai's Folks Obese, Population Shrinking." *China Daily News,* Feb. 19, 1998.

CHAPTER THREE

Westinghouse and Managed Care
Does the Emperor Wear Clothes?

"Gee, someone really should do something about this," exclaimed one of the health plan representatives at the conclusion of the consultant's presentation. The Medical Advisory Board of Westinghouse Electric Corporation (WX)—that is, the medical directors and account managers from the company's two health care plans, a Pittsburgh physician in private practice, and several staff members from the corporate human resources department—had just heard a summary of the results of an analysis of treatment patterns and costs of WX employees and dependents with cardiovascular disease. The goal of the analysis, which had been commissioned by Gene Clayton, VP of benefits in the WX corporate human resources department, was to examine cardiovascular-related claims data for WX employees to identify areas of opportunity to lower or maintain health

This case was originally written by the authors in 1997. Funding was provided by Astra USA. The authors express their thanks to Gene Clayton for his interest and assistance in preparing the case. This case does not necessarily represent the views or conclusions of the Westinghouse Electric Corporation or of Gene Clayton.

care costs while improving patient outcomes. Gene and his staff decided to commission the analysis largely out of their concern that WX's managed care plans were missing many opportunities to improve quality and reduce costs. According to Gene:

> Our per capita medical costs have been flat for four years but that's not good enough. We have been building an integrated claims database for years. It has been part of our overall health care strategy—making data available that can be analyzed to develop interventions. We have been asking the vendors to take the data and use it. But none of them have used the data at all. In fact, we even *gave* the medical claims data to one of our vendors in 1994, but they never did anything with it. So finally we thought *we* had to do something. We decided to take the ball and analyze the data ourselves, with the help of outside consultants. Westinghouse should not have to be mucking about with this data— that's the job of the managed care vendors—it's what we hire *them* to do. But we have been so frustrated that we knew we had to be proactive. And we found lots of opportunities to improve quality and reduce costs in just the small piece of the data we looked at. Our hope is that if we can lead the horses to water, maybe they will drink. But the edge of the water is about as far as we have gotten them so far.

THE FINDINGS OF THE CARDIOVASCULAR ANALYSIS

WX decided to focus on cardiovascular disease because it accounts for a significant proportion of total corporate medical expenditures, and pharmaceutical costs in particular. The cardiovascular analysis looked at four issues: use of beta-blockers following acute myocardial infarction, high-cost employees, the drug-taking behavior of hypertensive patients, and the appropriateness of physician prescribing. These issues were selected for analysis because of evidence, from a range of sound clinical sources, that these areas offer opportunities to improve quality and avoid costs. In addition, existing analytical methods could be used in the WX analysis.

Use of Beta-Blockers Following Myocardial Infarction

The use of beta-blockers after acute myocardial infarction (AMI) is one of the most scientifically substantiated, cost-effective preventive medical services. Many controlled studies have found that beta-blocker use following AMI decreases mortality and reinfarctions and increases the chances of survival by 20–40 percent. National cardiology committees strongly recommend the use of beta-blockers in eligible AMI patients. Despite these recommendations, physicians currently exhibit a low level of compliance with guidelines for use of beta-blockers after AMI. There are, therefore, substantial opportunities for improving care by increasing use of beta-blockers.

The WX analysis found that 43 percent of AMI patients with no contraindication are not on beta-blockers. In addition, some of the 38 percent of AMI patients who had some contraindication are also probably appropriate candidates for beta-blocker therapy. The overall conclusion of the analysis is that less than 50 percent of eligible patients currently use beta-blockers post-AMI. The WX results were very consistent with published studies showing estimates of eligible and untreated AMI patients ranging generally from 33 percent to 52 percent, and as high as 80 percent in some studies of elderly AMI survivors.

High-Cost Patients

The second part of the analysis found that WX has a small number of high-cost employees, defined as patients who had expenditures greater than $10,000 over the two-year study period and for whom cardiovascular costs represented more than 50 percent of their total costs. (There were 139 such cases, accounting for $4.9 million in total costs, with a mean expenditure of $36,000 and a maximum of $239,000.) The purpose of this analysis was to identify potential opportunities for better coordination of care and case management of patients with cardiovascular disease.

Drug-Taking Behavior of Hypertensive Individuals

The WX claims data was analyzed to detect patients with hypertension who had stopped taking their hypertension medication or who appeared to take it inconsistently. Research shows that compliance with drug therapy is often a problem with hypertensive patients; hypertension is an asymptomatic condition, and as a result patients may not take medication consistently or may stop drug therapy entirely.

In the WX analysis, 32 percent of approximately sixteen thousand individuals with hypertension were identified as potential problem patients because they did not take medications properly, either discontinuing drug therapy or taking their medication erratically. This analysis leads to the conclusion that opportunities for intervention to increase compliance with hypertensive drug therapy are significant.

Appropriateness of Prescribing

Hypertension is one of the most common conditions treated by the clinician, yet selection of appropriate treatment is often challenging, particularly because recommendations regarding treatment have changed significantly. Current national guidelines for treating hypertension recommend diet and exercise for the initial treatment of mild hypertension. Prescribing guidelines suggest starting hypertensive patients on diuretics and beta-blockers as initial therapy. Newer, more expensive antihypertensive medications, such as calcium channel blockers and angiotensin-converting enzyme (ACE) inhibitors, are recommended for use mainly as second-line agents except when the special circumstances of an individual patient justify their use as initial therapy. In addition, because of potential risks of treating patients with multiple medications, the recommended protocols are to begin with *monotherapy* (treating with one drug), and if needed, *sequential monotherapy* (first trying one drug, and if that drug does not work, replacing it with another drug), instead of using *stepped care* (beginning with a diuretic as the first step and then adding other agents as needed for blood pressure control) or *combination therapy* (starting the patient initially on two or more drugs).

Substantial evidence shows that many physicians do not follow these guidelines. In particular, the costs of treating hypertension could be reduced, and quality of care improved, if diuretics or beta-blockers were used more frequently as initial monotherapy. The results of the WX analysis confirmed that these opportunities exist for WX as well. The analysis found that although monotherapy or sequential monotherapy was the initial treatment regimen for 84 percent of hypertensive individuals, 8 percent of patients received either stepped therapy or combination treatment. Almost half of hypertensive patients (45 percent) were using either calcium channel blockers or ACE inhibitors, equal to the proportion of patients who were using beta-blockers or diuretics. Again, these results were consistent with the findings of research in other population groups. The findings suggest significant opportunities for cost saving if prescribing patterns can be changed. (The average cost per prescription for WX was $6 for diuretics and $11 for beta-blockers, compared with $23 for ACE inhibitors and $31 for calcium channel blockers.)

In summary, the consultants pointed out significant opportunities in the WX population to improve quality of care for individuals with cardiovascular disease while containing medical costs. The analysis estimated potential first-year cost savings at $1.6 million to $2.1 million, based on what the consultants believed were very conservative assumptions. The analysis suggested a range of possible interventions that could be implemented by WX and its managed care partners: physician education and feedback on appropriate prescribing; more effective aggressive identification and intervention in the care of patients who are candidates for beta-blockers by health plan discharge planners; better case management and coordination of care; and more proactive intervention, through means such as mail, phone, and fax, with patients who discontinue medication or have low compliance.

WX's Demand for Action

After the Medical Advisory Board heard the presentation of the results of the cardiovascular analysis, there was some discussion. Although representatives of WX's managed care vendors raised a few methodological concerns about the analysis, none of them really questioned either the data or the results. So, after throwing down the gauntlet by describing the results of the analysis as "really low-hanging fruit to the point that a midget could reach it," Clayton asked each vendor to develop a detailed action plan to address the study's findings, and to present the action plans to WX within thirty days.

WESTINGHOUSE ELECTRIC CORPORATION: FROM AIR BRAKES TO AIR(WAVES) JORDAN

In the words of one business directory, "industrial giant Westinghouse is changing channels" (*Hoover's Handbook of American Business*, 1997, p. 1438). Westinghouse, long an industrial mainstay, has undergone one of the most dramatic restructurings in American business in the last few years, transforming itself into a media and industrial conglomerate by a range of acquisitions and divestitures, including the purchase of CBS in 1995, Infinity Broadcasting in 1996, and the Country Music Television (CMT) and the Nashville Network (TNN) cable networks in 1997.

From its founding in 1886 by George Westinghouse, inventor of the train air brake, until the 1970s, WX expanded its businesses to include electrical generation and distribution, the manufacture of a range of electric products and appliances, and broadcasting. George Westinghouse entered the electric industry after developing a method for transmitting electric current over long distances. The success of his system resulted from a decision to use alternating current instead of the direct current favored by Thomas Edison. Westinghouse purchased the patents for AC from Nikola Tesla, an eccentric Croatian inventor, for $1 million. The company set up KDKA, the nation's first radio station, in Pittsburgh in 1920.

But by the 1970s, WX was struggling. It had lost a large part of its important utility generator business to General Electric (GE) in the mid-1970s. The company also sold its appliance business, which had always operated in the shadow of the market leader, GE. This sale was the beginning of a series of divestitures that would continue through the 1980s. These sales were combined with the acquisition of complementary businesses and joint ventures with foreign companies.

Although these actions had some positive effect on WX's financial and market position, by the early 1990s, the company was under extreme financial pressure. In 1991 and 1992, WX had a net loss of over $1 billion per year, mainly in its commercial credit and real estate businesses. It was forced to sell off a number of business units to generate cash, in some cases for prices that were considerably less than book value. In 1993 a new management team, headed by former PepsiCo executive Michael Jordan, took over the company. The new management continued the sale of WX businesses but at the same time initiated an aggressive—and expensive—media acquisition strategy, paying $5.4 billion for CBS and $4.7 billion for Infinity Broadcasting. In a continuing effort to pare down debt, the company sold several industrial units, including its electrical distribution and control business in 1994 to car parts maker Eaton, its WESCO division to CDW Holdings in 1994, its Knoll furniture division to E.M. Warburg Pincus in 1996, and its defense electronics unit to Northrup Grumman in 1996.

These sales and acquisitions have fundamentally changed the composition of WX's revenue and profit streams. The media and broadcasting segment, which includes CBS TV, CBS cable, Group W/CBS Radio, and various TV and radio stations, accounted for half of 1996 revenues and most of the corporation's operating profits. The industrial and technology group, which includes power generation, energy systems, government operations, and the Thermo King refrigerated transport unit, produced 50 percent of revenue but, with the exception of Thermo King, struggled from an operating income standpoint.

Later in 1997, WX plans to undergo a fundamental restructuring by dividing into two separate companies. The industries and technology group businesses (other than Thermo King) will be spun off into a company that will keep the Westinghouse Electric name, while the surviving media entity changes its name to CBS Corporation. In September 1997, WX announced its intention to sell Thermo King to Ingersoll-Rand Company. Each company will have its own board of directors and officers and its own publicly traded stock. The media company, which is estimated to have a much higher per share value than the industrial company, will assume all WX debt obligations, which are substantial after recent acquisitions, and retain the substantial and underfunded pension and retiree health care obligations. The new industrial company will be debt-free, but it will have potentially sizable product warranty liabilities.

WX's Health Care Strategy

When Gene Clayton assumed responsibility for health and welfare benefits in 1990, most WX employees were enrolled in a first-dollar coverage indemnity health plan. The indemnity plan was administered by a few carriers, depending on the type of charges (for example, hospital and physician benefits were administered by different carriers). Mental health, vision, and dental services were integrated into the indemnity plan. WX also contracted with more than a hundred HMOs in various portions of the country, and approximately 20 percent of employees were enrolled in HMOs.

Since 1990, WX, with the leadership of Gene and his staff, has fundamentally changed its health benefits approach. The traditional unmanaged indemnity plan has been eliminated, as have HMO plans. In their place, WX has adopted a comprehensive health care strategy, based on working in close collaboration with only a few managed care partners. Westinghouse regards these elements as critical to its health care benefits strategy:

- Convenient access to the highest quality of care at a manageable cost
- Systems that improve quality of care based on measurable standards
- Financial and quality incentives within a flexible format to change employee behavior and evolve toward a more effective set of programs

The company has undertaken a wide range of strategic initiatives and actions to fulfill this mission. It has redesigned health plan options, encouraged employees to enroll in managed care plans, developed a central data warehouse, and encouraged managers of individual business units to assume more accountability for the health care costs of their own employees. See Figure 3.1 for an overview of

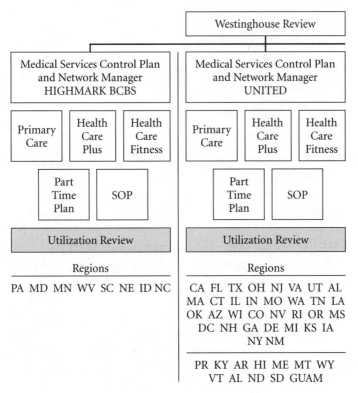

Figure 3.1.   *(Continued on page 56)*

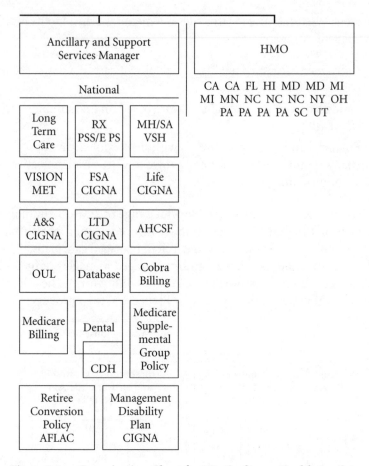

Figure 3.1.   Organization Chart for Westinghouse Health Services.

the way Westinghouse has organized its relationships with its health care vendors.

Although described by some of its managed care partners as "a high-maintenance account," the company generally receives praise for its efforts. According to one health plan representative:

> Westinghouse is more strategic than most other purchasers. The company has more of a plan for where it wants to go; we don't see that from other employers. The folks at Westinghouse are sophisticated, they know the jargon, they understand more about the clinical aspects of care, and they want to get from this point to that point and have no

problem telling you how to do it. They are innovative; for instance, Westinghouse asked for open access to OB/GYN services five years ago, before anyone else. But they also don't necessarily buy into the current fads. For example, Westinghouse refuses to allow carriers to use capitation payment arrangements for their plans because we can't demonstrate that they will save money.

Another independent observer remarked, "It's quite something to watch Gene and his people interact with the managed care plans. It's obvious that the plans are not asked to be this accountable by any of the other employers they deal with."

WX Benefit Design

The benefit plans WX offers to its twenty-three thousand active employees and twelve thousand early retirees are unique and complex. One outside consultant who works with many large employers recently commented that he had "never seen such a complex benefit plan." Some of the highly detailed nature of the WX benefit package is dictated by union contracts, although one observer commented, "I think it's partly a vestige of the fact that the company used to process its own claims—they are still in that micromanagement mentality sometimes."

Plans for Active Employees and Pre-Medicare Retirees

Most WX employees and pre-Medicare retirees have a choice of two medical plan types, an indemnity plan (called "Health Care Plus") or a point-of-service (POS) managed care plan (called "Primary Medical Care"). Benefits for vision, mental health and substance abuse, and prescription drugs are provided through national carve-out arrangements. Westinghouse employees who live in geographic areas where no provider network is available do not have the option of Primary Medical Care. In these areas, another managed care plan, called Total Care Management, is offered. This plan, which is administered by United Healthcare, requires members to consult by telephone with an individual care manager, generally a nurse, before obtaining certain types of services.

Health Care Plus is a traditional freedom-of-choice medical plan, with preadmission and emergency admission certification requirements in certain situations. After the covered person meets an annual deductible, the plan pays 80 percent of covered expenses; the patient is responsible for the other 20 percent, up to an annual out-of-pocket maximum. Both the deductible and the out-of-pocket maximum vary by the annual pay of the employee. Health Care Plus is administered by Blue Cross Blue Shield or United Healthcare, depending on geographic location. About 20 percent of WX's covered lives are enrolled in this plan.

The other 80 percent of covered lives are enrolled in Primary Medical Care, WX's managed POS product. This plan provides two alternative levels of benefits: in-network and out-of-network. Members are required to choose a primary care physician from a list of participating in-network doctors. The PCP provides and, when necessary, arranges referrals to other network providers, although self-referral to network specialists is permitted in some instances for obstetrical and gynecological services, and for chiropractic services.

Primary Medical Care members can decide whether to receive services in the network or out of the network each time they use medical care. Patient cost-sharing and administrative responsibilities are significantly lower if benefits are received within the network: office visit copayments are $10, with a 10 percent coinsurance for other services, up to an annual out-of-pocket limit. Network providers are responsible for meeting any care management requirements. If services are obtained out of network, the patient must meet an annual deductible and also pay 40 percent of the allowed charge (plus any balance billing beyond the allowed charge), up to an annual out-of-pocket limit. (As with Health Care Plus, deductibles and out-of-pocket maximums vary by the employee's annual pay.) The patient is also responsible for meeting all preadmission or emergency admission precertification requirements for care that is obtained out of network.

NETWORK MANAGERS. WX contracts with two network managers for Primary Medical Care, United Healthcare (United) and Highmark Blue Cross Blue Shield (BCBS), the plan that resulted from the merger of Blue Cross of Western Pennsylvania and Pennsylvania Blue Shield. Each network manager is responsible for administering Primary Medical Care in certain states. BCBS serves Maryland, Minnesota, Pennsylvania, South Carolina, North Carolina, West Virginia, Idaho, and Nebraska, areas that account for 60 percent of WX's covered lives;

United has responsibility for networks in thirty-four other states, serving the other 40 percent of WX employees and retirees.

The network managers are responsible for a range of activities including provider selection and credentialing, medical management, quality improvement, and claims payment. Although WX operates its health plans on a self-funded basis, and the network managers are not at financial risk for medical costs, since 1990 its contracts with all managed care vendors have contained detailed performance standards, including cost trend guarantees (which, in recognition of regional differences, vary by state). The vendors have significant financial risk for cost increases above the guaranteed trends. "Some of the vendors have not been able to deliver what they promised, and have had to pay some significant penalties as a result," one member of the human resources staff noted.

WX contracts with different vendors to administer its national drug, mental health, and vision care carve-out arrangements. The company's PPO-type prescription drug program is managed by Diversified Pharmaceutical Services. Although WX has been successful at containing its overall medical costs, its expenditures for prescription drugs have risen steadily in recent years, and WX has become particularly skeptical about the value of managed pharmacy programs. "We have decided that Pharmacy Benefit Management is a commodity business," according to one WX manager, "and that we will select vendors solely on price and access. No PBM vendor has been able to show us any real results from its care management activities. So we have concluded 'to hell with the clinical stuff,' at least for the next five years. We think the PBMs are that far away from demonstrating any real value added in terms of managing costs or quality."

Mental health and substance abuse services are offered through a PPO-type program managed by Value Behavioral Health. WX believes its behavioral health program has produced some positive results on the quality front, in addition to helping control costs. "We have clear evidence that recidivism and readmission rates have declined since we adopted our managed mental health and substance abuse program," a WX manager told us. "In fact, if anything, we get complaints that the program is managed too tightly. But we think the care management is improving quality. We see a real difference between our vendors that are run by clinicians and those that are run by businesspeople. The clinicians understand the clinical side, they know more about where the opportunities are and about how to make things work for the patients." She added, "But the downside is that some of their administrative processes are often not handled as well as by the businesspeople."

WX is currently seeking a new manager for its vision care program, after terminating its relationship with its previous vendor. "When our vendors have not performed up to our expectations, we have had no hesitation in looking for new partners," Gene said.

ELIMINATING HMOs. In the early 1990s, approximately 20 percent of WX employees belonged to HMOs. But in 1992 the company decided to begin phasing out its contracts with HMOs for a number of reasons. One frustration was the inability of the HMOs to provide account-specific data. WX also found it administratively complex and costly to deal with so many separate plans. In addition, the company concluded that contracting with HMOs was not cost-effective, and most likely resulted in higher costs. "We never saw the cost savings with HMOs," one manager said. "The company's trend was always lower in the indemnity plan than in the HMOs," said another manager. "And the HMOs attracted the younger, healthier employees, and were paid a community rate. If there were any savings, they were retained by the HMO instead of being passed along to Westinghouse." Between 1992 and 1995, WX continued to offer HMOs in geographic locations where Primary Medical Care was not available. In 1996, when networks had been established in all locations, HMOs were eliminated entirely for the active employee population.

Plans for Retirees with Medicare

The options WX offers to its forty-eight thousand retirees over age sixty-five are also complex. WX offers two plans free of charge: a limited $600 hospital benefit and a drug program with unlimited coverage but a 50 percent patient coinsurance amount. Retirees may also buy one of two additional coverages provided by BCBS, a comprehensive product that costs $42 per month, or a more limited hospital indemnity product at a monthly cost of $2.80. "The comprehensive plans attract two types of retirees, those who travel extensively, and those who are very sick," according to one human resource manager. As an alternative, retirees can enroll in one of fifty-five Medicare risk HMOs, which are offered as part of a national employer coalition that Gene helped initiate in 1993. To be eligible to treat WX retirees, an

HMO must offer an unlimited prescription drug benefit that is substantially equivalent to the regular health plan. In addition, since WX does not make a premium contribution to the HMOs, HMOs must have the ability to bill retirees directly for any premium. Approximately 14 percent of retirees are enrolled in HMOs.

Employee Cost-Sharing

The move to managed care has been accompanied by significant increases in cost-sharing for WX employees and retirees. "I think one of the reasons we are so demanding of our managed care vendors is that we want to help employees, who in recent years have felt the effect of increasing premium contributions," said one WX manager. "Although cost-sharing increases are hard from an employee relations standpoint, we consoled ourselves with our belief that there was a fair trade-off because employees would be getting higher-quality care in managed care plans."

The corporate goal is to have employees share approximately 25–30 percent of total health care costs, including premium and deductibles and copayments. Employee premium contributions vary by income, type of coverage (single, two-person, or family), and plan selected. Lower employee premium costs provide an incentive to join the managed care plan. For example, an employee making $40,000 per year in 1997 makes a monthly contribution of $50.50 for family coverage under Primary Medical Care, and $74.56 under Health Care Plus. (This compared with a monthly contribution amount in 1995 of $39.28 for Primary Medical Care and $57.96 for Health Care Plus.)

Employee Response to Health Plan Changes

Opinions about the reaction of WX employees and retirees to the company's managed care strategy range widely. "In general, I think the move to managed care went pretty well from an employee perspective, although many people still hate 'the referral thing,'" concluded one manager. "The biggest concern was access and if a person's doctor was in the network, they were happy." But network access was viewed by others as a problem, at least initially. "If you were in a big area like Pittsburgh, the networks were fine," according to another WX executive. "But in other areas, the networks were small or otherwise inadequate. For example, we had to deal with one network that looked like it had enough doctors within a few miles of all of our employees, but it turned out you had to drive fifty miles around a lake to get to the doctors who were shown on the map as only two miles away."

Opinions also vary about the effect of benefit changes and increased cost-sharing. "I think employees understand the reason why cost-sharing is increasing," said one staff member. "They read the papers, they know it's happening all over." Added another, "I think people are inured to benefit cuts. If they have a job, they are happy in these times." Many credit the WX unions with doing an excellent job in educating their members about the reasons for benefit changes.

But other observers disagreed with these assessments. "Although Corporate is still convinced that the benefit package is competitive, I don't think employees feel that way. They are skeptical and have real trust concerns," said one manager. Clearly the changes have not occurred without some pain for employees. "The biggest issue for employees is that Westinghouse, in its pursuit of lower costs, has had continual change in its benefits and its vendors," asserted one person. "People are often confused about who they have to call for which benefits—there's always a new phone number, a new process, a new name. Employees have reacted more negatively to these administrative changes than to the cost-shifting or to managed care."

An example cited by several managers of one administrative change that met with some negative reaction from employees was a recent decision by WX to outsource benefits administration. The company contracted with Wellspring to operate a central "Benefits Access Center," which employees can call via a toll-free number to obtain information on benefits. According to one manager, "The initial transition to the Benefits Access Center was rough—it was brought up too fast, and the staffing was wrong—the representatives were transaction oriented, not problem solvers. Those problems have been resolved. But many people miss the personal connection and trust they had with the on-site benefit administrators. They liked being able to go to someone where they worked to talk about benefits problems."

More Accountability for Business Units

Another component of the WX health care strategy is to attempt to get the managers of the corporate business units (power generation, Thermo King, broadcasting, and so on) to become more active in managing and controlling medical costs for their employees. As a first step, in 1992, the corporate human resources department began to provide each business unit every month with information about the *actual* health care costs of its employees, rather than an arbitrary allocation of corporate health care costs. Although useful, this change evidently had limited effect. "It was good for us to realize how much we were spending on health care and what the trends were," according to one business unit executive. "But there was so much talk about medical care costs in the press at that time that I don't think anyone found the data surprising. The time lag in getting the information was quite long—when we got the data it was already six months or so old. It just did not have the immediacy of other costs that were reported to us in a real-time way."

The reports were revised, and cost and utilization data are now reported more promptly, and in more detail. (See Exhibits 3.1 and 3.2 for samples of the types of information provided to the business units.)

Some business units have developed interventions based on the cost information. According to one manager,

> In my unit, we saw some seasonal trends in our costs. For example, back injuries went up in the spring and summer. So we instituted a stretching program in the factories. We also found a concentration of wrist injuries in one work area, and were able to reengineer jobs to deal with it. But although these were good programs, we could never really assess if they had much impact because our costs were still escalating and there were so many other things going on at the same time as our interventions, like benefit changes, that it was hard to isolate the impact of any one action.

One hope of WX's corporate human resources staff was that the business units would also experiment with other types of approaches to encourage employees and management to take more responsibility for medical costs and to reward health-promoting behavior. For instance, Gene and his corporate colleagues would like the business units to adjust their health plan premium contributions based on the performance and objectives of each business unit. The effects of this could be massive, as 85 percent of WX employees are covered under the corporate flexible benefit plan, under which they receive credits that can be used to purchase benefits from a range of offerings; the

Exhibit 3.1. Health Care Cost Report to Business Units, by Disease Category.

Major Diagnostic Category	INDEMNITY			POS			TOTAL		
	Total Claims	Benefits Paid	Benefits per Claim	Total Claims	Benefits Paid	Benefits per Claim	Total Claims	Benefits Paid	Benefits per Claim
Nervous									
Eye									
Ear, Nose, Mouth									
Respiratory									
Circulatory									
Digestive									
Kidney and Urinary Tract									
Musculoskeletal									
Skin & Breast									
Endocrine and Nutritional									
Kidney and Urinary Tract									
Male Reproductive									
Female Reproductive									
Pregnancy & Childbirth									
Newborns and Neonates									
Blood and Immunology									
Liver and Pancreas									
Infectious & Parasitic									
Mental Health									
Substance Abuse									
Injury & Poisoning									
Burns									
Other Factors									
Multiple Significant Trauma									
HIV									
Ungroupable									
Drugs									

Exhibit 3.2. Health Care Cost Report to Business Units, by Lifestyle Category.

Lifestyle Category	EMPLOYEES			SPOUSES			DEPENDENTS			TOTAL
	Paid Claims	Count	Average Cost	Paid Claims	Count	Average Cost	Paid Claims	Count	Average cost	Paid Claims
Tobacco Related										
Cardiovascular										
Chemical Dependency										
Injury Related										
Pregnancy Related										
Sexually Transmitted										
Arthritis and Rheumatic										
Cancer Related										
Stress Related										
Nutrition Related										
Tuberculosis										
Immunization Related										
Total Lifestyle										
Total Non-Lifestyle										
Total Paid Claims (No Rx)										
Lifestyle as Percentage of Total										

other 15 percent of employees are in union bargaining units. But so far, the business units have ignored this idea and have continued to adopt the contribution recommendations developed by the corporate human resources department. "We are used to the parent company doing everything," said one business unit manager. He added, "Besides, it's much easier to defend the corporate contribution recommendations to employees and the unions. It's a lot harder to say, 'Hey, we had a bad year financially in this business unit, so we want you to pay more for your health coverage.'"

Observers have a number of explanations for the failure of attempts to engage the business units in these types of initiatives. Ironically, one reason cited by a number of WX managers is their company's recent successes in holding the line on health care costs. "There was more immediacy a few years ago, when cost pressures were greater," said one business unit manager. "But health care costs are just not high on the radar screen anymore. They are not that significant in terms of overall costs for most business units and they are not rising." The outsourcing of benefits administration by creation of the Benefits Access Center was also given by some as another reason for business unit inaction. "It has created additional distance between the business units and health benefits," observed one human resource staff person.

Some managers have been discouraged by the need to show immediate results from any initiatives, particularly in the recent period of cost-cutting and downsizing at WX. "I know the human resource people have a sincere belief that if we take care of our employees better, we will have a better resource for the company, and that it's the right thing to do as well. But they know strategically that their initiatives need to be tied into a financial argument about the bottom line and return on investment. The problem is that if we can't demonstrate an immediate and adequate ROI to the corporate financial people, they won't support new programs. For instance, despite the sincere belief of the folks in human resources about the value of prevention, there is a lot of debate and disagreement about whether prevention and exercise really work, in terms of reducing medical costs." WX did undertake a significant worksite wellness initiative beginning in 1993, with the goal of reducing medical, disability, and workers' compensation costs and improving the quality of workplaces. Although the program was well received and participation rates were high, corporate funding for the program was eliminated in 1996. "Our strategic plan always was to provide the seed money for the program, and then get the business units to assume financial responsibility over time," said Gene. "But the only business unit that picked up the ball when our funding was cut was the one that hired the corporate wellness person we laid off."

The general level and pace of corporate change at WX have obviously also affected the success of this initiative. "Health care costs are really just lost in the shuffle of everything else going on around here," one manager noted. "There are layoffs, downsizings, restructurings— it's crazy. It's easier not to mess with benefits with everything else we have to do. And, frankly, when everyone is worried about whether they are going to be the next unit to be sold, it's hard to get excited or motivated about controlling health care costs," he said.

Some business units also question their potential to really affect health care costs and quality. According to one manager:

I am not too sure how much impact one individual business unit can have on costs. We don't have any control over the benefit design itself, although that's a change many of the business units would like to see. We can do prevention programs, but they probably really don't work too well. Our employees are dispersed geographically, so we don't have any real clout with providers. We also don't really have the expertise to develop interventions. There may be things that can be done in manufacturing plants, particularly to deal with reducing work-related injuries. But health care costs are really not our world, and we are not really engaged. I think it's reasonable that we need to rely on HR to deal with costs.

The corporate human resources staff remains frustrated by its inability to engage the business units in this initiative. According to Gene, "We have hit the business units over the head with data, and there has been very little effect. We have seeded programs but they won't grow. We have encouraged ownership in cost sharing, but the business unit managers have turned their backs. But we are still convinced that there are lots of opportunities for them to be creative and show results."

Central Data Collection

The ability of WX to hit vendors and business units over the head with data is the result of another corporate health initiative: the development of an integrated medical data warehouse. The goal of the data warehouse is "to allow us to have one version of the truth," says Gene. This effort, which is administered by Corporate Health Strategies (an outside vendor now owned by United Healthcare), collects claims data from all WX health benefit plans, including the indemnity product, the point-of-service plans, the pharmacy, mental health, and dental carve-out plans, and the short-term disability plan. The data is used to calculate the charge-back to the business units of the actual costs of medical services used by their employees, as well as to produce a regular series of monthly reports for the corporate human resources department and the business units.

Corporate staff are strong supporters of the data warehouse initiative, but they believe it has not realized its potential as a tool for change. "We have lots of data," said one staff member. "In fact, in a way we have too much data. The quality of the data is good but we don't know how to use it. And the people who work for our data vendor are data crunchers, not analysts or producers of information." Although the purpose of sharing the information with the business units is to "get a continuing dialog going," it is unusual for the business units to ask for more information or analysis. "I think the business units are drowning in data," according to one unit manager. In fact, it is more common for the corporate human resources department to get requests for data from its managed care vendors. "Vendors call us and ask, 'Can you get this report for me?'" said the manager in charge of the data warehouse. "When I say, 'But it's your own data that you are asking for,' they say, 'Yes, but you can access it easier and faster than we can.'" But corporate staff remain frustrated that vendors request the data for administrative purposes and have not used the data warehouse as a resource for identifying opportunities for clinical or programmatic interventions. "So we are just left with interesting data and useless information," said Gene.

"MANAGED": MISSING FROM THE CONTENT OF MANAGED CARE?

WX has been successful at controlling costs; its per capita health care costs have been flat for the past four years. (See Figure 3.2.) But despite this success, Gene and his colleagues have increasingly questioned the value added of managed care. In particular, they question

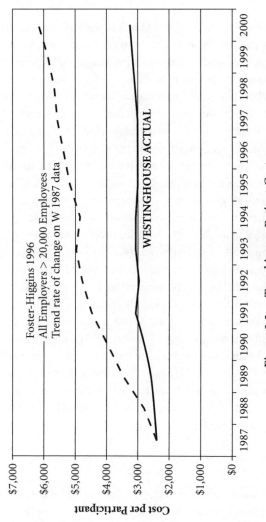

Figure 3.2. Trend in per Patient Cost.

Source: Unpublished data provided to the authors by Westinghouse.

Note: Figures cover all plan participants: actives, retirees under age sixty-five, COBRA, and surviving spouses.

the ability of the WX network managers to actually *manage medical care,* as opposed to managing costs. They believe whatever cost savings the vendors have produced have resulted almost entirely from price discounts.

According to Gene:

> When Westinghouse began its efforts to reduce medical costs, we knew we had to alter the process and content of care, and the behavior of providers, employees, and health plan administrators. We knew this would take a long time but we believed we could be successful if we worked in collaboration with our managed care vendors. We view our vendors as our partners. And we are very clear about the accountability of partners: A partnership is a relationship where the independence is equal, the dependence is mutual, and the obligation is reciprocal. We thought all of us were on the same track and working together. Some of our partners didn't make it, but we were committed to our objectives of managing costs while improving access and quality.
>
> So, over the last six or seven years, we changed our plan design, put in place strong financial incentives to drive our people into managed care plans, and almost all of our covered lives are now in a managed care environment. We have really pushed and confused our employees in terms of cost-sharing and administrative hassles to make these changes. But now we wonder what is really being managed? Where is the *managed* in the content of managed care? Our people are straining under the weight of trying to navigate the managed care systems—they are not getting the support they need, not the care management nor the connections. All we seem to get are higher administrative fees from the vendors but no real results. And when the vendors do develop new initiatives, they want us to pay more—I always thought that's what we were already paying them for.

Another manager added,

> We pay the vendors to think, to manage costs. The administrative fee is $5 or $6 per member month higher in the managed care plans than in the indemnity option. We have seen some savings: provider discounts, reduction of inpatient days, and elimination of some specialty visits. But we don't see any proactive initiatives. They aren't looking at the whole picture. The carriers just develop boutique products that may take a tiny bite out here and there but definitely add on costs. It's

like dealing with the phone company. We think all the add-ons should be part of the basic service package.

In commenting specifically on the cardiovascular analysis, one manager said, "We cannot believe that the vendors are so passive. Our analysis shows clear evidence of a problem. You would think the managed care plans would be *anxious* to do something about it. There are lots of possible approaches: educational efforts directed at physicians, case management, physician profiling. Maybe the carriers have competing priorities, but we sure don't know what they are."

Not surprisingly, the managed care vendors disagree with WX managers' assessment of their performance, although tactfully. In the words of one vendor:

Westinghouse is very aggressive compared to other purchasers, and rightfully so. The company is at the leading edge in terms of presenting data and asking us to do something about it. But we think our medical management strategy is very closely aligned with the needs of Westinghouse. We have been collecting, analyzing, and using claims data to identify clinical issues worthy of medical management for years, and have developed a variety of new programs in response . . . including new medical programs for ischemic heart disease and congestive heart failure. We plan to continue to investigate and develop new programs as our profiling tools direct us to new opportunities. While we understand the concern that we are not using Westinghouse-specific claims data to develop programs specific for Westinghouse, we believe the programs we currently offer and the programs we have in development will deliver significant value to all of our members, including those who are Westinghouse employees and dependents.

Managed care plans also denied that they are asking WX to fund their research and development efforts. "We use our own resources to pilot medical management programs," commented one plan. "In the rare instance that a customer has come to us with a unique, specific request for a program which clearly would be applicable only to that customer, we do ask the customer to work with us as a partner, including managing some of the expense of development. But that's not the case with any of the initiatives that apply to the WX account."

However, some managed care representatives did concede that some of WX's frustration was understandable. "Our reflex is to be defensive," said one plan executive. "But Westinghouse is right. In the past we either did not have the data we should have, or we didn't use it. But we are changing that and making great strides in developing data-driven interventions." Another vendor also sympathized, "We understand the frustration; none of these initiatives are moving as quickly as anyone would like. But it's hard to bring about a 'new order of things,' as Machiavelli said."

The managed care vendors pointed specifically to several factors that they claim have impeded their ability to manage costs, including the fragmented structure of the WX benefit plans. "Carve-outs are an obstacle to more effective care management," asserted one vendor. It's hard to create effective interface mechanisms; coordination and administration is more complex. Another remarked, "It was our own fault that purchasers adopted carve-outs, because we were slow to develop expertise in some areas, especially drugs. But it's very hard to integrate care when purchasers have three or four or five different carve-outs. For example, we don't have the drug data without a hand-off. And we can't make changes in someone else's formulary."

But one WX staff member disagreed. "We don't think the carve-outs have any impact on quality. Plus, the economics are compelling. For example, in the drug area there is no way a regional vendor can get the same discounts as a large national pharmacy benefit manager." At one point in the last few years, WX did consider reintegrating mental health and substance abuse services into the medical plans, but found that the medical plans could not offer a deal that was competitive financially with its carve-out arrangement.

The managed care vendors note that WX has derived financial benefits from other arrangements as well. "Westinghouse has saved millions of dollars just from our provider discounts," said one vendor. Ironically, WX believes that the vendors' provider discounts, at least in some locations, are definitely a two-edged sword. "It's hard economically for us or any other purchaser to walk away from any vendor that has market dominance, because no one else can match their provider discounts, even when we are completely frustrated by service levels or lack of response to our concerns about care management," noted one WX manager. "We want it all: lower costs, quality care, and broad access," said another. "Westinghouse wants a Cadillac for a VW price. Employees are used to access and its hard politically to break them. The only alternative we have to our current arrangements is to contract with HMOs. But we are not willing to accept the limitations of HMOs in order to break the power of the dominant carriers."

In fact, WX managers believe that the recent restructurings and consolidations in the managed care market are impeding progress and weakening the bargaining power of purchasers. "BCBS has been reorganizing, United merged with MetraHealth, our data vendor has been taken over by United, our mental health vendor is being bought by Columbia/HCA," said one WX manager. "We have to spend lots of time reeducating people."

Another observed, "Vendors are not as hungry anymore because of the industry consolidation. They used to be willing to lose some money on big accounts to get market share, but they don't need to anymore. The little guys were more customer oriented, but they have been swallowed up by huge, bureaucratic entities that are arrogant and adversarial." She added, "It's frustrating to pay these companies millions of dollars in administrative fees and have their first answer always be no." But at least one managed care representative disagreed, "The industry numbers simply do not bear out WX's consolidation theory. There are still lots of vendors and the market is getting more and more competitive. Plus, there are lots of HMOs in many accounts as well."

WX staff also believe that the company's acquisition and restructuring activities have had an adverse effect on its health benefits strategy and operations in a number of ways. "We have had to devote a lot of our time to divesting and absorbing new companies and merging and restructuring benefit plans," said one WX staffer. "It's made it hard to focus on more proactive initiatives," observed a manager. "Our workforce has shrunk from seventy-two thousand active employees in 1990 to only twenty-three thousand active employees today," a WX employee said. "So we aren't as prestigious anymore and we don't have nearly the market power we used to have with vendors. And the carriers sometimes like to remind us of that in subtle ways. Like the first thing they say during a meeting with us is, 'So, any more downsizing rumors?'" Another staff member said, "All the reorganizing and divestitures have shaved our big stick down to a nub."

But others questioned how much impact or power even a large purchaser could have on managed care vendors. "Even in our heyday, we were a small player, although we are big locally in Pittsburgh," one person observed. "We only accounted for a few percent of total covered lives then, and we only account for a few percent of covered lives now." He noted also that corporate downsizing is "depriving companies of the resources and expertise they need to manage vendors." WX has been involved with a coalition of other purchasers in Pittsburgh, but so far this effort has produced no tangible results. "I don't hold out a whole lot of hope for these efforts, at least in Pittsburgh," sighed a manager. "BCBS covers 60 percent of Pittsburgh-area residents—it is simply too big and too powerful here. And although the providers are consolidating like crazy, BCBS still has the upper hand."

This observation may have been somewhat prescient: Highmark BCBS recently announced that it will contract only with individual hospitals, not hospital networks or systems. According to a BCBS spokesperson, "Highmark can hold down costs better with individual negotiations. . . . The networks are being formed by tertiary hospitals to meet their needs. . . . There is little evidence that hospital-led provider networks have served their members in a more cost-effective way . . . or have been successful at reducing costs or improving quality. . . . In other parts of the country, some providers who have built integrated delivery systems are now taking them apart" ("War on Networks," 1997, p. 16).

THE NETWORK MANAGERS' RESPONSE TO THE CARDIOVASCULAR ANALYSIS

A month after the meeting of the Medical Advisory Group, Gene and his staff met with each of its two network managers to review the action plans they had developed in response to the cardiovascular analysis. One of the vendors produced no specific action plan steps to deal with the problems identified in the WX study, engaging instead in what WX staff characterized as "a rambling discussion which resulted in no specific action or management of Westinghouse cardiac cases." In response, WX sent this vendor what Gene termed "a nastygram," demanding within two weeks a "structured action plan to address the data, including action items, parties responsible for managing the targeted action, due dates, and measurement tools that will allow us to measure the success of the program." The vendor then provided information about a pilot "Congestive Heart Failure Management Program," that it had just implemented for a small number of its Medicare HMO members. Although the program was not developed specifically for WX, the vendor noted that it "will ensure that appropriate WX employees and retirees are included in this and other interventions."

WX's other vendor developed an action plan in response to the analysis. One component of the plan was a description of the vendor's existing cardiac disease management program, which had been implemented on a pilot basis with good results and is scheduled to be available to most WX employees in early 1998. The program has a longitudinal rather than episodic focus and relies on a proactive case management approach, with active identification of at-risk patients through a variety of means; the development of an individual care plan (including drug management and goals for lifestyle modification in smoking, exercise, diet, stress management, and other areas); patient education and training; and regularly scheduled focused contact with patients to assess progress, compliance, and needs. The cardiac care managers in the program are specifically trained in adult learning and education. Because coordination and accountability for care is often a problem, a lead physician is designated for each patient; the program uses information from patients to maintain contact with that physician about patient progress and any needed changes. As the vendor explained:

> We are trying to identify patients early enough to make a difference through modest interventions. Those interventions rely on getting doctors to manage well and then to steer patients to those providers and share savings with them. But our tools for doing high-risk assessment and patient identification are not precise enough yet—they identify lots of the wrong patients and miss others. So we need to keep working on new methodologies and refining our approaches before we adopt programs on a bigger scale. Some of the new approaches will work, some won't. We need to keep experimenting and it's not fair to want an ROI on every single effort.

The vendor planned to charge an additional fee for the program, probably on a per-patient basis. "If you can't demonstrate that it works, why should we pay for it?" responded WX. A case manager pointed out sharply,

> That should be your own R&D. You are nickel and diming us to death. This should be an inherent cost of case management. We already pay for case management. We were told years ago that you had programs like this—what have we been paying for all this time? If you have now decided that this more disease-specific approach is the one you should take, why don't you just change the mix of services in your case

management area and lay off general case managers and bring in specialists—why should we purchase new and different case management on top of what we already purchase?

"If you are still evaluating this approach, let Westinghouse be a pilot site at no charge," another WX manager suggested.

"We did not look at Westinghouse data to develop this approach," responded the network manager. "We designed the program based on our overall population. We think the program will be of value to Westinghouse. But generally we can't develop programs for just one account. It's not cost-effective."

The vendor also proposed implementation of a beta-blocker pilot program designed specifically for WX patients that would attempt to ensure the initiation of beta-blocker therapy within thirty days of AMI in those WX-covered patients for whom the therapy is not contraindicated. (See Figure 3.3 for details on this pilot.) The pilot would use existing care management processes to identify WX patients with AMI, ideally while still in hospital, and document drug therapy at discharge. Patients will be contacted individually within one week of discharge by a care manager to confirm medication regime and assess compliance. Patients who are not receiving beta-blockers or who have compliance needs will be referred to the medical director. The medical director will also contact the attending physician of patients not on beta-blockers to provide education and to follow up on any other issues. Patients will be contacted by care managers after three and six months to assess their compliance with prescribed medication.

WHERE SHOULD WX GO FROM HERE?

As WX continues its plan to split into two companies later in 1997, the new companies will have the opportunity to renegotiate their managed care contracts and rethink their health care approach. This puts Gene and his colleagues at a crossroads. According to Gene:

I feel like we are having to take a cattle prod to the managed care organizations to get even the most modest actions out of them. We believe in data analysis and developing interventions based on that analysis. We broke barriers and took on all kinds of problems at Westinghouse to push managed care. . . . We sold the employees and the unions on the benefits of managed care from a quality standpoint. . . . We have

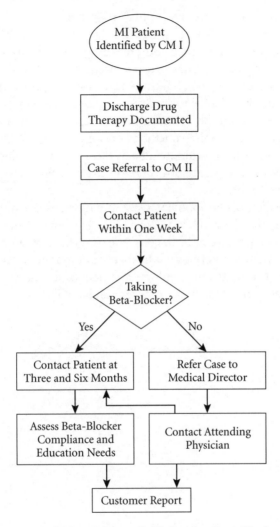

Figure 3.3.   Work Flow: Myocardial Infarction Beta-Blocker Patient Interventions.

produced all types of information that the vendors are just not using. We have given them the data, we brought them a full plate, but they refuse to eat. I will be hanging on a wooden cross soon.

Several WX managers think that the company's medical costs might actually be lower if everyone were in the indemnity product. "The discounts are the same as in the managed care plans, and the employee cost-sharing is higher," maintained one.

But Gene refuted this viewpoint strongly. "We are out in front on costs," he said. "Costs are not the issue. The data already demonstrate clearly that there is a financial difference between managed care and the indemnity plan." WX has a clear consensus that the managed care approach should not be abandoned, if only for political reasons. "We don't think we can eliminate the managed care plans—we would lose all of our credibility with the employees, and with senior management as well probably," concluded one of Gene's staff. "After all the work we have done to promote managed care, we would look schizophrenic. But while we are out there on the managed care limb, the vendors are sawing away."

Despite their disillusionment, Gene and his staff have not lost their commitment to their mission. As he said, "Even in the midst of all of the craziness here, we need to continue to push to change our costs and improve the quality of medical care and quality of life for our employees. If our current vendors can't help us do that, we will find someone else and some other approaches that will."

⧫ Epilogue: Westinghouse and Managed Care—Is the Emperor Dead?

Gene Clayton
Vice President, AutoNation
(formerly Vice President, Corporate Benefits, Westinghouse)

Who would have guessed a major U.S. industrial institution such as Westinghouse Electric Corporation would simply dissolve? That is what followed in late 1997. Westinghouse Broadcasting Company was renamed CBS Corporation, and British Nuclear Fuel purchased the nuclear business, while Morris-Knudsen purchased the government operations. These two industrial entities were all the manufacturing left in Westinghouse at this time. Subsequently, Sumner Redstone and Viacom purchased CBS Inc.

Following this time, my professional journeys allowed me to spend several years working inside other major corporations as a benefits consultant. My continued push for more focused meaning to managed care still met with resistance from health plan administrators.

Note: AutoNation, Inc., headquartered in Fort Lauderdale, Florida, is America's largest retailer of new and used vehicles. A Fortune 100 company, AutoNation employs approximately thirty thousand people and owns and operates 371 new vehicle franchises in seventeen states. For additional information, please visit the corporate site section of http://www.autonation.com.

Nothing was changing regarding the actual management of care. Only one last frontier of opportunity was as yet unleashed on this battle: the individual consumers themselves.

While working on a contract with Craig T. Monaghan, CFO of AutoNation, we were able to settle on a new benefit strategic course: Leverage qualified health plans and establish them as a base to price the medical products to employees. Unleash strong consumerism on this population and let employees vote with their own dollars regarding price, product, and service. Cast against this insured best of the best regional market, we added a self-insured medical option as well. The key is still to push for managed care, which tends to be the keystone of HMO and POS products, but to base the pricing for employer subsidies on the HMO products.

A lot has changed on the U.S. medical landscape over the past five years. But medical costs are on the rise once again. The forecasts are ominous, quality is still being challenged, and aspects of POS are being eroded and discarded. With the advent of the Internet, more and more medical data is provided to consumers, medical record management systems are springing up, and physicians themselves are subscribing to more of the efficiencies of Internet transactional usage.

But I would offer that we in the employer industries are still dealing with the processes and not the content of the problems surrounding quality, access, and costs. However, several legitimate and productive organizations in the employer sector have given rise to changes by the providers and health plans. Many regional employer coalitions and even the new Leap Frog national employer coalition are seeing positive results in improving medical quality and cost profiles. And several organizations are also providing relative and regional comparative information on medical facilities: mortality, morbidity, access, costs, and the like.

Since I accepted the invitation to remain at AutoNation, we have begun to ignite the new strategies and over the past year have seen great strides in managing costs while improving the strategic relationships with our various health plans across the United States. One such new relationship has developed on the West Coast. With the leadership of professional Jack Bruner of Hewitt Associates, AutoNation offers two insured health plans simultaneously. After annual enrollment, a retrospective risk adjustment arrangement is in place whereby each plan can be reevaluated depending on the risk of the employees who enrolled, and the premiums are adjusted accordingly. No losers, the plans compete based on their products and service as judged by the consumer-employee.

At the core of these new strategies is the notion that consumers— that is, our employees and their spouses—can help control the quality and delivery of health care with our health plans. We have established a new Medical Advisory team consisting of several practicing physicians from the provider community; we are working with health plans to begin to share utilization information; we are installing a central data warehouse to collect medical encounter data; and we are restructuring all existing provider contracts to reflect meaningful performance around the satisfaction measures our employees value, while changing the model of negative reinforcement contracts to one of positive reinforcement for positive performance. Engaging the district leadership in design, delivery, and pricing issues has been a critical element in this turnaround benchmark strategy. Corporate tends to establish health policy and other medical matters with some disregard for the field. Now there is a new collaborative process that takes place prior to major changes in structure and content of benefits. Districts are now charged for utilization costs. Before being acquired by Auto-Nation, all the dealerships purchased and managed their own health care programs. As we continue to expand and grow, it is imperative that corporate and the dealerships continue to work in an integrated management style toward the same objectives: reducing the medical costs, improving the competitive value, and reducing the risks while satisfying the expectations of AutoNation employees.

References

Hoover's Handbook of American Business. Austin, Tex.: Hoover's Business Press, 1997.

"War on Networks." *Modern Healthcare,* July 28, 1997, p. 16.

CHAPTER FOUR

Enhancing Access to Pharmaceuticals in Brazil

T he country of Brazil is widely hailed internationally for its efforts to make pharmaceuticals more accessible to its population. The government has been very active in a range of areas, including expanding public production and distribution of HIV drugs, price controls, and developing programs to make essential drugs universally available. As a result of these initiatives, many other countries are looking to Brazil for leadership in the pharmaceutical policy area.

Some of Brazil's initiatives have been controversial, particularly for threatening to break patents for several drugs and to engage in compulsory licensing. Despite many successes, the government is also criticized for its failure to reduce disparities in access to drugs, for omitting coverage for many chronic and noninfectious diseases, and

This case was originally written by the authors in 2002. Funding provided by Astra Zeneca. Many thanks to Carlos Felipe and Nancy Featherstone of Astra Zeneca for their support. Kudos to Tim Donohue of Boston Market Strategies, bodyguard, apprentice case writer, and traveling companion extraordinaire.

for public policies that some observers believe have stymied innovation and retarded the development of appropriate private sector market approaches for promoting drug access and containing costs,
particularly for middle-income individuals.

Being both rich and poor, Brazil provides an interesting case study
of the challenges involved in promoting access to pharmaceuticals in
a developing country: balancing public and private coverage, targeting limited public resources most effectively, finding the appropriate
blend of market forces and regulation, controlling prices while still
promoting foreign investment and technological innovation, and
determining the role that transnational drug companies might play in
promoting access to drugs, particularly among poorer populations.

SOCIOECONOMIC BACKGROUND

Brazil is the third-largest democracy in the world, with a population of
approximately 170 million. It is organized as a federal republic, and
comprises twenty-six states and the Federal District, the seat of the
national government, with a further subdivision into 5,508 municipalities *(municipios)* or counties. It is the second-largest economy in the
Americas, after the United States and followed by Canada and Mexico.
Brazil's federal budget is roughly 30 percent of the GDP, and 60 percent
of federal spending is on debt service for internal and external debt.
GDP as of 2000 was just under $600 billion, down from a peak of $801
billion in 1998 and reflecting a 40 percent devaluation of its currency in
1999. Roughly 10–11 percent of federal spending is on health care.

The country reestablished civilian democratic rule in 1985, after
two decades of military dictatorship. Since that time, Brazil has experienced many years of extreme economic and political upheaval,
including nine plans of economic stabilization, five price freezes,
dozens of calls for renegotiation of foreign debt, several currency
devaluations and changes, and multiple changes of government,
including one presidential impeachment. The late 1980s and early
1990s were particularly difficult years, when Brazil was plagued by
inconsistent growth and periods of extraordinarily high inflation. Since
the enactment of an economic stabilization plan in 1994, Brazil has
successfully reduced inflation and inflationary expectations, resumed
growth, reduced poverty, and increased private investment, particularly foreign investment. The country has also made enormous strides
in the past two decades in reducing poverty, increasing educational

levels, decreasing illiteracy, and improving many other socioeconomic
indicators. (See Table 4.1.)

Despite this progress, Brazil remains an extremely diverse and
unequal country, by virtually every social, economic, and health status
measure. The country is divided into five major regions: the North,

	Brazil	United States
1. People		
Population, total	170.1 million	281.6 million
Population growth (annual percentage)	1.3	1.2
National poverty rate (percentage of population)	22 percent	N/A
Life expectancy at birth (years)	68.1	77.1
Fertility rate, total (births per woman)	2.2	2.1
Mortality rate, infant (per 1,000 live births)	31.7	7.1
Mortality rate, under age 5 (per 1,000 live births)	39.0	8.7
Births attended by skilled health staff (percentage of total)	88	95+
Malnutrition prevalence (percentage of children under 5)	6	N/A
Urban population (percentage of total)	81	77
Prevalence of HIV, female (percentage of females 15–24)	0.3	0.2
Illiteracy rate, adult male (percentage of males 15+)	14.9	N/A
Illiteracy rate, adult female (percentage of females 15+)	14.6	N/A
2. Economy		
GDP (current US$)	593.8 billion	9.8 trillion
GDP growth (annual percentage)	4.4	4.2
Inflation, GDP deflator (annual percentage)	8.5	2.2
Structure of economy (percentage GDP)		
• Agriculture	7	
• Industry	29	
• Services	64	
3. Technology and infrastructure		
Personal computers (per 1,000 people)	50	585
Internet users	5 million	95 million
Paved roads (percentage of total)	6	59
4. Trade and finance		
Present value of debt (current US$)	223.8 billion	N/A
Short-term debt service (percentage of exports of goods and services)	90.7	N/A
Aid per capita (current US$)	1.9	N/A

Table 4.1.   Brazil Socioeconomic Data Profile, 2000.

Source: World Bank (http://www.worldbank.org/data); Data by Country, Brazil
(access date March 26, 2003).

with 45 percent of the land but only 7 percent of the population; the Central West with 18 percent of the land and 6 percent of the population; the Northeast, which has 18 percent of the land and 29 percent of people; the Southeast, with 11 percent of land and 43 percent of the population; and the South, with 7 percent of land and 15 percent of the population. Regional disparities are tremendous; the South, Southeast, and Central West regions of the country are in the upper ranges in many health indicators, while the North and Northeast are intermediate to poor by international standards. The country has undergone dramatic urbanization in the last forty years. In 1960 only 30 percent of the population lived in cities, compared to 80 percent today. This migration and growth of the urban population has created tremendous problems in major cities. Although the country's overall illiteracy rate was 13 percent in 1999, it ranged from 8 percent in the wealthier Southeast to 27 percent in the poor Northeast.

Brazil has one of the least equitable distributions of income in the world. An estimated 30 percent of population is poor (although this proportion has declined from approximately 44 percent in 1990). Nearly 35 million live in extreme poverty, often referred to by Brazilians as "below misery," and cannot meet their basic food needs. Nearly a quarter of the population live on a family income that is less than or equal to half the country's minimum wage (which is approximately $60 a month as of 2000). Poverty levels vary across the country. Close to 40 percent of people in the North and Northeast regions are poor, compared to 10 percent in the richer Southeast. Poverty is much higher in rural areas than in major cities.

There is, however, great wealth in Brazil and a large middle class. The richest 10 percent of the population receives almost 45 percent of national income, while the income share of the poorest half of population is only 12 percent. The mean income of the wealthiest 10 percent of the population is more than thirty times that of the poorest 40 percent. Wide income disparities exist across the country, with income per capita in São Paolo, the richest state, being more than seven times the income per capita in the poorest state. According to one government economist, "In Brazil, we know that people at the median income are a lot poorer than you would think looking at average income per capita. Surveys in the late 1990s showed that the mean average household income per capita was about $4,000, but the median was closer to $1,700. We have lots of poor people but lots of rich people too, and we're actually one of the better-off middle-income countries. Public policy is a challenge in a country of such great income extremes."

Not surprisingly, the diversity of Brazil in economic terms is mirrored in the diversity of common indicators of disease and health. The country has infectious diseases endemic in the developing world, and chronic noncommunicable illnesses typical of industrial countries. (See Table 4.2.) Malaria is the leading infectious disease in the country, with over 400,000 cases countrywide, mainly in the Amazon. Yellow fever, dengue, schistosomiasis, and tuberculosis are also problems, although the frequency of these diseases has been declining. HIV and AIDS have had a tremendous impact on the country, with over 530,000 individuals infected with the virus, although the rate of new infections has declined dramatically as a result of a variety of governmental initiatives.

Indicator	
Infant mortality (per 1,000 live births)	31.7
Mortality under age 5 (per 1,000 live births)	39.0
Maternal mortality (per 1,000 live births)	59
Percentage of women who get prenatal care	86
Life expectancy at birth (years)	68.1
Deaths due to communicable diseases (per 100,000 adjusted by age)	81.3
Deaths due to cancer (per 100,000 adjusted by age)	93.3
Percentage of population that smokes	18
Deaths due to circulatory disease (per 100,000 adjusted by age)	246.3
External causes (injuries, poisonings) (per 100,000 adjusted by age)	86.1
Immunization rates (percentages)	
DPT	75
OPV3	89
BCG	95
German measles	80
Prevalence of diseases (per 100,000 population)	
HIV	74
Tuberculosis	29
Leprosy	70
Diabetes	7.6 percent of population
Lung cancer	20.1 (males)
	5.9 (females)
Cancer overall	162 (males)
	176 (females)

Table 4.2.   Selected Brazilian Health Indicators (1999).
Source: Pan American Health Organization, 1999.

Brazil has made great strides in improving many health status measures in recent years, with significant declines in overall mortality rates, mostly as the result of dramatic declines in infant and childhood death rates. But regional variations are significant; states in the Northeast have much lower health indicators than states in the Southeast, in particular much higher rates of low birth-weight babies and higher death rates among young children.

With this progress has come a pattern of disease and death more typical of the developed world. The Brazilian population is aging rapidly, and most chronic diseases are on the rise. Cardiovascular disease is the leading cause of death in almost all areas of the country, followed by external causes (violence, accidents), cancer, respiratory disease, infectious diseases, and perinatal causes. (See Table 4.3.) Unreported deaths are very common in Brazil, particularly in the poorest areas. As many as 20 percent of deaths may be unreported. As a result, data on causes of death are quite unreliable in many regions. Obesity is increasing. Rates of smoking are high—and increasing among women and teenagers—which isn't altogether surprising, given that Brazil is the world's fourth-largest tobacco producer and the largest tobacco exporter. Regional variations abound in virtually every measure of morbidity and mortality, with poorer areas having a much higher burden of disease, higher rates of death from infectious disease, and higher rates of conditions such as diabetes and hypertension.

OVERVIEW OF THE BRAZILIAN HEALTH CARE SYSTEM

Brazil spent $51 billion on health care in 2000, approximately 7.9 percent of GDP, 41 percent of which was public spending, and 59 percent private spending. Eighty percent of the population receives care through the Brazilian public health care system, known as the Sistema Unico de Saude (SUS). There is also a private health insurance market, which covers approximately 30 million to 32 million people, or about 20 percent of population.

The Health Care Delivery System

Health care in Brazil is delivered by a combination of private and public providers (see Table 4.4). The three major provider types are those in the public sector, those in the private sector that work with the public system, and those exclusively in the private sector. The categories are further defined as follows:

- *Public sector providers:* This category includes mainly local primary care units and health centers and emergency services, which provide most basic and preventive care to those who seek care through the SUS. Only 30 percent of hospitals are publicly owned.

	Brazil	Ceara (Northeast)	Rio de Janeiro	São Paulo
Infant mortality (per 1,000 live births)	33.1	53.3	22.6	19.8
Cause of death (percentage of total deaths known)				
Infectious disease	6	10	6	6
Cancer	14	13	14	15
Circulatory	32	30	33	33
Respiratory	11	11	12	11
Prenatal	5	7	3	4
External	15	13	15	15
Undetermined cause	16	17	16	16
Estimated percentage of deaths not reported	15	30	11	7
Mortality rates (per 100,000 residents)				
Heart	46.8	22.3	79.8	68.3
Cerebrovascular	51.6	37.3	83.0	58.5
Transportation accidents	19.2	15.1	21.3	21.5
Homicides	25.9	13.5	55.3	39.6
Cancers				
• Lung	8.4	4.5	14.0	11.0
• Ovary and uterus	2.3	1.4	2.9	2.2
• Breast	5.0	3.3	9.8	7.3
• Stomach	6.6	5.8	9.0	9.6
• Colon and rectal	4.3	1.1	8.2	7.0
• Prostate	4.4	3.9	6.7	5.7
Diabetes				
• Men	14.8	10.7	31.7	17.1
• Women	20.1	14.5	39.1	23.0
Hepatitis and cirrhosis				
• Men	8.7	6.1	13.2	12.7
• Women	2.3	1.0	3.1	3.2
AIDS				
• Men	9.6	2.5	17.9	18.7
• Women	3.8	0.7	7.2	7.5

Table 4.3.   Mortality: Regional Variations (1999).

Source: Ministry of Health, Brazil. Data provided during authors' interview with Federal Ministry of Health officials, Dec. 2001.

Type of Provider	Number	Public (percent)	Private (percent)
Health care establishments	50,000	55	45
Outpatient facilities	24,000	65	35
Emergency facilities	8,400	38	62
Specialized diagnostic centers	16,400	25	75
Specialized treatment centers (radiation, chemotherapy)	7,000	28	72
Psychiatric care facilities	400	20	80
Hospital beds	544,000	75	25

Table 4.4.   Provider Capacity in Brazil.

Source: Ministry of Health, Brazil. Data provided during authors' interview with Federal Ministry of Health officials, Dec. 2001.

- *Private sector providers that contract with the public system:* These providers seek both public and private patients, and are most commonly specialists and hospitals.

- *Exclusively private sector providers:* These providers, which include doctors' offices, specialized care clinics (such as oncology) and hospitals (both for-profit and nonprofit), see only private patients. Most of this care is financed by private health insurance, although there is also a significant amount of out-of-pocket payment.

Nearly one quarter of hospitalizations and bed days occur in private hospitals. Most hospitals see both public and private patients. Most specialized care clinics see only private patients. Physicians often work part time for the government and part time in private practice to supplement their public sector salaries. "After thirty years in the public sector, I only make $420 a month," reported one physician in a public hospital in the northeast region of Brazil. "The pay is so low that I have to work in a private hospital, even though I would prefer to work here and the need is much greater. But it's hard to find a doctor here after two o'clock because we are all seeing private patients."

Provider capacity and utilization rates vary significantly by region. Physicians, nurses, dentists, and hospital beds tend to be concentrated in more developed regions, in state capitals and in higher-income areas, while providers are in short supply in rural areas and poorer regions. For example, the Southeast has twice as many beds per capita as the North. Seventy-five percent of physicians practice in the country's cities. One-third of municipal districts have no health clinic or hospital. According to one industry source, it can take up to three months to get an appointment with a SUS physician in a clinic.

Brazil is the only country in the Pan American Health Organization that does not have compulsory civil service for physicians. The federal government has undertaken efforts to attract doctors and nurses to medically underserved areas and needy places (that is, those with a high prevalence of tuberculosis, malaria, and leprosy, or higher-than-average infant mortality) by offering much higher pay, housing, food allowances, and private health insurance.

The government is also encouraging the development of more general practice physicians. According to one federal health official,

> General practice is not high status and is badly paid, so most physicians specialize. But the government is finding out that GPs are cheaper so we are undertaking efforts to promote the development of GPs. . . . We are also developing family health teams, comprised of a physician, nurse, nurse assistant, and several community health workers, who can focus on low-income people in underserved areas. Each team is responsible for the health of thirty-five hundred people, and does prevention, visits, diagnostics, and delivers a supply of essential drugs to families. So far we have eleven thousand family care teams and we hope to have twenty thousand by the end of 2002. These teams will help us provide more appropriate, less costly community-based care—we spend too much now on hospital services because that is the only setting where many people can get care. The family program will also give us a much better epidemiological profile of the needs of the poor in many areas.

The Health Care Financing System

The Brazilian public health care system—Sistema Unico de Saude (Unified Health System)—has been reformed and remodeled several times in the last few decades. During the military dictatorship, Brazil's health care system was highly centralized at the federal level. Reform of the health sector was a major goal of the redemocratization movement, and the reform movement espoused a variety of objectives, including strengthening the public sector, increasing and diversifying financial support for health care, and decentralizing and rationalizing the delivery system. When democracy was reestablished in Brazil, a new Constitutional Charter on Health was enacted that defines health care as a universal, egalitarian right of citizenship and makes the government responsible for ensuring this right for all Brazilians. The SUS was created in 1989, as a universal, comprehensive system that would deliver services proportionate to the needs of the population.

"Our health system is *Unico*—Unified—because there is only one system for all levels of government and it is subject to the same standards in all of the country," according to a federal health official. Although unified in its design, the SUS is decentralized in its operation. Each of the three levels of government—federal, state, and local—has a defined role in the health care system. The responsibility for financing SUS is shared, with the federal government providing 78 percent of funding, states 14 percent, and municipalities 11 percent. Federal funds for health services come from general revenues and three social funds, which are financed through earmarked taxes. States and municipalities generally raise money from property and services taxes. Virtually all state and municipal funding goes toward primary care. Federal funding is allocated approximately 25 percent to primary care, 60 percent to secondary care, and 15 percent to tertiary care. The federal share of primary care costs has been rising in recent years as a result of the implementation of a program of basic primary care for the entire population of the country.

The three levels of government are knit together through an elaborate and democratic network of government and institutional arrangements. The major roles of each level of government are outlined in the following sections.

FEDERAL. This level is responsible for macro level functions, including formulating national health priorities and policy, planning, implementation and assessment, and regulation. The federal government has a limited role in the provision of services, although it does operate some tertiary facilities and a number of national programs relating to communicable diseases, nutrition, and health promotion. The federal level also provides most of the SUS's funding, and makes payments to states, municipalities, and directly to certain providers.

The federal government discharges its responsibilities through three major bodies:

- *The National Health Council* (CNS), which is responsible for strategic planning and monitoring, and comprises representatives of federal, state, and municipal government agencies, providers, labor, industry, and SUS users. CNS is chaired by the minister of health.

- *The Tripartite Intermanagerial Committee* (CIT), which approves operating rules for SUS, and comprises representatives from the Ministry of Health, National Council of State Health Secretaries, and the National Council of Municipal Health Secretaries.

- *The Ministry of Health,* which manages the allocation of federal funds under supervision of CNS and proposes operating rules to CIT.

This same structure is mirrored at the state (State Health Secretariat, Bipartite Intermanagerial Committee, and State Health Council) and at the local levels (Municipal Health Secretariat and Health Councils). The federal Ministry of Finance also has an important role in the health care system, including enforcing price controls and antitrust law.

Every four years, Brazil holds a National Health Conference, which is attended by thousands of delegates elected from the state and municipal health councils. "The National Health Council is a vital part of our system," said one federal official. "Its composition is democratic—half from institutions and half from civil society—including representatives from all major groups—the disabled, elderly, business, unions, agricultural workers, community groups. Its decisions guide our national health policy. It is a bottom-up process, from the municipalities to the states to the national level. Each conference considers one topic—the 2000 conference was about equity and access to services. Every line of the report is voted on by the entire conference—it takes about ten hours."

STATE. This level plays largely a coordination, support, and evaluation role. States also manage certain types of tertiary care and facilities (for example, cardiac surgery, transplants), and are responsible for medical education and training. States provide some funding to SUS and also are the intermediaries for the flow of money from the federal government to the municipalities.

The roles for the states have evolved and changed with the move to decentralization. "The states' roles are less developed and often overlapping with the municipalities," according to one municipal official. "But many people are concerned about inequities among the municipalities and the need for strong state support and health planning processes."

Since 1999, the states and municipalities have been responsible for the purchase and distribution of basic drugs. In earlier years, this function was done by a federal agency, CEME, which was perceived as "ineffective and corrupt," putting the interests of manufacturers over those of the poor needing drugs.

MUNICIPALITY. This level is responsible for most direct patient care, including primary care services, health promotion, prevention, and rehabilitation. Municipalities also have responsibility for planning, organizing, and monitoring primary and secondary care. They are also expected to allocate 10 percent of their municipal budgets to health care, although, according to one federal official, "this is not required and the practice varies widely, based on the income and politics of the *municipio.*"

Municipalities receive two major types of payments from the federal government. The first is $4.20 per person per year to provide "basic care" to their populations. The municipalities can spend this money at their discretion on a range of primary and preventive care services, including health education, immunizations, nutritional care, consultations with primary care physicians, basic dental care, home visits by nurses or community workers, basic emergency care, and family planning. The federal government also allocates money to each municipality to finance national program priorities (for example, public health, nutritional deficiencies, environmental health).

Some municipalities have also been qualified as "full management" areas, which means they have the delegated authority to manage a broader range of health care services. They receive money directly from the federal government to pay local health units, hospitals, and other providers. The rest of the municipalities have "full management of basic care," which gives them more restricted responsibilities and means that provider units continue to receive funding directly from the federal government.

PRIVATE HEALTH INSURANCE. Approximately 30 million to 35 million Brazilians, or about 20 percent of the population, have private health coverage. Most people with private coverage live in the more affluent Southeast region, mainly in the larger cities. The majority of private coverage is offered through employers, although many people purchase private insurance directly. Tax exemptions for private health insurance premiums are estimated to be as great as 25 percent of all federal expenditures on health care.

Four major types of private health insurance operate in Brazil:

- *Group medicine:* These plans are similar to HMOs. A prepaid premium is paid to a group of providers, and this group or other contracting providers deliver all care. Approximately 10 million people are enrolled in this type of plan, mainly through employers.

- *Medical cooperatives:* Structured like staff model HMOs, medical cooperatives provide services through physicians who are also usually owners. Other services are delivered by contracting providers. Providers are paid on a fee-for-service basis, with fixed fee schedules. As many as 10 million people belong to medical cooperatives.

- *Employer-based plans:* More than two hundred employers in Brazil offer their own health plans, on either an insured or self-insured basis. These companies tend to be the largest firms in Brazil (for example, airlines, energy, steel, banks, utilities). Employer-based plans generally have a provider network, and providers are paid on a fee-for-service basis. Many plans use some types of care management techniques. Approximately 9 million people are covered by these plans.

- *Health insurers:* These plans provide indemnity coverage, with freedom of choice of provider. The insured must pay the difference between the provider's charge and the indemnity amount. Six million people are covered by health insurance plans.

Most private insurance offers comprehensive benefits for hospital and physician services, but generally does not cover prescription drugs. Insured people often receive discounted prices at pharmacy networks.

Private health insurance grew rapidly over the past two decades, largely as a result of perceived problems in the SUS and the tax incentives. "The public and private systems are different worlds," according to one consumer. "Everyone wants to have private medical insurance so they can get out of the public system. People make enormous financial sacrifices to pay for private health insurance coverage—at least for their children if they cannot afford it for the entire family." However, one academic noted, "the growth of private insurance has not reduced the use of SUS. There was lots of pent-up demand and many people with private coverage still use the SUS for some services."

According to several health insurance executives, the number of people with private health insurance declined recently—by almost 10 million—because of regulatory changes in the individual market. "We now have to take everyone and we are severely limited in our ability to use medical underwriting, waiting periods and preexisting condition exclusions," according to one insurance company official. "HMOs traditionally were able to have very limited coverage, so they were able to take almost everyone and still have low prices. They were particularly attractive to low-income workers. But now the same lenient underwriting rules have been applied to everyone because the government wants more people to have private coverage. . . . We are moving quickly to develop network products and do other things to try to restore our profitability. But the government has made a monster in the private health insurance market."

Mixed System, Mixed Results

Table 4.5 presents the World Health Organization ranking of the Brazilian system compared to those of the United States and France. Compared to the developed world, it has a way to go; however, agreement is widespread that the health reforms of the last decade have had a significant impact.

In particular, decentralization appears to have improved access, particularly in rural and semi-urban areas that were badly served by the previous centralized system. Nearly 100 percent of the population now has access to basic medical care, and care has shifted from the hospital to outpatient and community settings. Impressive improvements have been made in many measures of health system performance, including prenatal care, infant mortality, maternal mortality, rates of routine immunizations, use of contraception, and proportion of deliveries occurring in hospital, although concern is growing about the high rate of cesarean section, which is over 35 percent in SUS and as high as 75 percent in the private system in many parts of the country. Significant drops have occurred in mortality from acute complications of diabetes and hypertension in people under twenty-five years old.

Ranking (of 191 countries)	Brazil	United States	France
1. Overall health system performance	125	37	1
2. Overall level of health	111	24	3
3. Distribution of health	108	32	12
4. Overall responsiveness	(130–131)	1	16
5. Distribution of responsiveness	(84–85)	(3–38)	.995
			(3–38)
6. Fairness of financial contribution	189	54–55	(26–29)
7. Overall system achievement	125		6
8. Health expenditures per capita in international dollars	54 ($428)	1 ($3,724)	4 ($2,125)
9. Performance on level of health	78	72	4

Table 4.5.   WHO Ranking of Health System Performance: Brazil, United States, and France.

Source: World Health Organization, 2000.

Note: Explanation of measures:

1. Overall Performance = Relationship between overall achievement and overall expenditures.

2. Overall level of health = disability adjusted life expectancy.

3. Distribution of health = distribution of the risk of child death.

4. Responsiveness: Based on key informant interviews in each country. (Also applies to item 5.)

6. Fairness of financial contribution: Distribution of the ratio of total household income to amount spent on health.

7. Overall achievement: Composite score based on weighted average of score on overall health (25 percent), distribution of health (25 percent), responsiveness (12.5 percent), distribution of responsiveness (12.5 percent) and fairness of financial contribution (25 percent).

9. Performance on level of health: comparison of achieved levels of health with levels that could be achieved by most efficient health systems—measures relative efficiency.

However, the World Bank Operations Evaluation Department conducted a study in the late 1990s that identified four problems in the health sector:

• Severe underfinancing of the public system, resulting in regional inequalities and a perceived decline in quality

• Weak incentives for cost-effectiveness and quality

- Tension between decentralization and maintaining the quality of care
- Overemphasis on curative services

These problems appear to continue into the new millennium. "The system is quite erratic in its organization. It works well in some places and not in others," according to one academic. "We have extremely modern hospitals and care in places like Rio and São Paulo and then a lack of resources in poorer parts of country. . . . The system is plagued with regional inequities and inadequate resources. Richer municipalities can supplement federal resources and poorer areas cannot, even though they often have greater needs. The financing system is regressive and unfair. And the rich can buy out so they don't care." "Brazil has islands of tremendous quality in health care," agreed a specialist physician. "Some of our cancer hospitals and cardiology facilities are world-class and are available to any citizen. But there is a lot of treacherous water between the islands, particularly at the state and municipal levels. And citizens are rightly unhappy."

But many officials reject the idea that lack of money is the major issue in the SUS. "We have other sectors in Brazil without lots of money and they work quite well," said one federal official. "The problem in Brazil with health care is not the level of the spending but the quality of the spending. There is lots of corruption, waste, and mismanagement in the health system."

BRAZILIAN INITIATIVES TO PROMOTE ACCESS TO PHARMACEUTICALS

Brazil is the sixth-largest pharmaceutical market in the world, with annual sales of over $10 billion—about 3 percent of the world market as of 1997. Total drug spending has more than doubled since 1994, contributing to Latin America's status as the fastest-growing regional pharmaceutical market in the world.

The SUS and most private health insurance plans provide coverage for drugs used on an inpatient basis. Most private insurance provides little if any coverage for outpatient prescription drugs. As a result, over 80 percent of prescription drug costs are paid out-of-pocket by consumers. According to several observers, the disparity in coverage for drugs on an inpatient and outpatient basis used to create incentives for physicians to hospitalize patients who needed pharmaceuticals. "This was a huge problem in the early days of HIV," according to one physician. "But it's not as true anymore since the government programs were enacted. Still there are some incentives to put people with certain chronic diseases into the hospital if they cannot afford medicines that are not covered by public programs. This happens at SUS hospitals, but not usually at private hospitals where patients are wealthy and can usually afford the drugs."

Although the law requires a prescription before a drug can be dispensed, this requirement is widely ignored. "Most people in Brazil cannot afford to see a doctor to get a prescription," said one executive from a private pharmacy benefit management company. "But many of them do have enough money to get a drug directly from a pharmacy. We estimate 80 percent of drugs in Brazil are dispensed with no prescription." Furthermore, most private pharmacies do not employ a pharmacist, so self-medication is common—as are antibiotic-resistant bacterial infections.

Drug spending is among the most uneven areas of health care spending in Brazil. The top 15 percent of population in terms of income account for nearly half of drug spending—an average of roughly $86 per person per year in 1998, equivalent to spending in Spain or the United Kingdom. The bottom half of the country in terms of income accounts for only 16 percent of drug spending, or just over $8 per person per year. This group relies on public drug programs. "There are at least 30 million people in Brazil who essentially have no access to drugs because of economics or distribution problems," said one physician. Reminders of the problem of drug access seem to arise in unexpected ways. For example, on the authors' recent trip to Brazil, we encountered a poor man outside the Ministry of Finance who was begging for money by showing passers-by a copy of a prescription that he said he needed money to be able to fill.

The access problems include long waits for SUS physicians (besides long waits for appointments, it can require a long trip and missing a day of work to get to a SUS clinic in some parts of the country), as well as a limited supply of basic drugs, even those covered by SUS. The government's initiatives to promote access to drugs have been among the most publicized—and controversial—areas of recent Brazilian health care policy. In 1998 the country adopted a National Drug Policy that had several major components, including adoption of a list of essential drugs; promotion of drug production; promotion of rational drug use; scientific and technological development; safety, efficacy, and quality assurance; and development and training of personnel. These are described in more detail in following paragraphs.

Public Funding

The SUS has three major public programs to make outpatient drugs available to its population: the "Basic Drug" program, which provides access to a range of essential drugs; the "Strategic" program, which distributes free drugs for the treatment of selected prevailing diseases; and the "High Cost" program, which funds very expensive medications for certain infrequent conditions. As shown in Table 4.6, the federal government spent R 1,419 million ($570 million) on public drug programs in 2001, two and a half times the federal spending in 1997.

"The government had made major commitments to increasing spending on pharmaceuticals in the last five years," according to a federal health official. "The increases are even more significant when measured on a per capita basis. We are helping many more Brazilian citizens and we have also made substantial progress in reducing regional disparities in drug spending."

BASIC DRUG PROGRAM. This program was established in 1997 to ensure free access to drugs on a "National List of Essential Drugs," which is developed by the federal government through an extensive consultation process with providers and state and local government. The Basic program was a response to the lack of affordability of drugs for much of the Brazilian population. "We were seeing a growing problem with nonadherence to drug regimens and a recurrence or lack of cure for many diseases that were curable or controllable with drug use," said

Program	1997	2001
Basic	R 69	R 166
Strategic	R 313	R 780
High Cost	R 170	R 450
Essential drugs for mental health	R 16	R 23
Total	R 569	R 1,419

Table 4.6.   Federal Spending on Public Drug Programs (Reals millions).
Source: Ministry of Health interview, Dec. 2001. Does not include state and municipality contributions.

one municipal official. "Elderly people were particularly disadvantaged. . . . Many of them were spending one-third or more of their incomes on drugs."

The Basic Drug program is funded jointly by federal, state, and municipal government. The federal government contributes approximately $0.40 per person per year, an amount that is matched by the states. The municipality share is $0.25 per person per year, an amount that is subsidized by the federal government for municipalities that have fewer than thirty thousand people or that cannot afford to pay.

The procurement and distribution system has been decentralized since 1999. The municipalities develop a list of essential drugs for their area, based on the federal essential drug list. According to one state official, "There is not wide variation in the basic lists across the country, less than 10 percent, but local officials do somewhat customize their lists to the prevailing pathologies in their local region." It is the responsibility of the municipalities to purchase and distribute drugs to their populations, through SUS health clinics and other SUS providers. Procurement is done through a competitive bidding process. As described by one municipal official who handles drug purchasing in a large, affluent city: "We forecast demand for each drug based on historical use plus a factor of up to 25 percent to avoid having shortages. We do purchasing of every drug every year and get semiannual delivery. In this way we can take into account the economic situation of the country, which changes often. The contracts usually specify a minimum amount we have to buy and a maximum range, at a guaranteed price. The degree of competition varies by drug. Some companies will not follow this type of bidding because they aren't willing to guarantee prices for an unknown quantity for a year. We buy from both public and private manufacturers. In general we have tremendous market power and success. On average we pay about one-fifth of the retail price and many drugs are even cheaper."

Although decentralized purchasing was undertaken in reaction to a centralized system that was viewed as ineffective and corrupt, there remained some concern that, as a World Bank analyst phrased it, "most local governments in Brazil do not have the human and institutional capacity to manage the procurement and distribution of pharmaceuticals effectively" (Cohen, 2000, p. 17).

STRATEGIC DRUG PROGRAM. The federal government finances, procures, and distributes for free drugs designed to treat certain

Disease	Spending (million)	People receiving drugs
HIV/AIDS	$216 (R 515)	131,000
Diabetes	$40 (R 95)	5 million
Endemic diseases	$7 (R 17)	30 million
Hansen's disease	$1.7 (R 4)	90,000
Kidney failure	$58 (R 137)	7,600
Tuberculosis	$5 (R 12)	130,000

Table 4.7.   Strategic Drug Program Spending in 2001.
Source: Federal Ministry of Health. Data provided during authors' interview with Ministry officials, Dec. 2001.

prevailing diseases: several STDs, HIV/AIDS, Hansen's disease, tuberculosis, malaria, leishmaniasis, schistosomiasis, hypertension, diabetes, cerebral palsy, and cystic fibrosis. The program also includes some blood products and immunobiologicals that are cheaper to buy centrally. Spending on the strategic drug program has more than doubled in the past five years. Nearly 70 percent of spending goes to drugs for HIV/AIDS. (See Table 4.7.)

Some of these drugs in the strategic drug programs are manufactured in one of the sixteen public laboratories in Brazil; most are purchased from private pharmaceutical companies. The government engages in aggressive negotiations to obtain favorable prices for many drugs covered by the strategic program. "We buy from private companies, if they will accept our capped prices, and if we cannot handle our estimated demand in federal and state labs," said one federal official. "We review data on the international cost of production and we negotiate price reductions, based on raw materials prices, our costs to produce, cost of clinical trials, prices in other countries. . . . We don't allow marketing, advertising or other costs designed to lure or seduce doctors. . . . Some of us worked for the drug industry for years and we know how much they inflate the costs of research and development."

HIGH COST DRUG PROGRAM. These drugs are selected by the federal Ministry of Health, and include immuno-suppressive drugs, interferon, and many cancer drugs. The drugs are either purchased directly by large hospitals or bought by state governments. The federal government bears 70 percent of the cost, and the states pay the rest. Federal spending on the High Cost Drug Program has nearly tripled in the past five years. According to a federal official, "We have devoted many more resources to the program and we are reaching many more people. Nearly 110,000 Brazilians received drugs through the High Cost Program in 2001, compared to fewer than 8,000 in 1995 and only 23,000 in 1997."

These public programs are widely regarded as having been enormously successful in enhancing access to drugs for many Brazilians, and as having reduced morbidity and mortality from many diseases. For example, the availability of free drug treatment for people with HIV, combined with outreach and other community health supports, is credited with dramatic declines in hospitalizations, a halving of the incidence of tuberculosis in HIV-positive patients, and significant reductions in transmission rates of the virus.

Yet the public system still has sources of tension. One commonly heard theme is a concern about widespread disparities in the availability of drugs across local areas. One official who handles drug purchasing in a large city in a poor region said, "Cities in our area often do not pay their share and then people in those cities may not get their drugs, although sometimes they can go to health units in other cities. . . . Every government does not have the resources to meet all the demand. Access depends on where you live." A hospital physician in the same city agreed:

> We are not always well supplied with drugs, and the quality of the drugs is highly variable because the contract always goes to the bidder with the lowest price. . . . There is always something missing. For example, we have an excellent osteoporosis program and we have developed excellent protocols to ensure rational drug use and make appropriate decisions about which patients should get which drugs. But we often run out of the necessary drugs for days and people have to keep coming back day after day after day to see if we have them yet. This makes compliance very difficult. We cannot meet all the demand for drugs. . . . To practice medicine with what we have is almost a miracle.

However, when the municipal official from the richer city was asked about shortages of drugs, he responded, "We have guaranteed inventory because of our contracts and money is not a problem—if we run out, we just buy more. We always have resources."

The government is undertaking a number of new initiatives to help improve access to essential drugs. One is the family health program, described earlier, in which primary care teams visit poor households to check health and distribute kits of essential drugs. Another pilot program is targeting hypertension, which is estimated to exist in approximately 9 percent of the Brazilian population. Residents in ten municipalities with a combined population of more than 2 million are being screened for hypertension by local health units. When hypertensives are identified, they are stratified into one of three categories, low, moderate, or high. Appropriate medications are then mailed to these individuals for two months, followed by follow-up clinic visits. There is active follow-up if appointments are missed. The government hopes to eventually register the entire population with hypertension and ensure they receive appropriate medication.

Another expressed frustration with the public programs is the slow diffusion of newer drugs. "It can take six or seven years after FDA approval in the U.S. for many drugs to get to Brazil. The national branches of pharmacy in this country must answer to and address this delay," said one physician. Another physician working in the SUS said, "Even though the Basic Program has expanded access, patients are often not getting the best treatments. For example, the essential drug list has only beta-agonists for asthma care, not steroidal anti-inflammatory drugs. It is also very hard to get new drugs or drugs for unusual cases."

Tensions also exist over which drugs and diseases have been excluded from public drug programs. Brazil has a growing consumer movement that includes organized groups for patients with autism, cancer, diabetes, and renal failure, to name a few. These groups engage in a variety of lobbying and advocacy activities to pressure the government to increase support for their conditions. "One of our major goals is to get more resources from all over the world for treatment," said the head of a national group of cancer patients, adding,

> We are fighting for more resources and respect for people with cancer. The Ministry of Health is not hearing the voices of cancer patients. They think we are just troublemakers. Fighting is always misinterpreted. But we must dare to show the failures of the health care system because patients are dying because there are not enough resources—not enough drugs and hospitals and physicians to treat people. Cancer is one of the leading causes of death in Brazil, second only to cardiovascular illness. But cancer is a slow and silent killer, while heart disease kills in twenty-four hours—and it kills white powerful men so there is more respect for cardiac services. . . . People with AIDS were active, organized, and violent, and they got the leaders to

change the laws and to make HIV services and drugs available. Today
AIDS is respected. We need to do the same for cancer. There is money,
but so much is wasted on corruption . . . and preferential treatment is
given to people who are famous or who have connections. And the
very rich can just go to the United States for treatment. . . . The average Brazilian cannot afford the price of the drugs for cancer. So we
need to fight to force the government to make us a priority too.

A government official acknowledged that "in Brazil, it is common
to see someone in a Mercedes stop off at a health station for his AIDS
medication." An academic commented,

The government has created a double standard, one for AIDS and
another for other serious disease. AIDS activists were very well organized—they saw the opportunity and made their case. So the government started making HIV drugs, and there were no patent issues then.
But it's obvious that the AIDS drug program was much more expensive than government thought it would be—nearly 5 percent of the
total health budget—and that is why they threatened compulsory
licensing with HIV drugs. The government will find it gets increasing
pressure to do the same with other drugs for other well-organized
patient groups.

Federal officials had a ready response to this concern: "The simple
answer to this criticism is that infectious diseases have externalities
because they can be transmitted," said a Ministry of Health executive. "The government has obligations with infectious diseases that
it does not have with other diseases. But that does not mean that we
should ignore other diseases, and we do not. The federal government
sends the states 70 percent of the cost of high-cost drugs, including
cancer drugs. We are taking action in other areas, including undertaking a new process for producing or obtaining essential cancer
drugs—this new program will be implemented soon by the Ministry
of Health." An oncologist at a leading national cancer hospital
observed, "If I think of how much money is being spent on AIDS
care, I know many more lives would be saved if we spent that money
on family care and prevention than on treating advanced HIV. But
I also think that a lot of the patient advocacy in cancer is being
fueled by the drug companies who want to get faster approval of
their own drugs."

Public Production and Patents

Until five years ago, 90 percent of the drugs consumed in Brazil were imported. Today, after significant investment by the government in its public manufacturing capability, most of the drugs distributed in the Strategic Drug Program are produced in Brazil, many by national laboratories that now produce sixteen different drugs, including eight of the twelve most commonly used to treat people with HIV/AIDS. These labs also produce some of the drugs on the National List of Essential Drugs. (See Table 4.8 for a list of the drugs produced by Far Manguinhos, the National Institute for Technology in Pharmaceuticals.) Public production is now the source of 20–30 percent of drugs purchased in Brazil.

Public production of drugs brings up the topic of intellectual property and patent protection in Brazil. The country resumed patent protection in 1996 after twenty years without it. The change was made to comply with the rules of the World Trade Organization's Agreement on Trade-Related Aspects of Intellectual Property Rights, Including Trade in Counterfeit Goods (called the TRIPS agreement). TRIPS makes patent protection mandatory for all types of technology, including drugs that meet prerequisites for patentability. Under Brazil's drug patent law, anything commercialized anywhere in the world before May 1997 remains forever unpatented in Brazil. To date, this covers close to 90 percent of drugs consumed in Brazil. Any drug commercialized after that date is subject to the patent law, although exceptions from patentability can be made under TRIPS and Brazilian law in certain situations, including in a national emergency.

Most of the drugs produced in Brazil's national labs are exempt from the country's patent law because they were patented before 1997. But the country has threatened to seize the patents for several drugs that are subject to the country's patent law through a process called "compulsory licensing." This process would permit Brazil to manufacture or import a generic version of a drug patented in Brazil if it determines there is a national emergency. A reasonable royalty must be paid to the patent holder when a compulsory license is issued. While it hasn't had to issue a compulsory license yet, Brazil has successfully used the threat of compulsory licensing to obtain significant price discounts for many brand name drugs, particularly newer AIDS drugs under recent patents. Recently patented drugs for the treatment of hepatitis C and newer versions of some cancer drugs may be the next target. Brazil also recently passed a new law that issues a

Category of Drug	Drugs
Analgesics	• Acetaminophen
Anti-anxiety	• Diazepam
Anti-anemia	• Folic Acid
	• Iron Sulfate
Antibacterial agents	• Sulfadiazine
	• Sulfamethoxazole with Trimethoprim
Antibiotics	• Neomycin and Bacitracin
	• Tetracycline
Anti-convulsives	• Carbamazepine
	• Phenobarbital
Anti-diabetes	• Chloropropamide
	• Glimepiride
Anti-gout	• Allopurinol
Antihypertensives	• Captopril
	• Enalapril
	• Methyldopa
Anti-inflammatories	• Ibuprofen
Anti-malaria	• Chloroquin
	• Primaquin
Anti-micotics	• Ketoconazole
Anti-parasite	• Diethylcarbamazine
	• Metronidazole
	• Praziquantel
Anti-ulcer	• Cimetidine
Anti-virals	• Didanosine
	• Lamivudine + Zidovudine
	• Estavudine
	• Ribavirine
	• Lamivudine
	• Zidovudine
Cardiovascular	• Digoxin
	• Propranolol
	• Dipyridamole
Corticosteroids	• Dexamethasone
	• Prednisone
	• Dexamethasone Cream
Diuretics	• Hydrochlorothiazide
Leprosy	• Dapsone
Anti-psychotics	• Chlorpromazine
	• Haloperidol
Tuberculosis	• Ethambutol
	• Isoniazid + Rifampin
	• Ethionamide
	• Isoniazid
	• Pyrazinamide
	• Rifampin

Table 4.8.   Drugs Produced by Far Manguinhos National Lab (as of Dec. 2001).

Source: Far Manguinhos. Data provided during authors' interview with Institute staff, Dec. 2001.

compulsory license for any new drug that is not issued a patent in Brazil within three years of being patented elsewhere in the world. However, compulsory licensing is only possible when there is an independent source of raw materials, which is not the case for some of the newest drugs. Brazil imports 60–70 percent of its raw materials from India and other countries.

Drug companies have strenuously opposed the government's threat to use compulsory licensing. According to one drug company executive, "When the new patent law was approved, there was significant new investment by drug companies in plants and research and development in Brazil. Drug companies took the law seriously. We initially thought that the delays in approving patent applications were just due to a lack of inspectors and inefficiency. But there have been almost no approvals of new patents since the law passed and there are fifteen thousand applications pending. There is no time period during which government has to act on a patent application. It's clear now that the Ministry of Health just wants to break patents and lower prices. But these actions will hurt innovation and limit access to the best drugs for the Brazilian population." Most of the pending patent applications are by transnational drug companies, particularly from the United States.

An academic agreed, at least in part:

Failure to approve new drugs has tremendous effects on access and health. The government has made access to some drugs very easy and impossible for others. Look at the strategic initiative, for example. Many of these drugs have terrible side effects and complicated regimens, so they don't have as much adherence as we want to. It's hard to respect patents when diseases are killing people. But compulsory licensing is not a solution to Brazil's overall economic problems. Even with compulsory licensing, many of the newest drugs are going to be too expensive for most people in Brazil, or the government, to afford. We need to discuss how we are going to make these drugs available . . . and it's going to get harder because many of these diseases are increasing because of poverty and there are so many new drugs being developed.

Federal officials defend the government's actions on several grounds. "The invisible hand of the market does not work well in the drug area," said one Ministry of Finance official. "The market left alone does not produce a socially fair level of prices because it is ruled by patents, which give a monopoly to the patent holder. But patients must take the drugs and there are often no substitutes for the drugs.

Government must therefore intervene. We respect intellectual property and the rights of business but access to drugs is more important than patents. We need to do our own production and find other ways to lower prices."

Some health policy analysts agree. "Transnationals account for 75–85 percent of annual drug revenues in Brazil," said one observer. "Our internal companies cannot really compete, particularly because we have to import most of our raw materials. We are overly dependent on foreign companies . . . and at their mercy. Patent protection in Brazil has created monopolies for transnational companies. Thus we need to have government production and other initiatives, such as compulsory licensing, to keep prices at reasonable levels."

Price Controls

Brazil has a system of price controls for drugs. The government establishes a list of maximum prices, called the *Brasindice,* which specifies the most that can be charged for each drug by both retail pharmacies and hospitals. It specifies two prices for each drug: the "maximum price that can be charged to the retailer" (for example, pharmacy, hospital), and the "maximum price that can be charged to the consumer." (See Table 4.9 for a list of sample drug prices from a retail pharmacy in Rio de Janeiro, compared to prices for the same item in Boston.)

In addition to the Brasindice, most drug prices have been frozen since August 2000. "There was widespread concern about drug price levels," said an industry representative. "So in the summer of 2000, the government formed a working group to examine this issue and develop a new regulation. The industry agreed to voluntarily freeze prices while the working group deliberated. But then the government was very fearful that prices would really rise when the freeze ended, so they extended the freeze for a year, and then another year. While we can appeal if we think we need a price increase, this appeals process exists only so we cannot sue the government."

The overall effectiveness of price controls as a means of containing costs and improving access to drugs is a topic of lively debate among policymakers, payers, and drug companies. Many top officials in the Ministry of Health think drug prices are too high and need to be reduced by any available means: "Drug companies have had a seat at the policy-making table and we have listened and we understand their viewpoints," said one senior policymaker. "We think there is a lot of

Drug	Dose	Quantity	Price in Rio de Janeiro Pharmacy (December 2001)	Price in Boston Pharmacy (May 2002)
Brand Name				
Adalat	20 mg	30	$4.35	$49.69
Amoxil	500 mg	21	8.32	13.49
Atenol/Tenormin	50 mg	28	5.46	43.19
Capoten	12.5 mg	30	5.02	45.49
Celebrex	200 mg	10	6.23	30.19
Claritin D		12	6.54	45.89
Cozaar	50 mg	28	20.67	54.59
Keflex	500 mg	8	5.68	37.59
Monocordil/Imdur	20 mg	20	1.76	51.59
Nexium	40 mg	14	17.40	68.99
Nexium	40 mg	7	9.90	36.69
Synthroid	0.1 mg	30	5.13	15.75
Trental	400 mg	20	9.01	19.49
Uprima/Apomorphine	2 mg	2	14.73	Not available
Viagra	50 mg	4	25.76	41.39
Vioxx	25 mg	7	5.72	22.09
Zovirax Cream	10 mg		5.05	93.59 (15 gm)
Generics				
Acyclovir Cream	50 mg	10 g	2.84	Not available
Amoxicillin	500 mg	15	3.45	$9.99*
Ampicillin	500 mg	6	1.48	$9.99
Atenolol	50 mg	30	2.92	9.99
Atenolol	100 mg	30	4.97	10.69
Captopril	12.5 mg	30	2.65	9.99
Captopril	25 mg	30	4.19	9.99
Cephalexin	500 mg	8	3.59	9.99
Ranitidine	150 mg	20	3.30	24.69
Potassium Chloride	50 mg	20	2.11	13.29
Enalapril	10 mg	30	4.96	29.19
Enalapril	5 mg	30	3.47	26.89
Omeprazol	10 mg	14	4.42	Only available as brand name Prilosec $61.59
Omeprazol	20 mg	7	4.30	Only available as brand name Prilosec $34.09
Simvastatin	10 mg	10	3.75	Only available as brand name Zocor $28.99

Table 4.9. Comparative Retail Pharmacy Prices, Rio de Janeiro and Boston (US$).

Source: Data gathered by authors on visits to retail pharmacies in Dec. 2001 (Rio de Janeiro) and Jan. 2002 (Boston).

Note: *Boston pharmacy has minimum price of $9.99 per prescription.

fat to be trimmed in their companies, and that even with much lower prices, they would still make a fair profit margin."

Private health insurers are also concerned about drug prices, particularly for drugs used by hospitals. Hospital managers concede that drugs are a major source of profits on privately insured patients. "We set our drug prices at the Brasindice, regardless of how much we paid for the drugs," said a hospital pharmacy director of a private hospital. "The Brasindice sets the price assuming a 30 percent profit margin, but ours is much higher than that because we get such good prices from the drug wholesalers and drug companies. Pharmacy is a very important source of profit for the hospital—it subsidizes other non-profitable services." The director of a cancer hospital agreed: "We buy drugs for $1 and charge up to the maximum of the Brasindice to privately insured patients, which is often five times as high. Drugs are just the biggest example of the way in which private patients subsidize SUS patients overall. For example, our hospital has 140 beds but we only use about 80 of them—about 50 for SUS patients and 30 private patients. We do not have enough resources to open them all, even though there is demand. But we would need to have more private patients so we that we could afford to care for more SUS patients." The waiting time at this hospital for inpatient cancer treatment was one month for cancer of the breast and uterus, two months for prostate cancer, and three months for stomach cancer. According to the director, "Most people get here at Stage 3, so the wait is not affecting the outcome. But people are upset about the wait."

Although they recognize this problem, private health insurers have made little progress in dealing with it. "We know that hospitals make extraordinary amounts of money on drugs. We have been taking aggressive action to reduce the costs of inpatient drugs and medical supplies because we realize the markups are so high," reported the medical director of a large insurance company. "We buy many medical supplies directly from the manufacturers and either give them to the hospitals or have implemented fee schedules that set prices at no more than the price at which we can purchase the supplies. This program saved us $10 million last year. But it's much harder to do with this with drugs because there are so many of them and they are harder to distribute. Also hospitals and drug companies are very powerful politically and it's hard to take them on."

The Ministry of Finance is not in favor of price controls for drugs and would like to look to other policy alternatives. "Brazil has a drug access problem, not a price problem," asserted one economist at the Ministry of Finance. He added,

> Our prices in Brazil are not very different from other countries. Most of the price increases are due to currency changes and devaluations, not monopoly power. . . . Our drug problem is the one-quarter of the population that is poor. Price controls don't help the poor because they can't afford the controlled price—even a price of one *real* [at current exchange rates, US$0.42] would be too much for them. In the last twenty years many of our social policies have benefited the middle class and not the poor. If we flew in a helicopter and threw money for social programs out of it we would target our spending better to the poor better than we do now. . . . The middle class knows more about social programs and benefits from them more than the poor. . . . Price controls are inefficient—they benefit mainly the middle-class and upper-income groups and they also reduce foreign capital in Brazil.

Drug companies agree that price controls have been damaging. Reported one industry executive,

> When combined with currency devaluation and the push for generics, we have lost profit margins in Brazil. Most research and development–based companies are losing money in Brazil. . . . But frankly we are not as worried about price controls and the price freeze as about ensuring patent protection since we are an innovator. If the government starts to target more drugs for compulsory licensing, that will be a much bigger problem for us. . . . We think the price freeze will be temporary, but that there will be permanent price monitoring. But we think it's important to target subsidies to the poor and also to support policies to promote overall increases in personal income, since those will help our demand.

Promoting the Use of Generic Drugs

The Brazilian government has recently begun a variety of efforts to increase the use of generic drugs as a way to make drugs more affordable. Generics are a relatively recent phenomenon in Brazil, with a law enacted only in 1999 to regulate their licensing, inspection, and distribution in the Brazilian market. Approximately four hundred generic drugs have been registered in the country, and they are, on average, 40–60 percent cheaper than their brand name equivalents. Generics account for less than 5 percent of total drug sales in Brazil. Pharmacies are permitted to substitute generics unless a physician specifies otherwise.

A number of barriers must be overcome to increase the use of generics. "There is a lot of concern about the quality of generics," said one pharmacist. "There have been a number of problems with counterfeit drugs and drug effectiveness. People will not be willing to use generics, even if they are much cheaper, until they truly believe that generics are equivalent." The head of pharmacy at a private hospital agreed: "Our doctors will not use generics. They are concerned about quality and we need to prove to them that generics meet the same requirements as all of our other formulary drugs. The efforts of the Ministry of Health will help give credibility to generics and help us get doctors and patients to accept them." The head of a PBM also concurred: "The owner of the biggest drug store in Brazil told me recently that he was tired of seeing people come back to his stores with infections when they took generic drugs."

Drug quality has been a major problem in Brazil, with several highly publicized cases of drug counterfeiting, including drugs for prostate cancer. An oncologist at a federal cancer hospital expressed some concerns about the quality of many cancer drugs:

> We have to go through a public bidding process to buy drugs. It's the same process as for buying bricks: if you're the cheapest bidder you win. Plus there is no real assurance of quality once [the manufacturers] get a license to sell the product. [The manufacturers] can change suppliers and not have to submit the change to the government for approval. So a company can switch from a supplier in Poland to Bangladesh with no new testing. . . . These suspicions about quality are pushed by the major drug companies to the doctors—they tell us, "who knows what is in the vials?" One solution is that we should do our own testing with chromatography. So far, I have not been too worried because I know the major drug companies are testing their competitors and no one has blown the whistle yet.

Similar concerns were expressed by the drug purchasing staff of a major municipality:

> We have had problems with quality for a number of drugs—oral contraceptives, cancer drugs, and others, including package failures, stability, lack of active ingredients, even some sabotage. Generic drugs

are a big problem—therapeutic effects are not clear and we often have concern about active ingredients based on reports from doctors and patients. We recently did a contract for cyclosporin for patients with renal disease, and got bids from a major manufacturer and a generic company. The clinical committee had concerns about the therapeutic effectiveness of the generic product, based on a review of all the evidence. But the generic company won because the law favors the lowest price. We had the same issue with EPO [erypotin], so in the RFP we required proven experience with a certain type of distribution system so that we could ensure a certain major manufacturer would win. In our municipality we are developing independent quality control standards and a testing program because the central government does not have the staff or resources to follow up all of this and usually nothing is done. . . . I don't know what smaller or poorer municipalities can do.

Another challenge to promoting the use of generics is the existence of "similars," which are therapeutic substitutes for brand name drugs but not bioequivalents. Similars have a long history in Brazil and are generally 10–20 percent cheaper than brand name drugs but more expensive than generics. If consumers are interested in lower-cost alternatives to brand name drugs, pharmacists and clerks often have a financial incentive to recommend similars rather than generics because they receive higher commissions because of the higher price. Consumers often do not know that they received a similar and not a generic drug. To address this problem, the government has required companies to mark generic drug packages with a large yellow "G" so that consumers will be able to easily identify generics.

Drug quality remains a problem, although in 1999, the Brazilian Congress established the National Health Surveillance Agency (ANVS) to oversee pharmaceuticals as well as medical equipment, cosmetics, and hospital services. It both registers products and licenses manufacturers of pharmaceuticals. As of 2001, the agency did not have the manpower to do independent testing of drugs or any postregistration or postlicensing surveillance. Problems with drugs in the system are required to be reported to ANVS, which will then sample the batch in question.

Although there is no real opposition to the government's efforts to promote generic drugs, many doubt that wider generic use will have a major impact on improving access to drugs for the poor: "Substitution may work well for upper- and middle-income people, who have the education and can shop to get the benefits," according to one observer. "But generics have not increased consumption among the poor because poor people cannot afford these drugs either."

Phytotherapy

Homeopathy is well established and accepted in Brazil, particularly in many poorer regions. Several initiatives are under way across Brazil to produce phytotherapeutics and homeopathic remedies as cost-effective alternatives to prescription drugs for many conditions. Fortaleza, a poor city in the northeast region of the country, has a major program of plant cultivation to produce eight drugs for a range of illnesses including dermatitis, an ointment that helps heal wounds from Hansen's disease, several cough medicines and bronchodilators, and treatments for depression and a number of parasitic diseases. "For many nonserious illnesses, these plants can be quite helpful," said a municipal official. "Our biodiversity in Brazil is immense and we can make more use of this for many conditions. . . . The program can also be a means of economic self-sufficiency for some of the poor in our communities." In Fortaleza, these medicines require a prescription and are distributed by the pharmacies at SUS health units, as well as at day care centers and social welfare departments. According to local officials, the government provides strict oversight of growing and production of the drugs, along with extensive education of consumers and providers about their proper use. "We want phytotherapies to complement pharmaceuticals," said an official. "We absolutely hope this program will save money. . . . Some studies show 50 percent savings from preventing bronchitis and resultant hospital stays. . . . We work actively with physicians, boards of health, social action councils, and others before we introduce any new product. Doctors are resistant initially but then they come around. One of our major marketing challenges is packaging. With our limited resources, it's hard to develop packaging that can compete with the drug companies. But we are having good success."

PROPOSED NEW INITIATIVES
Improved Distribution

The Ministry of Finance and drug manufacturers have been working to develop alternative approaches to improve access to drugs for the poor in Brazil at an affordable cost for the government. The National

Bureau of Economic Research was recently retained by the drug industry to design what the manufacturers called the "National Program of Access to Medicines." This program proposes to replace the government's Basic Drug program with a plan to distribute drugs to the 50 million poor people in Brazil through the country's approximately forty-five thousand retail pharmacies.

The retail drug industry is highly fragmented; the few chain stores are regional in scope and quite small. Although pharmacies are required to have a pharmacist on site to dispense drugs, this requirement is frequently ignored because of a shortage of pharmacists. Several pharmacists interviewed for this case reported that clerks do much of the dispensing and counseling, and that it is quite common for a pharmacy to have a pharmacist who visits just once a month to review and authorize relevant paperwork.

In the proposed program, patients would fill their SUS prescriptions for any drugs on the essential drug list at retail pharmacies (rather than at SUS clinics), which would then bill the SUS. The prescription would still have to be written by a SUS physician. The plan would be financed by obtaining significant discounts from drug companies and reductions in the current markups taken by drug distributors and pharmacies. Drugs in the program would also be exempt from taxes, which now account for over 19 percent of the average retail price charged to consumers.

Table 4.10 shows the industry estimate of the typical pricing structure and markups for prescriptions purchased in retail pharmacies in Brazil. As shown, if a prescription costs the consumer $10, the pharmacy keeps approximately $2.55, the distributor makes $1.12, the government collects $1.93 in sales tax, and the drug company gets $4.15.

The Ministry of Finance has been supportive of the industry proposal. "Under the industry plan, it would cost about $2 billion to actually provide the entire population with the drugs on the essential drug list," said one Ministry official. "So we would need an additional $1.8 billion because we are already spending $200 million on the Basic Drug program [federal, state, and municipality shares].... That's a lot of money but doable from a cost standpoint."

Expanding Private Health Insurance

The Ministry of Finance, among others, is also supporting the growth of private health insurance coverage as another way to improve access

	Mark-Up	Dollar Amount	Percentage of Consumer Price Retained by Each Party
Maximum price to consumer at retail (established by federal government)		$10.00	
Pharmacy margin	25.5	(2.55)	25.5
Manufacturers price		7.45	
Distributor charge	15	(1.12)	11.2
Invoice sales value		6.33	
Sales tax	30.5	(1.93)	19.3
Freight, insurance	4	(0.25)	2.5
Cash value of sale to drug manufacturer		$4.15	41.5

Table 4.10.   Typical Pricing Structure for Drugs in Retail Pharmacies in Brazil.

Source: Data provided during authors' interview with Abifarma officials, December 2001.

to and affordability of drugs. "More than half of the population will never be able to afford drugs and the government needs to provide free drugs to these people," said one official. "But the government does not have the resources to provide free drugs for everyone, so we need to find ways to bring more private money into the system. . . . If the number of people with private coverage goes from 30 million to 60 million, the number who use the SUS goes from 130 million to 100 million. The math is simple. Private coverage will not solve the efficiency problems in the SUS but it could free up more resources to expand public services."

Advocates of increasing private coverage face a considerable challenge. Fewer than a million privately insured people have insurance coverage for outpatient prescription drugs. Another 10 million people receive significant discounts through programs offered by their health insurers. Any move to mandate drug benefits is opposed by insurers and employers, who fear that rising costs will make insurance unaffordable for many people. Many health insurers are reluctant to offer broader drug coverage on a voluntary basis because of concerns about cost and the potential for adverse risk selection.

As of December 2001, the government was debating a proposed law that would offer tax benefits to employers who provide drug coverage to low-income workers. The law would permit employers to deduct the cost of drug coverage provided to any employee whose wages are at or below five times the federal minimum wage (which is, as noted earlier, roughly $60/month), up to a maximum amount of 4 percent of the employer's total income tax liability.

Among the proposal's supporters are Brazil's Pharmacy Benefit Management (PBM) companies, a fairly new but growing industry. "We hope this new law will be a boon for us," said the president of Brazil's largest PBM. He added,

Historically, health insurers have not managed cost or health, and they saw no need to cover medicines. When diseases became chronic, patients just shifted over to the SUS. Diabetics are a classic case—when they need insulin, or dialysis, or transplants, the state pays the bill. But we think there is an opportunity to show employers that if they cover drugs, they will save money in other areas of expense, such as hospitalization, which accounts for nearly 50 percent of health insurance premiums. PBMs can use information technology to help identify potential drug interactions and errors—there are lots of preventable hospitalizations and expensive side effects from poor prescribing. But drugs have to be a covered benefit before we will have the information we need to take advantage of these opportunities for cost savings. . . . We also think there could be a role for us in the public delivery system. Right now, drugs are delivered to the government units, but there are lots of problems with storage, theft, and distribution. There are even hijackings of some drugs, like Viagra. The SUS could use PBMs as a model of delivery to make drugs available through retail stores, just like Medicaid does in the U.S.

Another PBM executive was optimistic but a bit more cautious:

Our major competitive advantage now is that we can offer significant discounts to patients—an average 25 percent discount off retail prices. We've also been somewhat effective at dealing with fraud and abuse, which is rampant among pharmacies. But there's not much more we can do by contracting because people in Brazil don't like limited networks—they are used to convenience and just going around the corner to get drugs. So we've had to offer open networks, home delivery, and mail order to be competitive. A drug benefit will cost lots of money, so we will need to find new ways to control costs. Since we are a poor country, our plan is to start small and offer a limited benefit that covers drugs for chronic illnesses—diabetes, COPD, hypertension, anti-cholesterol, hyperlipidemia—places where we know there are effective drug therapies and we should be able to reduce inpatient costs. We will also certainly have copayments, although not tiered copayments since we have no incentive to encourage the use of generics; we make our profit on the price spread from the drug manufacturer to the retailer, and if prices are lower, so is our profit. But it's going to be hard to tell employers or individuals that even though they are already paying lots of money for private insurance and taxes to support the SUS, they need to pay more for drug coverage to save money in the future. That is a difficult speech in any language.

FINDING THE RIGHT MIX OF ACTIVITIES

Brazil has a widespread consensus that it has made tremendous progress in improving access to pharmaceuticals for its population in recent years, and that significant challenges lie ahead. Many people have strong opinions about what the government's future priorities should be in the drug area. Here are a few examples:

> We need a much more transparent process for government drug policy, and much more citizen involvement, both in terms of patients' knowing their rights and in terms of setting and implementing policy. How are they deciding which drugs are approved? How do they decide which drugs are purchased by hospitals? Often there are shortages because the hospitals order the drugs but the state does not fill the order because they don't want to pay. There are decrees and formulas that say how the money is supposed to flow but it is never distributed. The government does not want to have manufacturers selling the newest drugs—it is keeping fifteen thousand patent applications pending. It is just pushing generic drugs and homeopathy.
> *—The head of a national patients rights group*

> We have limited resources and we have to use them much more wisely. Much more money must be assigned to prevention—there is very little money spent on prevention except in the Southeast, in the richest areas. Most drugs are prescribed for people who are symptomatic already— we need more proactive interventions. . . . We also need to focus on appropriate drug use. The education of Brazilian doctors is based on the U.S. model from the 1950s—it is disease oriented, specialist oriented, and students are influenced by teachers and taught to use brand name

drugs rather than to respect the formulary.... We need to retrain all of the 250,000 doctors in Brazil—doctors write whatever they want, even when there are protocols.... We also should not incorporate new drugs easily—we need to do much more cost-effectiveness work before we add drugs to formulary or approve existing drugs for use in new ways.... We are better off putting much more money into prevention and early detection than paying for second- and third-line therapies that are not proven any more effective. We know prevention and primary detection are cost-effective. Plus there are lots of opportunities to do better palliative and end-of-life care. Lung cancer is our biggest cancer killer but only in eighth place in terms of palliative care.

—A physician at a national cancer hospital

Our major problem is a political one. The Brazilian government invests very little in health—the equivalent of $300 per capita. The government spends more in other areas and wastes much of it on politics.... It is better to build roads from nowhere to no place than to put enough money into medical care. Bad medicine usually kills poor people and they don't vote anyway. Our long-term debt to the IMF is huge. It would take R 4 billion a year to extinguish misery in health, but we pay many times that to IMF. Education would change the politics but we spend even less on education than health.

—A physician at a public hospital in the Northeast

An organized and educated society is the only way to change this. If people don't have food and housing, medical care won't make a difference. One good part of the economic crisis is that middle-class people lost private insurance and they had to go to the SUS and they found out it was unacceptable and started to complain.

—An academic

Our vision is limited by our budget. Brazil cannot meet all the demand for drugs—no country can. There is no "right" amount to spend on drugs; this is an economic and political decision. Our negotiations with the private sector are made according of the logic of the private sector, but they also have to take into account political considerations. There is a growing awareness in Brazil about how to deal with public funds, public accountability, and public-private initiatives. We need to find the right mix of all of these activities.

—A Ministry of Health official

References

Cohen, J. C. "Public Policies in the Pharmaceutical Sector: A Case Study of Brazil." World Bank, LCSHD Paper Series 21064, Jan. 2000.

Pan American Health Organization. "Brazil: Demographic Indicators." *Basic Country Health Profiles, 1999.* Updated data available online: http://www.paho.org/english/sha/prflbra.htm (access date: March 26, 2003).

World Health Organization. "World Health Report," 2000. Available online: http://www.who.int/pub/en (access date: May 11, 2003).

PART TWO

Managing Care

CHAPTER FIVE

Moving from the Possibilities to the Practicalities

Health Care Reform in Krakow

F or the past ten years, Poland has experienced a profound ongoing movement from a centralized, planned socialist economic system toward a more market-oriented economy.

The overall economy has undergone what is often characterized as "shock therapy," with an extremely rapid pace of political, social, and economic change, but the pace of reform of the health care sector has in many ways been much more gradual and deliberate.

Nonetheless, Poland has undertaken a series of significant health care reforms, and the cumulative effect of these changes is dramatic. The administration of the health sector has been decentralized to a considerable extent, with significant power shifted from the central government to state *(voivod)*, county *(poviat)*, and municipal *(gmina)* authorities. In 1999, the financing of health services changed dramatically with the establishment of health insurance funds organized at

This case was originally written by the authors in 1999. Funding was provided by Astra Pharmaceuticals, L.P. The authors thank Andrzej Rys and Paul Campbell for their interest and assistance in preparing the case.

the state level, funded by payroll taxes rather than by general taxes to the central government that were then allocated out to the regions by a budgetary process. The sickness funds have assumed primary responsibility for financing health care services; they are beginning to use a variety of techniques, including provider contracting and capitation, to attempt to increase the efficiency and quality of the delivery system.

At the same time, the trend is toward privatization of providers, with an increasing number of physicians and dentists working in private practices rather than as employees of the public sector. There are also attempts to increase the power of consumers in the health care system, including allowing patients free choice of physician and collecting and publicizing provider-specific patient satisfaction information.

The city of Krakow has been at the vanguard of many health reforms, and has piloted a number of new approaches to health care delivery and payment. The overall impact of these changes on providers and consumers is beginning to be felt in very tangible ways. Although many participants in the reform process are optimistic about the longer-term potential for positive outcomes for patients and providers, the current climate is one of great uncertainty, lack of information, and a growing realization that there is, as one provider noted, "a big gap between the possibilities and the practicalities" of health sector reform.

GENERAL BACKGROUND

In 1990, Poland was the first country of the former communist Eastern Bloc to reestablish democracy and embrace radical economic transformation. After several difficult years in the early 1990s, with a mass contraction of output and a sharp rise in unemployment, the economy has begun to rebound, and Poland has experienced steady growth in its overall GDP and GDP per capita. Health indicators also improved during the transition (see Table 5.1), perhaps due to the rising standard of living. Inflation is high by Western standards but has moderated significantly in recent years. Private enterprise has expanded steadily, and the private sector now accounts for half of Polish GDP. Unemployment, officially nonexistent before 1990, has moderated considerably since 1994, although the official unemployment level of 10 percent in 1998 is assumed to understate the true

Indicator	1990	1992	1994	1996
Population (millions)	38.1	38.4	38.5	38.6
Population over 65 (percent)	10.1	10.4	10.8	11.3
Crude birth rate (per 1,000 population)	14.5	13.5	12.6	11.2
Infant mortality (per 1,000 live births)	19.3	17.3	15.1	12.2
Female life expectancy at birth	75.5	75.7	76.1	76.6
Male life expectancy at birth	66.5	66.7	67.5	68.1

Table 5.1.   Polish Demographic and Health Indicators.
Source: European Observatory on Health Systems, 1999, p. 3.

level. In addition, pockets of very high unemployment exist in many regions where agricultural and industrial restructuring has been particularly difficult. The number of Polish people living in poverty recently declined for the first time since 1990, although income inequality is growing. Poland became a member of the Organization for Economic Cooperation and Development (OECD) in 1996 and hopes to join the European Union early in the next century.

Despite this progress, pressure on the government budget is growing, as payments on external and domestic debt absorb an increased proportion of expenditures. In addition, significant resources are required to restructure and modernize important industries such as steel and coal, as well as to make other investments in infrastructure and human capital, particularly in rural areas where much of the poverty is concentrated.

Health Sector Reform

During the communist era, from 1945 to 1990, Poland had a strong centralized approach to health care. Health care was a government responsibility, in terms of both financing and delivery. Under Poland's national health system, all residents had access to a comprehensive range of services provided through government-owned and -operated facilities. These facilities were financed primarily by the federal government, although much of the money flowed through regional authorities who made decisions about budget allocations to specific providers. However, the regional officials were appointed by and accountable to the federal authorities. Figures 5.1 and 5.2 sketch the overall structure of the Polish health care system in the communist era and in 1999.

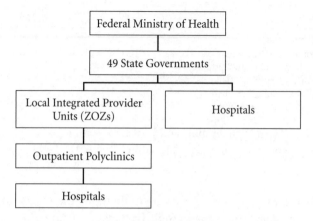

Figure 5.1.   **Polish Health Care System During the
Communist Era.**

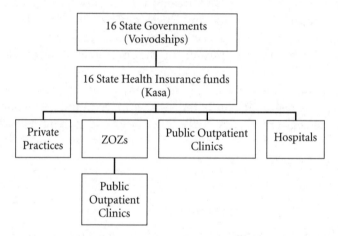

Figure 5.2.   **Polish Health Care System as of January 1, 1999.**

During this period, the government made significant investments in the health care sector, in terms of both personnel and capital. The Polish national health care system achieved impressive improvements in health, including significant reductions in mortality from infectious disease and decreases in the infant mortality rate, resulting in increases in life expectancy. But the national health system was also widely criticized for inefficiency, inattention to costs, uneven and often poor quality of care, indifference to patients, poor attitude and motivation among workers, dilapidated facilities, lack of modern equipment, limited choice of providers, lack of incentives to encourage providers to improve performance, and corruption.

In the years before and during the economic transition, the government resources allocated to the health care sector declined, particularly during the late 1980s and early 1990s. This contraction of spending, combined with the high level of fixed capacity in the Polish health care system (number of physicians, hospital beds, and so on) resulted in widespread access and quality problems, including inadequate maintenance and capital investment as well as shortages of medical supplies. As a result, an existing system of informal payments to public providers to obtain better access and care (often referred to as "envelope payments") grew significantly.

Although these informal payments were and are still illegal, they have become a significant component of health care spending and a major source of income for many providers. The official data on Polish health care spending indicates that spending is low by OECD standards, at approximately 5 percent of GDP. (See Table 5.2.) But recent research suggests that the level of spending is actually closer to 7 percent of GDP if informal payments are included, and rather more if one allows for the accounting issues that affect the official data, including the absence of totals for medical education. It is estimated that informal payments may account for as much as 50 percent of physician incomes. Total out-of-pocket payments, including informal payments, have become a significant burden for Polish consumers. According to recent estimates, total out-of-pocket expenditures for health care increased fivefold in real terms from 1990 to 1997, while real wages declined.

	1985	1990	1992	1994	1996	1997
Health care as percentage of GDP	4.0	4.6	5.0	4.6	4.6	4.2
Government spending as percentage of total	100	94	N/A	70	76	73
Spending per capita (US$)	N/A	N/A	$234	$219	$371	N/A
Spending by selected category (percentage of total)						
Inpatient	N/A	45	45	39	47	N/A
Ambulatory	N/A	18	19	27	13	N/A
Pharmaceuticals	N/A	13	12	18	9	N/A
Mental health	N/A	3	3	2	3	N/A

Table 5.2.   Trends in Polish Health Care Spending.
Source: European Observatory on Health Systems, 1999, pp. 17, 20, 24.

Health Care Delivery System

Poland has both public and private health care facilities. During the communist era, private practice was never eliminated, and since the government liberalized the laws on private enterprise in 1989 many providers have established private practices. Although some providers are fully private, it is more common for clinicians to operate private practices in addition to their employment as salaried employees of public facilities. The degree of privatization varies by type of provider; the proportion of providers involved to some extent in private practice is estimated to be 90 percent for dentists, 66 percent for physicians, and almost 100 percent for pharmacists.

Pharmacists are widely regarded as among the groups that have benefited most from privatization. According to one policymaker, "The nicest shops in Poland are the drug stores. They have sprouted up like mushrooms after the rain. Pharmacies have been paid on a fee schedule, with fixed margins that are negotiated with the Ministry of Health. . . . Doctors are unhappy that pharmacies are doing so well when the doctors are not."

So far, very few Polish hospitals are in private hands. Some hospitals that were taken over by the communists have been returned to their original owners. But by the end of 1998, only about forty Polish hospitals were private, out of a total of nearly seven hundred nationwide.

The number of health care providers in Poland has grown slightly over the last decade. (See Table 5.3.) The supply of most types of health care providers is generally regarded as adequate, although

	1980	1985	1990	1992	1994	1996
Hospital indicators						
Beds per 1,000 population	6.7	6.6	6.6	6.4	6.3	6.1
Admissions per 1,000 population	10.1	1.06	10.6	10.8	11.4	N/A
Average length of stay	14.0	13.1	12.5	11.8	11.0	10.6
Occupancy rate (percent)	84	78	73	71	72	72
Health care personnel (per 1,000 population)						
Physicians	1.78	1.96	2.14	2.18	2.27	2.35
Dentists	0.47	0.47	0.48	0.43	0.45	0.46
Pharmacists	0.43	0.43	0.40	0.43	0.49	0.52
Nurses	4.4	4.8	5.4	5.4	5.4	5.6
Midwives	0.45	0.53	0.63	0.62	0.63	0.64

Table 5.3.   Selected Measures of Polish Delivery System Capacity and Performance.

Source: European Observatory on Health Systems, 1999, p. 33.

geographic maldistribution poses some problems, with shortages particularly in rural areas. The substantial capacity of the system is the result of a financing system that for decades based payment on factors such as staffing levels and number of hospital beds. Under this system, resources flowed to facilities based on historical costs rather than following patients or service usage. Many observers of the Polish system believe that the country has insufficient resources to support its current capacity adequately to ensure quality care. In the words of one academic, "Poland has a developing country financing system trying to support health care service and population demands of a more developed country."

The major providers of outpatient services in Poland are the ZOZs (*Zespol Opieki Zdrowotnej* or "integrated health and services units"). When they were originally established in the early 1970s, the ZOZs were responsible for managing outpatient clinics, specialty clinics, school- and employer-based clinics, secondary hospitals, and some social services (such as community-based nursing and other supports to people at home). In the early 1990s, the responsibility for outpatient and hospital services was separated, and the ZOZs became outpatient management units.

Poland has approximately five hundred ZOZs, each of which has historically been responsible for providing care to residents of a specified geographic area of 100,000 to 200,000 people. Until the establishment in 1999 of the state health insurance funds, the ZOZs received budgets from government authorities at various levels (generally, county or city). For many years, the ZOZ budgets were based on historical costs but in the last few years payment became population-based, with adjustments based on the age distribution of the ZOZ's geographic service area.

The ZOZs operate a range of outpatient facilities. In most cities, physicians practice in large multi-specialty practices called *polyclinics*, which employ internists, pediatricians, nurses, some specialists, and often dentists, generally on a salary basis. Health care workers are relatively poorly paid, with even physicians making less than the countrywide average wage. Most physicians rely on private practice revenues and informal payments to supplement their government incomes.

For instance, according to Chawla, Tomasik, Kulis, and Windak (1997), the average salary of a physician in a government job in 1997 was 9,112 zloty per year ($2,330). Other benefits—social security, taxes, and bonus—add another 4,388 zloty ($1,122). Average annual earnings from the physician's private practice, which many physicians maintain in addition to their government job, are estimated to be 20,000 zloty per year, about $5,115. Finally, there are the "envelope payments," amounts that patients who are receiving supposedly free government care pay under the table to physicians for better attention and access to services and supplies; based on a 1994 Ministry of Health and Social Welfare survey, the average annual earnings from these payments are 30,000 zloty ($7,673).

Ironically, the *lack* of informal payments for some physicians has also become an issue. The majority of Polish anesthesiologists went on strike for several months in 1999 to protest base salaries that they complained are not rising fast enough to allow them to maintain an adequate standard of living. One observation of the anesthesiologists was that only doctors who deal most directly with patients, such as surgeons, obstetricians, and urologists, receive envelope payments. According to one anesthesiologist quoted in the *Washington Post*, "I love my job but many times when I get to the end of the month, I am not able to pay my bills. I don't need to live like a doctor in America. But I do want to be able to put food on the table" (Finn, 1999).

Overspecialization of physicians is also a problem, with a ratio of specialists to primary care providers of 3:1. "Primary care is very low stature and poorly paid," said one official. "Patients want to see specialists." Although primary care doctors are supposed to operate as gatekeepers to specialty care, they are regularly bypassed by patients who go directly to specialists, whom they perceive to be better trained and have better resources. Even when patients do initially see a primary care doctor, most primary care visits end in a referral to a specialist.

Poland did not have general practitioners or family practice physicians until 1996, when the federal government established a new family practice specialty training program. Training is available to new physicians and specialists in internal medicine. The government is promoting the growth of family practices as an alternative to polyclinics, and financial assistance has been available to family practice physicians who want to establish private practices.

Poland has no advanced practice nurses (for example, nurse practitioners). Although nurses are becoming more professionalized, they have less training and status than in many other countries, and a more restricted scope of practice.

Subacute and community-based services are also relatively undeveloped in Poland and, as a result, many patients are in acute care hospitals for nonmedical reasons or conditions that could be cared far more appropriately in less expensive settings. Hospital lengths of stay are very long by U.S. or even European standards.

There have been some recent moves to strengthen public health and health promotion in Poland. The country has implemented a National Health Program—with the aim of improving a variety of health measures over the next decade, including reducing tobacco and alcohol use and improving nutrition. Although Poland's public health program is better than those of most other countries in Eastern Europe, it is still not highly developed and has been hampered by a lack of funding.

HEALTH REFORM IN POLAND

Beginning in the late 1980s, Poland adopted a series of major health sector reform initiatives. As articulated by the government, the goals of these reforms are ambitious: improving health status, ensuring universal access to a wide range of high-quality services, improving quality, increasing effectiveness, stabilizing funding, controlling costs, and improving consumer choice. Although the pace of reform has been slowed, at least in part, by financing and resource constraints, the approach has been deliberately incremental, with a concern about putting in place the laws and structures needed to support competition before market forces are unleashed.

Health reform has had four major components:

- Decentralization of government accountability for the health delivery system

- Fostering independent managerial autonomy of publicly owned units

- Development of pluralistic "ownership" structures for providers

- Separation of the provider and payer roles by the establishment of regional sickness funds (health insurers).

Decentralization of Government Accountability for the Health Delivery System

Over the last ten years, political and budgetary accountability for the health care sector was shifted from the federal government to state and in some cases county and municipal authorities. Accountability for most outpatient facilities, including polyclinics, specialty clinics, and public health providers, was transferred to the states and, in the case of the forty-six largest cities (including Krakow), to the municipal level. The largest cities also took responsibility for the general (secondary) hospitals, while the state government assumed responsibility of secondary hospitals in other regions. The states also organize and finance most tertiary services. The federal government is responsible for certain tertiary facilities, including the national centers for cardiology and maternal health. Medical schools have day-to-day autonomy but report to the Ministry of Health.

According to one health policymaker, the decentralization of health system accountability is intended to address the problems of limited accountability and inefficiency that resulted from centralized control of the health care system. "A focus of the reforms is to devolve ownership and control to the local level. . . . Local communities will be able to run the health care system better than the central government. . . . They know better what is needed and citizens have more influence on local officials than on federal officials. . . . Communities will act as real owners of the health care system."

Managerial Autonomy of Publicly Owned Units

The second major component of Polish health reform was allowing publicly owned health facilities to become independent or self-managing units. In 1995, the federal government set standards that health care organizations could meet to become self-managing. Several hundred hospitals, polyclinics, and ZOZs have been approved by the Polish government as independent units.

The self-managing units are still supervised by the government. The assets of the facilities remain government-owned, and the units cannot incur debt on behalf of their supervising governmental body. But the units are subject to commercial laws rather than the laws applying to government bodies. As a result, they have more autonomy in personnel practices, including authority over hiring and firing and staffing levels, the freedom to shift resources among different line items of their budgets without government approval, the ability to borrow for short-term purposes, and the authority to enter into contracts (for example, with the sickness funds). As of January 1, 1999, the primary source of revenue for the independent units is the sickness funds rather than government budget appropriations.

However, some ambiguities about the real meaning of being an "independent" unit remain. For example, although the units do have hire-and-fire authority, many question whether they will be able to use this authority effectively because of the political power of unionized health care workers. Also, while in theory the units could conceivably go out of business if their financial performance is poor, that possibility may be offset by the fact that the local governments have a legal responsibility to ensure access to health care for their residents. Thus it is possible that local governments would end up funding deficits or other financial requirements of financially troubled units. There is also concern that provider competition, both among the self-governing units and between these units and the traditionally managed units, will make it increasingly difficult to achieve systemwide health care objectives.

Based on interviews conducted by the Harvard-Jagiellonian Consortium for Health (Campbell and others, 1999) with a number of independent and traditionally managed units, the managers of the independent units report that they believe they have more authority in personnel and financing compared to the traditional units, although they rarely use it. The independent units appear to have been more aggressive at introducing new services, reducing staffing, and making improvements, although they have not yet begun to make widespread use of financial management tools such as pro forma budgets, cash budgeting, or capital investment analysis. The independent managers express a need for more capital investment, and for the establishment of governing bodies that have meaningful oversight and policymaking authority.

Pluralistic Ownership of Providers

Many different forms of provider ownership are now possible, including private, cooperative, local government, regional government, and federal government. Despite these changes, most providers in Poland remain publicly owned, and debate continues about the privatization of providers and how much the country should rely on competition among providers to achieve its health care goals. Some observers believe this reflects uncertainty about whether health care should be treated differently from other sectors of economy. "Many of us are concerned about what type of system we will get if we rely more on market forces," said one observer in Krakow. "We have concerns in particular about equity and costs. Most people already believe that inequity in the health care sector has increased with the development of private physician practices. We also see how expensive health care is in countries such as the United States that rely on a competitive model. It is vital that Poland has an equitable basic health care system for all in place to support all of our other economic reforms. Such a system is a critical component of a stable democratic society."

Separation of Providers and Payers: State Health Insurance Funds

Poland was slow to adopt a new financing system for health care, debating the issue for more than six years before enacting the new financing law that became effective on January 1, 1999.

In the past, the central government was the major payer for health care. The Ministry of Finance allocated money for health care to the various government entities responsible for providing health care services, including the federal Ministry of Health, the states, the counties and cities, and certain other government agencies that provide health care for specific population groups (for example, the military, prisons). These entities then appropriated money to the health care providers. The distribution of resources among regions was based largely on historical budgets until 1995, when the federal government changed the distribution method to take into account regional differences in demographics and selected health indicators (such as mortality rates). Additional revenues in some cases also came directly from state or local government. As described earlier, out-of-pocket payments by consumers were a major source of revenue for many providers.

The new financing law established a system of seventeen state health insurance funds, one in each of the sixteen states *(voivods)* and another for the existing separate health systems (military, prison). The funds are autonomous and self-governing, although their governing boards are appointed by the state government. Many sickness funds are governed by political appointees from the powerful labor unions, as well as from government agencies such as the Ministry of Finance. As health insurance is a new experience for Poland, most sickness fund leadership and staff are learning on the job about contracting, actuarial estimates of costs of a defined population, claims processing, consumer education, network development, payment methods, and other standard tools of the health insurance trade. These funds now provide health coverage to all residents of Poland, as the country does not permit voluntary private health insurance. (The financing law contemplated the possibility of private health insurance beginning in 2002, but as noted in the Epilogue, that has not emerged.) The funds do not compete against one another but provide exclusive coverage for the residents of their geographic area.

Financing for the health insurance funds comes from a 7.5 percent tax on wages and salaries, which is deducted by employers from paychecks or pensions and paid to the funds by the federal government. The self-employed make payments directly to the funds. Children and students are covered by their parents, while local governments make payments to the funds to cover orphans. The federal government pays the funds for coverage of individuals who are unemployed, and a national mechanism redistributes revenues among the regional funds to spread resources more fairly across Poland according to where the population is rather than where historical expenditure levels have been incurred. Under this mechanism, 60 percent of the revenues collected are distributed directly to the funds and the other 40 percent are distributed by the national body according to a formula.

The average payment for health insurance is approximately $200 per year. An interesting by-product of the law is that the unemployment rate in many parts of Poland, including Krakow, has increased significantly in the last few months as many individuals have officially registered as unemployed so as to be eligible for government-paid health insurance coverage. The government estimates that only 60 percent of those who are required to pay the tax are actually doing so. The other 40 percent of employed individuals—referred to as "nonparticipants"—are not paying the tax and therefore are not insured by the funds. "Many people who are in good health are just paying for health care out of pocket because it's cheaper than paying the tax," said one ZOZ manager. "We are concerned that those people are going to private practices, while those who are in bad health are paying the tax and using the polyclinics." Roughly one-third of all outpatient care is paid for by patients, that is, in the form of participants' copayments, or by nonparticipants and by participants who either request services not covered by the sickness funds or go to providers who do not have a sickness fund contract to provide such services.

The sickness funds cover a broad range of services with a few exclusions (alternative medicine, cosmetic surgery, abortions except in certain circumstances). However, copayments are required for certain services, including prescription drugs and many types of dental care. The cost-sharing for drugs ranges from about $0.50 for any drug on the basic list to 30–50 percent for other prescriptions. Out-of-pocket payments for prescription drugs can be substantial. According to one consumer, "Most drugs are not covered on the basic list. The list really includes only life-saving drugs. Physicians are not sensitive to the cost of drugs, so they prescribe the most expensive drugs. The public thinks the doctors have deals with the pharmaceutical companies and that the doctors benefit if they prescribe certain drugs."

The federal government continues to fund public health programs and certain specialized services (organ transplants, immuno-suppressive drugs) as well as to pay for capital investments of public facilities and for medical training and research.

The state sickness funds negotiate contracts with hospitals, physicians, ZOZs, and other providers for the provision of services. They are permitted to contract with both public and private practice providers. Provider payment methods are not specified in the law, and it is expected that the funds will use a variety of payment methods and financial incentives to change provider and patient behavior. Beginning in 1993, the government permitted some experimentation with provider payment methods, and some counties and cities have tested a variety of payment methods, including diagnosis-related groups (DRGs) for hospitals and capitation and fee schedules for primary care physicians.

Proponents believe that the new system will bring new sources of revenues into the health care system, improve equity by replacing informal payments with insurance payments, encourage local accountability, and increase the efficiency of the delivery system. However, others have concerns about the creation of an entirely new payer. "The county and city governments should have remained the payers," argued one city official, citing experiences since 1992 in provider payment reforms and public education about health reform, and continued,

> The insurance funds now have the money and the power. But the city still has the legal, financial, and political responsibility. . . . If the health insurance funds underpay the providers, the city will have the account-ability. . . . It is the guarantor of the health care facilities. . . . The split between the payers and providers makes no sense, but it has become

almost a religion. For years we had only one ideology, communism. Nothing else could be discussed. Now we have just adopted another single new idea—the market. The free market is seen as solving all of our problems. . . . Many of us argued that we should create and test many ideas and solutions. But we lost out to the people saying we must separate the payer and provider roles. But this is a mistake—there is no monolithic solution for Poland.

THE SITUATION IN KRAKOW

Krakow is a city of 780,000 people in southern Poland. The third-largest city in the country, it has long been Poland's intellectual, educational, and cultural center. After World War II, Stalin had a huge steelworks built at Nowa Huta, just a few miles away from the historic center of Krakow, in an attempt to break the traditional intellectual fabric of the city. Although the steelworks produced massive pollution, it was not successful in achieving its social reengineering purpose, and today, with the six-century-old Jagiellonian University and eleven other institutions of higher education, Krakow has more than seventy thousand students. As the best-educated city in Poland, Krakow has done relatively well during the period of economic transition, and has a much lower unemployment rate than the rest of Poland.

Health Reform in Krakow

Krakow has been at the forefront of many health reform initiatives in Poland. Since 1995, the city has been receiving assistance from the Harvard-Jagiellonian Consortium for Health, a project funded by the U.S. Agency for International Development, to help Krakow and other local areas develop and implement health reforms and study and share results and lessons learned with health leaders throughout Poland.

The city of Krakow is responsible for providing outpatient care to residents of the city and nearby suburbs. Krakow has four ZOZs, which employ approximately 370 physicians practicing in forty-nine outpatient clinics. The first family practice physician practices in Poland were established in Krakow, and the city now has approximately a dozen family practices. In addition, it has more than fifty private practices of varying size.

The city is also responsible for providing and financing primary and secondary hospital services. Four small hospitals in Krakow have become independent units, and three of the larger hospitals are due to become self-managing by the end of 1999. There are four tertiary hospitals in the city, one owned by the state and three by the federal government. The central government also operates several specialty facilities, including a pediatric hospital and a cardiology institute.

In 1997, the health services budget for Krakow was approximately 72 million zloty ($18 million), of which 62 million zloty ($15.8 million) came from central government and 10 million zloty ($2.6 million) from the city budget. In 1998, the budget for health care was 93 million zloty ($23 million), with 13 million zloty ($3.3 million) from the city. In both years, health care spending represented approximately 20 percent of the city budget. In addition to providing outpatient and hospital care, the city carries out a range of public health programs (such as alcohol and drug awareness and rehabilitation, and breast and cervical cancer awareness campaigns). The city's health care budget for 1999 was not available as of March 1999. According to one public official, "Now that the health insurance fund controls the money, we don't know how much spending will be. It is possible it will be less than before because the sickness funds have money only from the central government according to the tax formula and no contribution from the city . . . and the city is not intending to add more money initially."

Health reform began in Krakow, as in the rest of Poland, in 1992 when the city separated budget and management responsibility for its four ZOZs from that of its hospitals. "This was a good decision on the local level," said one observer. "The ZOZs thought they were neglected and that the hospitals got all the resources, including the modern equipment. With the separation, the ZOZ director had to prepare business plans and cooperate with the Ministry of Health. But the ZOZs now had separate budgets and predictable finances so they could control the allocation of resources better within ambulatory services. But there was not really much change at the service level."

In 1997, the city began to pay the ZOZs based on population size in their geographic areas, adjusted by age category. The age factors were 1.3 for children through age seventeen, 1.0 for adults aged eighteen to fifty-nine, and 1.8 for individuals aged sixty and older. "We picked these age groupings because that's what was done in the United States," explained one participant. "In the old system payment was based on historical budgets and the number of staff," she continued. "The best situation for any ZOZ under this system was for the ZOZ

ZOZ district	Krowadza	Nowa Huta	Podgorze	Srodmiescie	Krakow total
Over 65 (percent)	15	6	6	16	10
Female (percent)	73	73	69	68	71
College educated (percent)	81	67	71	76.8	73.8
Self-reporting poor health (percent)	38	31	29.7	32.1	32.6
One or more chronic diseases (percent)	47	44	37	40	42

Table 5.4.   Demographic and Case Mix Data, City of Krakow.
Source: Lawthers and Rosanski, 1998.

to have lots of people on its payroll but have 20 percent on sick leave so they weren't being paid."

The move to population-based payment was a major change for both providers and politicians. "The head of the city's executive board really loved this idea because it increased accountability," noted one policymaker. "But it was very painful. Some of the ZOZs benefited while others were losers. Two of the ZOZs have an older population based in the old city and two cover the younger population in the modern parts of Krakow and its suburbs. . . . The change was also shock therapy for the city council members. In the past, they all tried to get money for their friends and the ZOZs in their areas. The payment change was a way to change their thinking about the health sector."

Table 5.4 shows the distribution of key demographic characteristics of the various geographic areas covered by the four Krakow ZOZs.

Family physicians in private practices also began to receive capitated payments from the city in 1996. To be budget neutral, the capitation was based on average per capita spending in Krakow, adjusted for patient age using the same age modifiers as applied to the ZOZs' payments. The capitation included payment for almost all non-inpatient services, including primary care, diagnostic tests and laboratory services, specialist consultations, nursing and rehabilitation services, and minor surgeries. Some of the services were furnished directly by the practices and others were purchased.

As of 1997, a typical primary care practice in Krakow with responsibility for covering primary care delivered on site, specialty physician consultations, infant care, laboratory and diagnostics, limited rehabilitation care, and supplies was paid a capitation rate of roughly 82 zlotys per person per year ($21). Per capita variable medical costs (excluding primary physician and nurse salaries) were estimated to be roughly 13 zlotys per year (roughly $3.32). The remainder covers nurse and physician salaries, equipment costs, rent, administration, marketing, and miscellaneous other direct costs of the practice (Chawla, Tomasik, Kulis, and Windak, 1997).

In 1997, Krakow also began to allow patients to have access to any specialist in the city. Prior to this change, patients were required to see specialists affiliated with their ZOZ, and they frequently encountered problems with long waiting times for appointments. Primary care physicians (generally internists, pediatricians, and family medicine practitioners) are expected to continue to play a gatekeeping role for most referrals, although consumers have open access to certain specialties (such as gynecology and psychiatry). When someone takes advantage of the ability to go to another area, the patient's home ZOZ must compensate the specialist's ZOZ.

As of June 1998, patients in Krakow were also able to choose any primary care physician and are no longer assigned to specific polyclinics. Access to care after hours improved as of March 1, 1999, when the health insurance funds contracted with ten polyclinics in Krakow to be open twenty-four hours a day in an effort to stop unnecessary use of emergency services. The sickness fund will now pay for emergency care only in the case of a true emergency—one that a polyclinic can't handle.

During 1997 and 1998, the city government in Krakow pursued a number of strategies designed to foster change at the provider units, including linking 30 percent of each ZOZ manager's compensation to the achievement of specific annual goals, and holding weekly meetings with all the ZOZ directors and city health department officials. One official explained the rationale for this approach:

> The problem with health care reform is that all change ultimately depends on human factors, not changes in the law, economy, or political system. . . . We have made changes on the macro level but not worked so much on the institutional or individual levels. But behavioral changes by providers, managers, and consumers are perhaps more important than financing changes. There has been lots of attention directed to making new financing and insurance systems, without developing the capacity to administer and manage the systems. . . . The

problem with the competition among provider units is that we are not sharing best practices across the ZOZs or developing capacity. We want to use competitive forces to improve health care for everyone. . . . The meetings with the ZOZ directors were a place where they could discuss their problems and share best practices . . . to explain how they managed to achieve such a high vaccination rate or how they trained the receptionists at their clinics. . . . We also made the ZOZ managers come up with strategic plans and then operational goals that fit those plans and the priorities of the city. They had to defend those proposals before the city health commission, as a way to increase their accountability and educate the commission. And we made sure journalists were there.

The View from Providers

Based on discussions with a number of providers in Krakow, views about the impact of the reforms implemented so far and prospects for the future vary widely. Some common themes do emerge, however: concern that resources are inadequate, frustration with the negotiations with the health insurance fund and the lack of information available from the fund, and the need to develop providers' capacity and infrastructure in many areas, including finance, contracting, information systems, organizational behavior, and marketing. Despite these problems, most providers are passionate about the need for reform and cautiously optimistic about the future. The following extensive excerpts from interviews with a number of providers are presented to give a sense of some of the issues, concerns, and perspectives present in the Krakow provider community.

PROVIDER #1: A ZOZ DIRECTOR

Only the payer changed as of January 1. We have had many changes in the ZOZs in years past, including the decentralized budget, the distribution of budgets to the clinics, and the change to independent clinics.

The biggest change is that patients can pick their own primary care doctor. They had to declare their doctor by the end of March. As of today [the first week in March], only 55 percent of our patients had declared. We have an implied patient list [that is, a list of all people residing in the geographic service area] and hope we can keep our patients until they pick a provider. They can switch anytime they want. But we can't begin to make any changes at the ZOZ until we have the real list and know what our resources will be.

We are trying to encourage our patients to pick a doctor. We have a list of doctors, along with their pictures on the walls of the clinics. Patients are picking doctors by the photos, as well as their qualifications and degree of specialization. The more specialized doctors are getting more patients.

Since our revenues from the health insurance fund are based on capitation, we need patients. The doctors are being much more available and friendly because they want patients. The ZOZ is also advertising on the TV, in home magazines, and on the Internet. Our marketing slogan is, "We want to perform services in the best possible way while using all available knowledge and experience." We do very limited quality improvement work but we hope to do more. Our major activities are a semiannual patient satisfaction survey at the clinic level (waiting times, registration, "did the doctor smile, was the doctor kind, responsive") and some education of the doctors on over- and underutilization.

Our negotiation with the health insurance fund was not really a negotiation. The ZOZ submitted a proposal by a certain date. But no one from the health insurance fund looked at it. The fund said it had limited resources and put a very low capitation rate on the table. This was a psychological approach. Then when they increased the capitation a little bit, we were supposed to think we got something. The capitation was 25 percent lower than last year's payment levels.

Under the payment arrangement with the health insurance fund, we receive a capitation for each enrolled patient. The capitation does not vary by patient age, which is a big problem. Out of the capitation, we must pay for all services except hospital care, nursing home services, and drugs. Approximately 50 percent of the capitation goes to salaries for primary care physicians and the other half goes to all other services.

We can negotiate again with the health insurance fund after three months. We have a whole list of things we want. For example, as of January 1, nursing homes no longer employ doctors. But neither the ZOZ nor any doctor gets paid to provide visits in nursing homes. So in our ZOZ service area there are fifteen hundred patients in nursing homes who are not receiving care from a physician.

Our ZOZ is planning to have our primary care physicians form an independent group practice. The practice will buy administrative services from the ZOZ—including transportation, supplies, technical services, equipment, and facilities management. Our specialists, imaging, rehabilitation, laboratory, and diagnostic services will all stay with the ZOZ. When the primary care physicians are independent, they will negotiate own financial payment with the insurance fund. The doctors might hire the ZOZ to negotiate with the fund for them or do it themselves.

We are going to move to a new payment method for our physicians in the fall: capitation for our primary care physicians and fee-for-service for the specialists. We think that primary care doctors should be at risk only for primary care in order to prevent any incentive for withholding referrals, but the insurance fund might agree to capitate the primary care doctors for specialty services also. This would be a way to reduce specialist referrals.

A big weakness is that we don't get any information from the insurance fund. For example, we do not know with whom the fund has contracted for specialty care and hospital care, so we don't know where to send our patients. The insurance fund is eventually planning to have separate departments for different types of services—primary care, rehabilitation and spa, hospitals, clinics, drugs—but it has almost no staff yet.

We have a very limited information system at the ZOZ. We can track referrals in general terms but not in any detail. But we are developing a new information system so that we can track patients, referrals, admissions, and other information on a physician-specific basis. One big problem is that we have no data on drug use on the system. The health insurance fund has that information but can't manage it and gives nothing back to the ZOZs.

To make up the shortfall in revenues from the health insurance fund, our ZOZ is looking for other revenue sources, including contracting with employers to do physicals, providing privately paid services like dental care and special lab tests and blood tests for patients who cannot get authorization from their doctor. We are also looking for outside support, for example, from the national disability council to help us improve the handicapped accessibility of the clinics.

Contracts for other services are another potential source of revenues. For example, the Ministry of Health is running a "competition" to select a vendor to provide breast cancer prevention and cervical cancer screenings for the city—only one provider will win. The ZOZs are getting together to bid jointly and agree how to allocate the money and business if our bid is accepted.

Although there are opportunities for cooperation among the ZOZs, we must also compete with the other ZOZs for capital funds from the city. I hope we can cooperate better with the city than in the past. The new city council is thinking in new ways but they are still learning.

Overall, there is confusion, chaos and a lack of information right now. The patients don't know where to go, what is covered, what is not covered and how to get a referral. But in general, I think the patients are getting better primary care, access has improved and the physicians' attitudes are better and they are making the patients feel more welcome.

PROVIDER #2: A ZOZ DIRECTOR

When the city first moved to population-based payment in 1996, it was a dramatic change. We had to reduce our staff by three hundred people, or about 30 percent. We tried to do this mainly by eliminating support staff and not physicians or nurses.

Now that patients can choose their providers, we are doing much more marketing—at meetings, in the newspaper, on television. So far we have a net increase in patients of about twelve hundred people. [This ZOZ serves an area of approximately 200,000 people.]

But the lack of risk adjustment in our payment from the health insurance fund is a big problem. For example, we have very good family nurses and we do a good job working with diabetics. Under the new payment method, we don't really want to enroll more diabetics as patients. But at least we will do a good job managing them if they do pick us.

We are also making a number of administrative changes to improve service and patient satisfaction. For years, the most important person at the health clinics has been the woman who registers the patients. But these people have been paid very poorly. We have set up our clinics so each group has a person who registers patients and we are using money from our capitation to pay these women better.

There is a tremendous abuse of referrals, caused by too many specialists, fee-for-service payment, and overworked primary care physicians. In our ZOZ, we have specialists that we know do too much but we have to be political about how we handle the management of referrals. We are preparing a list for our primary care doctors of who *not* to refer to. The primary care doctors are salaried but also eligible for a bonus at the end of the year if the ZOZ does well financially, so they have an incentive to want to control referrals and other costs.

We are afraid that there is not enough money to make the changes we need. If you want to change performance, you need to provide support and money. For example, we had a very long wait for ophthalmology appointments at our health centers—two to three weeks. This was because we did not have adequate equipment. We bought new equipment and now patients can get treatment the same day. We are afraid that the resources will not be there. Health insurance was supposed to increase resources. But our 1999 budget is 20 percent lower than in the previous year, and 30 percent lower if you correct for inflation. And this is just the beginning; resources will get tighter and tighter. We cannot make a great reform without money. We have reformed the delivery side without funding it.

But it is unlikely that there will be more money in the near future. The Ministry of Health doesn't want to increase the payroll tax. Raising copayments is a concern because people will not seek care. But we could have real access problems. The insurance fund pays providers on a monthly basis so it's possible that a ZOZ or hospital could run out of money every fourth week and curtail services.

The purpose of reform was to redirect money to primary care. But this is not happening yet. Seventy percent of spending is in the hospital. We need hospital budgets to follow patients too. There are too many hospital beds in Krakow, especially in secondary hospitals. But hospital payment is not affected by length of stay so there is no motivation to get people out and nowhere to put them. We need to reclassify some hospital beds and change them into geriatric beds and nursing home beds. But it will be hard to close or convert hospitals. The workers know how to fight changes and they can mobilize patients. Plus we have no objective data to measure quality so it is almost impossible to make comparisons that are meaningful. We need a restructuring program. But this will take time and money. The Ministry of Health should be making capacity decisions, not the health insurance funds.

The system is very unstable financially, and very unstable politically. We are still missing major pieces of the law and anything could change in the future. In Krakow, we will have an election in October, and there may be changes then. But for now the mayor and other politicians are trying to avoid talking about health care and health reform.

PROVIDER #3: A ZOZ DIRECTOR

We are learning a lot and gathering information. In the past, we had to spend money according to laws, regulations, and line item budgets, and no variation was allowed unless we got the approval of the central government. Now we are free from the central government and we can spend according to our own plans.

But the change to the insurance fund has been hard. I am still in a state of economic shock. All of our money this year is coming from the insurance funds and we will get very little money from the city—no money for repairs, just some help with financing some new equipment. So I have money only for salaries and for basics like utilities. There is no money for raises. The doctors want to earn more money, but we must become more efficient if that is to happen.

Fortunately, there are lots of opportunities to become more efficient. We have too many personnel—80 percent of my costs are salaries. And lot of duplication of services in different clinics that is unnecessary. I upgraded and centralized the lab and diagnostic centers—now all the clinics use the same diagnostics. This saved money and I laid off ten people.

We also introduced a productivity-based bonus system for doctors. If a doctor sees more than six hundred patients per month, they get a bonus. This was initially opposed by doctors, who are members of union. But is now accepted.

It is important for our primary care doctors to get patients because the money follows the patients. More than half of our patients have already signed up with us, but it is hard to get the patients to enroll and some of them never will. The only incentive for the patients to sign up is to get access to the new twenty-four-hour-a-day centers. We are hoping that the health insurance fund might accept a negative list.

It is essential that physician attitudes change since we have the same doctors as in the old structures. Based on our patient satisfaction surveys, the doctors can compete by improving service standards, improving their qualifications, increasing the range of services they offer, and establishing better links to entire families. Patients are protected by competition because they can change doctors any time they want. But physicians are not protected if they don't do a good job.

I encouraged the ZOZ's dentists to become independent. The dentists could make a lot of money by providing more primary care, which is cheap, than by doing restorative care. And the public thinks state-owned dental facilities are not of high quality. The dentists and other workers also did not always behave well when they were part of the ZOZ. For example, people did not respect the materials and equipment and many dentists would use state-owned material for their private practices.

At the Harvard-Jagiellonian classes we learned the economic and political model of reform, but the reality has been quite different. The necessary changes must come at the grassroots level.

Profile for Provider #4: Seven primary care physicians (three pediatric, four internal medicine) and ten nurses, and 14,000 patients (3,000 children aged fourteen or under; 3,000 students aged fourteen to twenty, 7,500 adults aged twenty-one to fifty-nine, and 500 aged sixty or older).

PROVIDER #4: A PRIVATE PHYSICIAN GROUP PRACTICE

We were the first physician practice to become independent in Krakow, as of September 1998. Although we split from the ZOZ for legal and management purposes, we have stayed in the same clinic space.

The negotiations with the health insurance funds have been a challenge. The nurses in our practice formed their own group and concluded their contract with the fund before the physicians did. We did not know what the nurses had negotiated before we negotiated our own contract, even though the nurses' pay comes out of our capitation. Our nurses are the only ones in the city with their own contract—it's supposed to be an experiment. The nursing community views the contract as a model one and it has been written up in the nursing journal. But the fund realizes it made a mistake doing this type of contract but says it cannot renegotiate the deal until next year.

We waited for three weeks to start our negotiation with the health insurance fund. We would go to the fund and they would tell us to come back another time. Finally after three weeks we sat down and had a short meeting. There was no negotiation. The fund told us that resources were limited, especially after the nursing contract, and we could not get any more money.

Under our contract with the health insurance fund, we are paid a monthly capitation per enrolled patient. The capitation does not vary by patient age. This payment covers all services except hospital care, nursing home services, drugs that we do not administer in the office, and certain tertiary diagnostic services financed by the city (such as CTs and MRIs). Thirty percent of the capitation goes to the nurses, 35 percent to the physicians, and 35 percent to cover all other services. Because we felt the capitation was inadequate, we tried to limit the scope of services it covered. The health insurance fund only agrees to limit our risk for OB/GYN care. We are at risk only for services related to pregnancy, and the fund pays for all other gynecological services. We asked for this exclusion because patients have open access to OB/GYN services and we didn't think we could control use or costs.

Our practice decided not to contract with the insurance fund to provide twenty-four-hour-a-day services because there were not enough resources to pay for it. The fund was proposing only 1 zloty per patient per year (about $0.20) to be open twelve more hours per day. This would not cover our costs.

We have had difficulty getting our patients registered with the practice so we can receive the capitation from the insurance fund. We started gathering the declarations from our patients last year and we got eight thousand of them. Then the sickness fund said we had used the wrong form, so we had to start all over again. We are spending a tremendous amount of physician time at night and on the weekends entering data into the computer to create a list of our patients for the fund. We tried to hire a data entry person to put the information into the computer but it would have cost us the equivalent of two physicians' salaries.

The administrative burden of running this practice is enormous. We are spending the equivalent of one full-time-equivalent physician on administration, split between the two doctors who are sharing administrative duties. This works out to one FTE for twelve hours each weekday and eight hours on Saturday. We are doing the same clinical work but we are now responsible for so many new things. We did not realize we would have to be concerned with so many things—how many responsibilities we would have. But we are learning day by day.

We were more financially secure in the previous system. We only had to worry about treating our patients. Now we have to worry about resources, supplies, relationships with other providers, rent, negotiating contracts, lawyers. We have realized that it is not so easy. . . . We do not have many of the necessary resources—no modern computer, no typewriter, no office equipment, no money for printing referral forms. . . . Our clinic was very poor before, and now we have to buy everything we need from the money we get from the health insurance fund. So equipment and supplies are our priority and there is no money for raises for the doctors. Our physicians are making only 700 zloty ($179) per month in salary. The clinic space is not good or efficient, but we have no money to modernize it. We lease equipment and space from the clinic but it is not modern.

We decided to become a private practice because we are trained in public health, and when we took part in the city's training, we came to the conclusion that the reform offered a possible way to restructure. But the reforms and discussions made us aware of the possibilities, not the practicalities. We hoped that we could improve motivation and gain enthusiasm because in the old system everyone was devoid of enthusiasm. Now the people in our practice are more enthusiastic although we may not survive. We are working more hours and even have homework. We don't have the resources to employ the support staff or the accountants or the data analysts or the other managerial capacity we need to improve our practice.

Patients don't know the details of the reforms. They don't know how to behave, where they can go for care. We don't know which hospitals and which specialists have contracts with the insurance fund, so we're not sure where to refer. The health insurance fund is not providing any information and no one answers the phones. So we have to take half-days away from our practice to go to the fund to try to meet with people and get our questions answered. We try to exchange information with another private practice that has more experience than we do. But we also have to use intuition a lot. Based on our experience so far, we have great concerns about the competency of the funds to perform many of their new functions.

Profile for Provider #5: Seventeen doctors, forty midwives, thirteen office locations, 350,000 patients in the geographic service area, 110,000 of whom are women of childbearing age.

PROVIDER #5: A PRIVATE OBSTETRICS AND GYNECOLOGY PRACTICE

Our practice was established in March 1999. We used to be part of the ZOZ, but we split off and now the ZOZ has no OB/GYNs. We are leasing some equipment from the ZOZ and purchasing other equipment.

There was no negotiation with the health insurance fund, just regulation. Our strategy was not to fight this year, but to work on building our patient base. Then next year our position will be stronger and if the fund will not negotiate, we will not contract with it.

Our group negotiated a fixed payment with the insurance fund, based on our historic costs for caring for our 110,000 women of childbearing age. But any woman covered by the fund can come to the practice for any covered service. The amount of money is very small because the fund assumed patients would not come for care. So we dream that the patients won't come this year, and that they won't be expensive if they do come. But next year our payment will be based on patient declarations, so we want to build our practice this year. The only motivation to get the patients now is to get declarations for next year.

The best marketing is word of mouth. The best way to attract new patients is to be kind to the ones we have. Our group is adopting a number of new policies designed to improve care and satisfaction. For instance, we are requiring that physicians must get coverage by another doctor in the group when they go on vacation. In the past, a woman would often arrive for an appointment or go into labor and discover her doctor was on vacation. Continuity of care was awful. The new coverage patterns and other changes will let us provide better care. This is important because patients are beginning to realize that next year their satisfaction will determine how well doctors do financially.

This is the first time in Poland we have been able to treat patients and get paid decently. We have always served people, but we could not be paid. The number of women seeking gynecologic primary care has been declining. And the poorest women could only come to the polyclinics while the richer women got care in the private practices. We must increase the awareness of women and doctors that now any woman, regardless of income, can come to our private practice and receive high-quality care for free.

We are also looking to develop other revenue streams that will provide self-pay, fee-for-service income for the practice. We will soon open a same-day minor gynecologic surgery in one of our offices. We can do a range of procedures there, including D&Cs, colposcopies, cervical biopsies, and cauterizations. We also hope to develop several comprehensive women's health centers, with osteoporosis clinics, mammography, and breast health services. If these new programs are successful, we will try to get funding eventually from the health insurance funds.

We are also evaluating our use of hospitals. At the moment, the practice admits to a number of hospitals. [Krakow has eight OB/GYN inpatient services.] Most often the doctor admits where they have other part-time jobs. But we are beginning to talk to one local hospital to see if we can get a better deal and better care for our patients. For example, we want to have more control over the anesthesiologists and a guarantee that beds will be available when we need them. The hospital is regarded as the best one in the area, with the best amenities, including double rooms and private baths, which are rare in

Poland. We have power because we control 110,000 women. The hospitals will have to pay attention to us.

If we can attract enough patients, we will build our own hospital. We hope to attract many patients from the three other ZOZs. We have the advantage of being the first big group and we have no competition because we have all the doctors, and there is no capital, no money, and no returns now for building a practice. Maybe in five years other practices will emerge, but right now we are investing, creating the infrastructure and trying to take over the market before competition emerges. Being first and being successful will create enormous barriers to entry.

One financial burden for our practice has been the number of midwives, which exceeds the need of the practice. But we have an ethical obligation to these women, some of whom have worked for forty years in their positions. We cannot neglect them in the reforms. In the next few years, ten or twelve of them will retire so we will keep them on and everyone will earn a little less until then.

Reform must be reflected not only in the law but also in people's minds. We have not gotten more resources, so our salaries are not increasing yet. In fact, salaries are going down right now because of the need to pay the midwives and to make investments. But money in the short term is not the issue. Obstetricians and gynecologists are not the poorest doctors in Poland, so we can afford to incur some costs, spend some money on personnel, and take out some loans. We can see a broader perspective and we have hope for the future for what we do. The money will come later.

Profile for Provider #6: Fifty-six dentists (twenty-three generalists, twenty-five specialists, and eight superspecialists) plus ninety other staff, practicing in nine clinics and thirty schools.

PROVIDER #6: AN INDEPENDENT DENTAL PRACTICE

We became an independent practice in November 1998. Before, we were employees of a ZOZ and practiced as part of a thousand-person polyclinic. We are still physically located at the ZOZ and we lease space and pay other expenses related to our practice.

When we became independent, we did not reemploy everyone. Twenty dentists were not taken and are still working at the ZOZ under the old structure. The health insurance fund did not contract with the ZOZ dentists for any but a few services—let's hope the contracted services included novocaine!

Now that we are independent, we have more flexibility to run the practice the way we want (for example, hire our own receptionist). We don't report to anyone so there is no bureaucracy. Before there were layers to get through before you could change anything: the clinic director, the medical director, the city health department. Now we can change whatever we want to improve practice and performance.

Under our contract with the health insurance fund, we are paid fee-for-service, not a salary. The contract specifies a limited number of points per month (80,000) that the health insurance fund will pay for—each service has a point equivalent. We wanted a cap of 100,000 points but the insurance fund said it had a revenue cap. So the more one dentist does, the less another can do. Our practice worked for one year before the contract with the point system on a phantom basis to see how it would work and how we needed to adapt. So unless someone changes their practice behavior, we have a good sense how it will work.

But not all services are covered by the fund. We estimate about 40 percent of our services will be covered, including orthodontics for children under fourteen. The other 60 percent of services will be paid by patients (such as crowns and bridges). We have increased our percentage of self-pay services from 50 percent before we became independent, and there may be more room for growth. For private-paying patients, the dentist gets 50 percent of the billings and the other half goes into taxes, utilities, support staff, and materials. So the dentists have a strong financial incentive to attract self-paying patients.

Our fee schedule has been structured to reward prevention—we are paid more to do prevention than to drill. We know an investment of 5 percent now will save 25 percent in the future. Ninety-three percent of kids in Poland need fillings now. If we did better prevention and got that number down to 50 percent, it would save a lot of money for other uses.

The biggest change is that there is higher risk for the dentists if they are not good and more financial opportunity if they are. This is motivation to do good work. Good performers and highly qualified specialists will do much better now. The fundamental issue is a change of mentality. The profit goes to the dentists now if we work hard. Before we could not be paid more if we did good work, because we were salaried. So people worked in the morning for the state and in the afternoon in private practice. Now the jobs are combined so it is less exhausting and more economical. Under the old system each public clinic patient was a potential enemy. Now for the first time dentists are interested in having lots of satisfied patients and in attracting new patients. This is good for patients—doctors are looking for patients and not patients looking for doctors.

We can already see the change in the attitude of the dentists—some are doing very well, eager to work, because they will be paid. Incomes for some dentists are up by 100 percent, while others are less popular and are earning less than before.

The biggest barrier we face is the lack of an adequate information system. Before we had nothing because we could not afford anything and did not need it. Now we have one computer in the practice, which we hope to upgrade but can't afford to do so far. We are focusing first on upgrading our specialty equipment. We lease equipment now from the clinic but it is very outmoded. We are funding this investment from operations because interest rates are so high.

Eventually we want to make more investment in the practice but for now we have to get money to dentists. The average dentist's salary is $300 per month, which is not enough to live on, so many dentists are moonlighting in other jobs. We have to increase wages—people won't invest until they see the idea works.

The biggest risk to us is the insurance fund—how will it do financially. If it survives, we will survive. If it goes bankrupt, we will just be running our private practices in the same place. There is no way we can fail—it can only be an improvement.

There are significant barriers to changing other dental practices: They have no vision and no leadership. Plus they are afraid of responsibility—you have to form a partnership to do this. Another group could compete if they had significant money for investment. But we do not really feel at risk—we have nine clinics and pretty much cover the area.

Profile for Provider #7: Beds—130, plus 12 in a one-day surgery (patients come in during the afternoon, stay overnight, have surgery, and stay another night before being discharged). Average length of patient stay in the main hospital is fifteen to twenty days from admission to discharge.

PROVIDER #7: A PRIVATE HOSPITAL OWNED BY THE CATHOLIC CHURCH

We were the first hospital in Poland to become independent. We have been an independent hospital since August 1996. As an independent, we had to lay off all our staff and rehire them. We only rehired the best workers, based on training, performance, and experience. Our overall staff was reduced by 10–15 percent. Ninety percent of the people we hired were former employees and 10 percent were new. Since then, we have instituted a new staff evaluation system to improve accountability. . . .

The hospital had an agreement with the province in 1997 and 1998, and just signed one with the health insurance fund. In the past, our payment was based on our historical budget, adjusted for inflation. The health insurance fund wanted a case rate by ward type (for example, general surgery, internal medicine, vascular surgery) regardless of disease. The case rate includes payment for room and board, anesthesia, and surgery. We wanted to be paid a case-based rate by procedure and/or diagnosis for the vascular surgery ward, and we analyzed the most recent two years of cost data by procedure to prepare proposed rates of payment. But the fund would not agree to our approach because it had no data. There was no real negotiation with the fund . . . the amount they are paying us will not cover all of our costs of providing care.

Because resources are limited, many hospitals do not want to treat elderly patients because they are expensive. But that is not the Church's philosophy so we won't discriminate, even if we incur more costs because of this. We are hoping to establish a nursing home for patients as a better and less costly alternative for patients who do not need to be in the hospital but cannot live at home.

We are also trying to increase our revenues from services that are paid for directly by patients. The hospital got 5 percent of revenues in 1997 from direct payment services, and 16 percent in 1998. We expect to do better in 1999. The insurance fund did not contract with us for our one-day surgery unit. The hospital started this unit as a means to generate profit to subsidize other services. We bill patients directly for the care, and try to attract patients based on patient satisfaction, as well as atmosphere and amenities, including private rooms and bathrooms, which are very rare in Poland. Patients like the unit and are very comfortable there. And their payments are tax deductible. . . . But we need more volume to break even and twice the volume if the unit is to be as profitable as planned. On this unit we are experimenting with a number of new approaches, including paying most nurses on a contract rather than salary basis so we can vary costs based on volume of surgeries planned.

Profile for Provider #8: Staff of 135, serving about 20,000 patients. The clinic offers internal medicine, pediatrics, rheumatology, OB/GYN, pulmonology, dermatology, endocrinology rehabilitation services, and dental care.

PROVIDER #8: THE EXECUTIVE DIRECTOR OF
A HEALTH CLINIC IN ONE OF THE ZOZs

We were recently voted the best health clinic in a city-sponsored competition. The results were based on patient surveys. Patients were asked to judge their health clinic based on a variety of factors, including clinician competence, attitude toward patients, waiting times, timeliness of lab and test results. The prize was 10,000 zlotys donated by a drug company. We divided the prize up equally among all the clinic staff and gave everyone a gift certificate (to save on taxes).

People like this clinic because the staff is competent and friendly, and the place is organized well. For example, patients can make appointments at specific times and there are no long lines and waits. We have worked hard at the clinic to change staff attitudes about patients. In the past, they did not see why they should be nice to patients because it did not affect their pay. But I have been trying to explain that changes are coming and we need to prepare. We have made a number of changes to change staff attitudes, including instituting a bonus system for physicians based on their qualifications, productivity in terms of the number of patients they see, and the results of the satisfaction surveys of their patients. The bonuses are small but they are changing people's attitudes.

We have gotten many new patients since the competition, both primary care and specialist referrals, but no new money. We hope the ZOZ will eventually increase our budget—the money should follow the patients.

Resources are tight, and we need to upgrade our facilities. So we have had to look for outside sources of support. Last year we got prisoners to paint the clinic. A local supermarket donated the paint and we got the curtains from a drug company. We also opened a fee-for-service (self-pay) densitometry service. We advertise this service in the local newspapers and we got publicity when we gave flowers and champagne recently to our twenty thousandth densitometry patient.

Our growth is constrained by our physical space. But there are three other clinics nearby and we don't want to be the only one providing excellent care. We would love to work with other clinics to help them replicate some of the changes we have made here. It is not a secret here what we do.

The dentists at our clinic have become independent and formed their own practice. In the long run we may go our separate way, but the time is not right now. We need to see how the new financing system works. Does the money really follow the patients?

The View from Consumers

Interviews with a number of consumers in Krakow suggest mixed reactions to reform, including confusion, suspicion, and indifference. "There is a lack of trust and credibility in the system," said one consumer. "We have heard promises in the past with no real results. Why will this time be different?" "There is a common belief among the public that the health insurance funds will go bankrupt," said another consumer. "I and everyone I know expect to keep having to pay large amounts out of my pocket, even with the health insurance contributions." People generally agreed that most consumers are very confused about many aspects of health reform. "Everything to do with health care has blurred edges. . . . Before, at least the rules were clear to people," said to one consumer. A local government official agreed, "People have lost their feeling of safety. There are too many new things and there was no information for people before changes took place."

While Poland has enacted a number of patient protections in the last decade, including guaranteed privacy, informed consent, and access to medical records, the country has no real organized consumer or patient movement, and no national emphasis on public information, social marketing, or any other type of activity to engage consumers in the issues of health reform.

But in Krakow, the city government has realized the importance of educated consumers and the need to change patient attitudes and behavior, and it has undertaken a number of actions designed to influence and mobilize public opinion. "The health care system is not really on the minds of the public except for heart transplants, helicopter lifts, or the anesthesiologists on strike," said one policymaker. "So we needed to come up with ways to get the public's attention."

Among the tactics pursued by city officials was a weekly TV news magazine on health reform, which used humor and props to engage the public. City officials also wanted to "open the eyes of public to the conditions in the clinics" so they went on tours of the clinics, accompanied by a newspaper reporter, and interviewed patients about their problems. "People talked about waiting lists, atmosphere, the attitudes of staff," said the official. "The stories were very interesting and resulted in changes . . . but it's hard to get the newspapers to sustain interest in the issue." The city also sponsors an annual competition for the "best health center in Krakow," based on a patient satisfaction survey conducted at each public clinic (see Table 5.5).

Quality of Outpatient Services, Krakow District

	District Average Response	Benchmark (best practice)
Access:		
Successful registration by telephone (percent)	73	95
Successful in-person registration (percent)	91	100
Waited less than 10 minutes at registration (percent)	87	100
Waited less than 30 minutes to see doctor (percent)	38	61
Waited less than 30 minutes to see doctor if patient rated problem as urgent (percent)	40	100
Average waiting time for registration (minutes)	11	5
Average waiting time for doctor on day of appointment (minutes)	53 minutes (min-max: 0–420 minutes)	26
Satisfaction:		
Rating of receptionist politeness (percent)	73	81
Perception of receptionist skill (percent)	75	86
Received sufficient information from receptionist (percent)	78	81
Clinical Quality:		
Doctor treated patient with respect (percent)	94	99
Doctor communicated with patient (percent)	95	99
Doctor gave patient sufficient information (percent)	77	91
Doctor was gentle during exam (percent)	98	100
My privacy was protected (percent)	95	100
Doctor examined me carefully (percent)	89	98
I had a chance to tell of my complaint (percent)	97	100
The doctor listened to me carefully (percent)	94	99
The doctor talked to me in a clear way I could understand (percent)	94	100
Received sufficient information about:		
Current complaint (percent)	71	87
Further management of current complaint (percent)	73	88

(Table 5.5 Continued)

Table 5.5 (continued)

	District Average Response	Benchmark (best practice)
The use of medication (percent)	87	97
Results of previous tests (percent)	72	89
Future recommended tests (percent)	75	93
Preventive health: percent of patients reporting blood pressure reading in last year:		
Patients over age 21	75	89
Patients over age 65	92	100
Patients with self-reported heart disease, hypertension, or diabetes (percent)	87	100
Pap smear in last three years for women over age 18 (percent)	51	58
Clinical breast exam by MD in last year, women ages 50–70 (percent)	37	75
Preventive health care counseling at routine periodic visit (percent)	56	83

Table 5.5.   Patient Satisfaction Survey.
Source: Lawthers and Rosanski, 1998.

Public officials express some frustration about being able to get people to distinguish what's going on in Krakow from events on the national level or in other parts of Poland. One official said, "For example, there was a big scandal in another area of Poland when it was discovered that the directors of the ZOZs negotiated very generous employment contracts with the state governments before accountability for the ZOZs shifted to the local level—high salaries and two to three years of pay if the contract was terminated. In Krakow, we have very good contracts with the ZOZs, with accountability and bonuses if performance targets are met. But the public thought the problems were everywhere, including Krakow. This undermines confidence and makes the public cynical about the possibility of reform."

A journalist in Krakow who is a long-time observer of the local health care system gave her assessment of how consumers feel about the health care reforms in the city:

Patients do not care about who gives the money for health care or who owns the health care providers. They only care about how they are treated and what services are provided. This has not changed for patients. Although some of the changes may, in the course of time, result in better health care, patients are confused and dissatisfied with the reforms. For example, patients did not applaud when family doctors appeared, although the majority of family practice doctors have nice, well-equipped offices. Patients do not like the family practice doctors because the doctors decide whether to refer or not and limit access to specialists. The bad organization of the clinics makes this worse, because there are long lines and it takes a long time to get the referral. . . . Many clinics won't make appointments by phone or for a specific time. . . . Doctors are also dissatisfied with the reforms because they are not earning more, so they are exaggerating the problems to the patients in an attempt to get the patients to rebel. I have never met a patient who would say that he is satisfied with the reform of the health care system, and everyone thinks they lost something.

—–∿– Epilogue: Health Care Reform in Poland

Nancy M. Kane

The health reforms of the late 1990s brought in four major components: decentralization of government accountability for the health delivery system, independent managerial autonomy for publicly owned provider units, pluralistic ownership structures for providers, and the separation of purchaser and provider through the establishment of quasi-independent sickness funds responsible for financing health care, supported by special payroll deductions.

As of November 2002, the fourth component has been repealed, and financial responsibility for health care returned to the central government. The road to repeal was fraught with difficulties, some of which related to the structure of the sickness funds, and some of which related to the plan of funding them with special payroll deductions. The remaining three components remain in place, but the "pluralistic ownership structure" is in jeopardy as the central government retrenches and reconsiders how to pay providers, and which providers to pay, for the delivery of a basic benefit package to all Polish citizens. The government has not been able to afford to keep its promises.

DETAILS

Between June 1999 and July 2000, public support for the reforms plummeted. By July 2000, only 9 percent of those responding to an opinion poll felt that the health care system functioned better after the reforms than before, while 68 percent felt that system performance had deteriorated (Bobinski, 2000). As many as 20 percent of people surveyed ended up going to private doctors and paying for the visit out-of-pocket because they could not get access to treatment that was publicly funded. Specialty care, in particular, required very long waits if a patient wanted to be covered by the public insurance fund. Many others simply coped with health problems without getting treatment, because they could not afford to pay privately and could not get access to publicly covered benefits.

Part of the problem lay in the fact that health care spending was funded at only 3.8 percent of the GDP in 1999 and 2000, leaving the system without enough resources to provide the level of benefits promised by the state. Contributing to the underfunding problem was a breakdown in the social security service (ZUS) that was responsible for gathering individual premiums and forwarding them to the sickness funds. Due to chronic underfunding, the sickness funds and the providers ended up incurring substantial debts, which the federal budget was expected to pick up.

In addition, the sickness funds were established with no infrastructure in place for setting prices and contracting for health services; many funds were overwhelmed and unable to implement their basic functions.

Parliamentary elections late in 2001 led to a change in governing party, from the "right-wing" AWS or Solidarity party that believed in market-based reforms to more "left-wing" parties that rejected the 1999 reforms. In particular, the new government passed legislation that will liquidate the sickness funds in January 2003 and redirect the funds for health care back under the control of the central government. Sickness funds were characterized in the media as "uncontrolled and accountable to no one. . . . Such a system could not function, especially since it was not isolated from its environment: the financial ambitions of the political-bureaucratic apparatus, the unfavorable attitude of the media, and the generally weak respect for the law" (Polish News Bulletin, 2002). The system of payroll deductions earmarked for health care was under debate as well, with the new government calling it unnecessarily costly, and critics complaining that the full amount of the payroll deduction never reached the sickness funds because intermediate parties kept taking their cut.

With the repeal of the sickness funds, the privately owned clinics are concerned that the government will not renew their contracts. The fear was articulated by the president of a private Warsaw clinic, Centrum Medyczne: "I assume that if local government has to support large unprofitable hospitals then it will be difficult for a private medical center to sell its services without links to local government" (Goodale, 2002). The head of the Association of Healthcare Employers commented that "it would be difficult for local governments to afford private medical services as pressure to support their own facilities, many of which are badly run and outmoded, would drain their budget allocations" (Goodale, 2002).

Meanwhile the original plan to introduce private health insurance into the health care market in Poland has been put on hold indefinitely, thereby eliminating what many policymakers had hoped would be a mechanism to bring new funding into a grossly underfunded system.

SUMMARY

The Polish market reforms of the late 1990s are currently in free fall, and it is not clear what will survive with the new financing scheme. However, the process and public reaction to the reforms illustrate the difficulties faced by former communist states, as articulated by Elias Mossialos of the London School of Economics in his presentation at the Polish symposium where the Krakow case was first discussed in the summer of 1999:

- Public policy is viewed with suspicion, with citizens convinced that some individuals will use it for enrichment and to favor some people at the expense of others.

- The attitudes, skills, and knowledge are not yet in place to adopt Western styles of power-sharing and democracy. In particular, people have a problem with accepting individual responsibility because of a widespread belief in "negative egalitarianism" (if I gain, someone else loses, so I should not gain), and that all actions are either good or evil, which does not allow compromise.

References

Bobinski, C. "The Switch to Private Primary Healthcare Has Been Met with Mixed Responses and Has Raised Thorny Issues About Who Should Foot the Bill for the Nation's Health." *Financial Times,* Apr. 17, 2000.

Campbell, P., Chawla, M., Klich, J., Bylanowska, B., Kautsch, M., and Kulis, M. "Enhancing Managerial Autonomy in Polish Health Facilities." Unpublished paper, Feb. 9, 1999.

Chawla, M., Tomasik, T., Kulis, M., and Windak, A. "Economics of a Family Practice in Krakow." Unpublished paper of the Harvard-Jagiellonian Consortium for Health, supported by USAID, Cooperative Agreement #: DPE-5991-1-00-1052-00, July 1997.

European Observatory on Health Systems. "Health Care Systems in Transition: Poland," 1999. Available online: http://www.who.dk/observatory/Hits/20020524_22 (access date: April 7, 2003).

Goodale, G. "National Healthcare Plan Worries Insurers." *Financial Times Information,* Feb. 11, 2002.

Finn, P. "Polish Health Professionals Balk at Reform." *Washington Post,* Feb. 8, 1999, pp. A11–A12.

Lawthers, A. G., and Rosanski, B. S. "Quality of Outpatient Services: Krakow Gmina." Unpublished paper of the Harvard-Jagiellonian Consortium for Health, supported by USAID, Cooperative Agreement #: DPE-5991-1-00-1052-00, May 1998.

Mossialos, E. "Health Policy in Eastern Europe, Past and Future." Presentation to conference titled "Health Care: A Global Perspective V," Wroclaw, Poland, Aug. 4, 1999.

Polish News Bulletin. "Poland Cannot Afford Hybrid Healthcare Systems." *Economic Issues,* Feb. 8, 2002, based on article by Pawel Szalamacha in Feb. 7, 2002, issue of *Rzeczpospolita,* p. A8.

CHAPTER SIX

Germany's Ode to Alain Enthoven

Is Managed Care New Wine in Old Bottles or a New Rhine Whine?

‐‐‐ "The people in the Jackson Hole Group never imagined conditions like this when they were designing their managed competition proposal," mutters Sabine Richard to herself as she ponders the somewhat daunting task before her. Richard's employer, the BKKs, the federal association of employer-based sickness funds in Germany, have decided to develop a new managed care plan in response to opportunities created by a national health reform law passed in 1992.

Although the BKKs are anxious to take advantage of the flexibility under the new law to experiment with managed care pilot programs, Richard knows it is going to be a challenge to design and successfully market a new managed care product. Serious competition among sickness funds is fairly new, and until recently most consumers have had little or no choice of sickness fund. Although the contribution for sickness fund coverage is split evenly between the employer and employee, most consumers are not cost-conscious, and Germans are

This case was originally written by the authors in 1996. Funding was provided by Astra USA.

long accustomed to comprehensive coverage with little or no cost-sharing. They are also legally entitled to free choice of provider. Enlisting provider support is also going to be a challenge. Although provider payment arrangements are highly regulated, German physicians enjoy a degree of clinical autonomy that has become virtually unknown to their U.S. counterparts. Strict financial and structural divisions separate the different sectors of the German health system, and German providers have little history of cooperation or coordination of care. In particular, they maintain a strict separation between ambulatory physicians, who are private contractors and practice mainly in solo or two-person offices, and hospital-based physicians, who are salaried employees of hospitals. In only limited circumstances can hospital physicians and ambulatory physicians encroach upon one another's turf. Physicians are highly organized and very powerful politically. Doctors are legally obligated to belong to a regional association of sickness fund doctors, which negotiates collectively with the sickness funds over payment. These associations, referred to as the KVs (for *Kassenärztliche Vereinigungen*), are widely regarded and referred to as a monopoly. The BKKs are legally required to develop their managed care pilot in conjunction with the local KVs. Although the BKKs are one of the larger categories of sickness funds in Germany, their total market share is only 12 percent of the German population, which limits their negotiating and bargaining power with providers.

But the most daunting obstacles facing the BKKs are the structural and legal limitations imposed on sickness funds interested in developing managed care pilots. Although the reform law relaxed certain provisions of the laws governing relationships between sickness funds and providers, significant constraints still apply:

- Participation in the pilots is voluntary for consumers and providers.
- Consumers in a managed care pilot have to continue to be permitted to have free choice of health care provider.
- Sickness funds can develop provider networks, but any physician must be given an opportunity to apply to participate, and contracting decisions have to be based on what are referred to as objective criteria. The BKKs have to continue to negotiate and contract with physicians through the KVs.

- Managed care plans must continue to cover the full range of comprehensive benefits mandated by law for all sickness fund members, although additional benefits can be offered.

- Consumers cannot be offered lower premiums or reduced cost-sharing (such as lower copayments) to enroll in a managed care plan or to use network providers.

- Sickness funds have to continue to pay ambulatory physicians on a fee-for-service basis, according to the same fee schedule that is used in the regular sickness fund coverage. The funds can, however, make additional payments to physicians for providing new services or participating in new activities (such as patient education or participation in quality improvement programs).

- Sickness funds negotiate budgets and payments separately with physicians and hospitals, within a system of national and regional global budgets. The managed care pilots will continue to operate within this framework. The ability of funds to redistribute money among the different health care sectors (such as ambulatory physicians, hospitals, and drugs) will continue to be very limited.

The data available to the BKKs to develop their pilot are also limited. Although the funds have detailed data on hospital and drug expenditures, because they pay providers directly for those services, the BKKs do not have access to data on utilization and costs for office-based physicians, who are paid by the KVs (which are in turn paid by the sickness funds). Although the funds are interested in working with the KVs to establish a more comprehensive and coordinated information system, at least for the pilot program serious nationwide concerns about protecting the confidentiality of patient information have led to strong resistance to permitting centralized organizations to create large comprehensive databases. Germany has recently adopted a new uniform ID card system for members of the statutory sickness system, which has the capability of containing encoded patient data on member ID cards. However, the card as adopted has only limited patient information and no clinical data, because of public concerns about confidentiality. Physician organizations have also been able to exploit the public's fear about privacy to resist providing their associations or the sickness funds with more detailed information on their practices.

Richard knows that any project the BKKs undertake will attract national attention and, with such a high profile, it is critical that it succeeds. The BKKs strongly supported the move to more competition among sickness funds as a means of containing rising costs. Perhaps more important, the BKKs believe that introducing managed care elements has the potential to help improve the quality of care received by members of the sickness funds. But not everyone is so supportive or optimistic. The BKKs know that the results of the project will be scrutinized particularly carefully by the Federal Ministry of Health, the agency responsible for all health-related issues in Germany, including overseeing the statutory health insurance system of which the sickness funds are a part. It is no secret that some Ministry officials are quite wary of the move to promote greater competition among sickness funds, and especially skeptical about the value managed care can bring to the German system. In the words of one Ministry official:

> It is not clear what managed care means for Germany. It sounded nice when it was first proposed: the flair of "efficiency" and "market orientation." But managed care is just old wine in new bottles; the German system already has all of the elements of managed care. I often ask myself, "Why are we doing this?" Germany has been rather successful at controlling costs. Competition among insurers and managed care will be counterproductive; the sickness funds will just play off against each other and skim. . . . Managed care has not worked in the United States. We do not want the U.S. system: all chaos and uncontrollable expenditures. That is the danger of managed care.

BACKGROUND

Germany has an enviable record of providing high-quality, comprehensive health care to all its citizens at costs far below those in the United States. During the 1980s and early 1990s, Germany controlled its health care costs more successfully than any other industrialized country; health expenditures grew at almost the same rate as the growth in national income. However, despite the successes of the German system, which has relied on regulation and global budgets, costs have increased steadily in recent years.

The health care system in Germany is part of a larger set of social structures designed to ensure the economic protection and social welfare of German citizens. The social support system is based on the principle of "solidarity": the belief that all members of the society have a responsibility to provide for each other to guarantee an adequate level of welfare for everyone. In the health realm, this principle is manifested in an emphasis on providing equal access to comprehensive care to all citizens.

However, tension and concern about the rising cost of the social budget, which includes costs of health care, unemployment benefits, and pensions, are growing in Germany. The share of GDP going to social spending has risen significantly in recent years, from 29 percent in 1989 to 33 percent in 1994. A number of socioeconomic, demographic, and political factors are behind this increase, including relatively high levels of unemployment; a rapidly aging population, which is shrinking the ratio of workers to retirees; the 1990 reunification of East and West Germany; and the changed markets that have resulted from the end of the cold war, increasing European integration, and market globalization.

Combining the health care systems of East Germany and West Germany proved a major challenge. In the former East, referred to now as the new *Länder,* both the financing and provision of health services were the responsibility of the federal government, and physicians were salaried employees of the state. Since reunification, a network of sickness funds oversees health services in the new *Länder,* and physicians are paid largely on a fee-for-service basis. One of the ironies about the development of managed care in Germany now is that the former East Germany had an extensive network of multi-specialty group practices or "polyclinics" that could have served as a base for staff model–type HMOs but were closed after unification at the demand of physicians' associations in the West.

The average hourly wage rate in Germany is among the highest in the world, as are average total labor costs. Employers have been among the major advocates of reforms to the health and social security system. According to a 1994 report of the Confederation of German Employers' Associations on "the welfare state at the crossroads": "Social security contributions and taxes have reached historically high levels which are no longer economically acceptable. . . . They will be driven even higher if energetic countermeasures are not taken." However, there is great concern in many quarters that any reforms not undermine the principles of solidarity.

THE HEALTH INSURANCE SYSTEM

The German health care system is a carefully designed structure in which each party has a distinct role. Although the system is largely decentralized, the federal government sets clear parameters in most areas, including membership rules, financing, benefits, and the organization and functions of the sickness funds. Operations are left to private players, including the sickness funds, physician associations, and other providers. The system operates by negotiation, consensus-building, and compromise, within formalized roles and rules.

Structure

Germany has a comprehensive statutory health insurance scheme that covers 90 percent of its 80 million citizens. Germans covered by the statutory system belong to one of approximately 960 sickness funds *(Krankenkassen)*, which act as intermediaries among employers, consumers, and providers. Membership in a sickness fund is mandatory for employees whose gross income is less than a threshold amount, which was $3,920 (DM 5,850) per month in 1995 in the former West Germany and $3,220 (DM 4,800) in the former East. The statutory system also covers farmers, students, apprentices, the unemployed, and most retirees. The self-employed and individuals who earn more than the threshold amount may remain in the sickness fund system, opt for private insurance coverage, or go uninsured. Approximately 10 percent of the population has private insurance. (Approximately 84 percent of those enrolled in the sickness funds have annual incomes below the threshold amount; the other individuals could opt out of the statutory system but have chosen not to do so.) An individual who opts out of the statutory health insurance system is never permitted to reenter it.

There are a number of different categories of sickness funds. Approximately 60 percent of the population is covered by so-called primary funds and 30 percent by the so-called substitute funds. Primary funds include local funds, called AOKs *(Allgemeine Ortskrankenkassen,* which are local or regional in scope and open to anyone), company funds (run by individual companies for their own employees), and craft funds (for members engaged in similar trades). Most states have only one AOK, but several regions have dozens of them, and Germany has eighty-four in all. All the AOKs belong to the Federal Association of the AOK, which acts on their behalf at the federal level. The company sickness funds number approximately 633, all members of the federal association known as the BKKs. An employer must have at least two thousand employees willing to join the funds before one can be established.

There are also special purpose funds, which cover miners and sailors, and agricultural funds, which cover farmers. The primary funds cater to both white- and blue-collar employees. The fourteen substitute funds are national in scope; seven are for white-collar workers and seven for blue-collar workers. However, 95 percent of substitute fund members are in the white-collar funds. (See Figure 6.1 for total membership by type of sickness fund.)

Sickness funds are self-governing quasi-public organizations authorized by law to negotiate with providers on behalf of their members. The boards of the local and employer sickness funds are composed of equal numbers of representatives of members and employers. The boards of the substitute funds are composed solely of members.

Until 1996, the choice of fund was limited for most individuals— only about 55 percent of Germans had a choice among two or more sickness funds. White-collar workers could choose a local fund, a substitute fund, or a company fund, if one was offered by their employer.

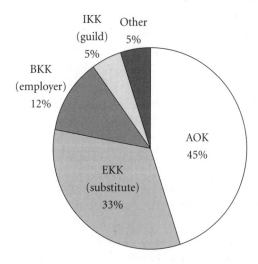

Figure 6.1.   Membership by Type of Sickness Fund (1995).
Source: Data from Schönback and Richard (1996), p. 189.
Note: Total population 80 million; sickness fund members, 72 million
(90 percent of population).

Most blue-collar workers had no choice of funds. A key provision of the 1992 reform law (discussed later in this chapter) was to permit individuals to select any sickness fund as of January 1, 1996, for enrollment beginning in 1997.

Benefits

Germans are permitted freedom of choice of provider. Sickness funds are required by law to provide standard benefits with little permissible variation. Although the funds can offer benefits above the federal requirements, few do. The required benefits are comprehensive, including unlimited hospital and ambulatory care. Sickness funds also provide cash benefits to workers on disability, maternity, or child sickness leave (see Table 6.1). Cost-sharing is minimal, with no copayments for any physician services. Patients are required to pay $7 (DM 11) per hospital day, up to a maximum of about $100 (DM 154) per year. Copayments for drugs vary by size of prescription, ranging from $2 to $4.70 (DM 3 to DM 7). Copayments cannot exceed 2 percent of income in any year, and many groups are exempt from copayments, including children, welfare recipients, unemployed persons, students, and others who meet financial hardship criteria.

The range and scope of benefits provided by the sickness funds have been the subject of considerable recent debate. Many employer groups and physicians have advocated changes to eliminate certain

Service	Payment (DM billion)	Percentage of Total
Hospital care	53.9	30
Physician services	28.9	16
Pharmaceuticals and dressings	27.1	15
Sickness benefits	12.3	7
Remedies and adjuvants	10.8	6
Dental treatment	10.2	6
Dentures	6.8	4
Pregnancy and maternity benefits	3.6	2
Sanatorium treatment	3.2	2
Intensive long-term care	2.3	1
Death benefits	1.3	1
Other services	7.8	4
Administrative expenses	8.7	5
Total	176.9	100

Table 6.1.   Sickness Fund Payments by Type of Service, Old *Länder* (1992).
Source: Federal Ministry of Health, 1994, p. 27, Figure 8.

"unnecessary" services (such as spa treatments) and to increase consumer cost-sharing. Many of the sickness funds have argued that greater discretion to offer different benefit structures would enhance competition and encourage consumers to be more cost-conscious. However, critics believe that it would be difficult to define what the minimum package of "necessary" benefits should be, and they fear that the principle of solidarity will be undermined if sickness funds have the ability to reduce benefit packages and tailor benefits (and contribution rates) more to individual risks.

Financing

The statutory sickness funds are financed through salary-based payroll deductions, split evenly between employee and employer. (Contributions for the unemployed, students, welfare recipients, and other nonemployed people are generally paid by public agencies.) The contribution rate is the same for all members of a fund regardless of age, sex, number of dependents, or other characteristics; it is a percentage applied to wages and salary up to a maximum annual income ceiling. Retirees generally remain members of the same fund they belonged to before retirement. The contribution rate for retirees is the same as for active employees, and the employer share is paid by the retiree's pension fund. These retiree contributions cover less than half of the actual costs of retirees. The balance is made up by a special contribution by employees and employers, with additional cross-subsidies by the federal government and retrospective adjustments to compensate for differences in the percentage of retirees covered by each fund and the cost of the retirees.

The sickness funds are fiscally independent and financed on a pay-as-you-go, self-supporting basis; they do not accumulate large reserves. Each of the substitute funds has a uniform national contribution rate for all members, regardless of the region where the member resides, while the local funds have regional contribution rates. While the uniform contribution rate for all members of a sickness fund is designed to result in cross-subsidies—females by males, lower income by higher income, older by younger, unemployed by employed—the contribution rate varies significantly across funds, based on the risk structure, age composition, percentage of families, and income of the fund's members, as well as the availability and use rates of medical resources in the fund's region. Growing concern about risk segmentation across sickness funds, and the resulting growth in the variation of contribution rates, was a major factor in the risk compensation scheme enacted as part of the 1992 reform law. For example, the local sickness funds, AOKs, have 40 percent of the population, but they have 50 percent of retirees and 90 percent of retirees from the new *Länder* (the former East Germany).

The sickness fund contribution rate is the major indicator that Germans use to track health care costs, and stabilizing this rate has been and continues to be a major goal of all major parties in the German system. Although the rate has increased steadily over the years, it has stabilized in the last two years. (See Figure 6.2.)

Private Health Insurance System

Approximately 10 percent of Germans have private health insurance. In addition, almost 8 percent of sickness fund members buy supplemental coverage for copayments and other noncovered services (such as private hospital rooms). The insurers in the private market are split evenly between nonprofit mutual companies and for-profit stock companies. The premiums and provider fee schedules of private insurers are regulated by law. In general, the fees paid to providers by private insurers are significantly higher than fees paid by the sickness funds. Premiums are based on age at time of purchase and family size, although premiums are derived from community rating rather than experience rating. Many insurers offer premium refunds to insureds who have no claims over a two- or three-year period. As a result of the differences in the rating structures used by private insurers and the sickness funds, private insurance appeals particularly to high-income individuals without children. However, as noted earlier, an individual who opts out of the statutory system loses the right to return to it.

THE DELIVERY SYSTEM

Historically, the separation between ambulatory and hospital-based physicians has been strict. Ambulatory doctors, who comprise approximately 45 percent of practicing physicians, are private practitioners who operate primarily in solo practice. Only 20 percent of ambulatory physicians practice in groups; 60 percent of ambulatory physicians are specialists, and 40 percent are primary care doctors. Physician offices are generally equipped with a wide range of expensive high-tech

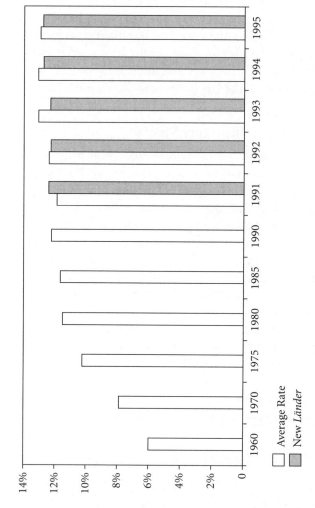

Figure 6.2. Average Sickness Fund Contribution Rate, Percent of Payroll.

Source: Federal Ministry of Health, 1994, p. 31, Figure 9, and unpublished data provided to authors by Ministry of Health officials during interviews.

Note: Contribution rates and ceilings have been different in the former East Germany since reunification, but will be the same by 1997.

equipment, including ultrasound machines. Hospital-based physicians, who comprise approximately 55 percent of practicing physicians, are salaried employees of the hospitals. Physicians are permitted to be employed only by hospitals or other physicians, and doctors are prohibited from forming group practices unless they are all in the same specialty.

Until recently, ambulatory doctors were not permitted to treat patients in the hospital (with a few exceptions), and hospital physicians could not treat patients outside the hospital setting. This separation, which was supported by the physicians, essentially eliminates competition between hospital and ambulatory physicians, and has resulted in serious problems of coordination and quality, including lack of communication among physicians and widespread duplication of tests by hospital doctors. As a result of this separation, day surgery is rare in Germany; only 5–10 percent of surgical procedures are performed on an outpatient basis. These restrictions were relaxed somewhat in the 1992 reform law, which permits office-based doctors to perform certain types of day surgery on their premises and to visit hospitalized patients at the end of their stays, and allows hospital physicians to provide outpatient care, including preadmission testing, prior to hospitalization.

Payment of Ambulatory Physicians

Every doctor who treats sickness fund patients must join the regional physicians' association, or KV. This membership conveys the legal right to treat and bill for sickness fund patients. Sickness funds may not contract selectively with physicians and must contract with any doctor who belongs to the regional KV, creating a monopoly by the KVs in the provision of care. In addition to the KV, physicians must also join the medical chamber, which licenses physicians and establishes education and quality standards. Most doctors also belong to specialty associations and professional political organizations.

Ambulatory physicians are paid on a fee-for-service basis, with the amount of the payment determined by negotiations between the sickness funds and the KVs. To establish payment levels, a relative value scale is first negotiated between representatives of the seven national sickness fund associations and the national physicians' association. All sickness funds use the same relative value scale, but the payment conversion factor or multiplier varies among geographic regions and among funds. The substitute funds have historically paid physicians more than other funds, in an attempt to increase fund membership by claiming that higher payments are associated with higher quality of care. There is also a negotiation in each region between the regional KV and the primary funds to determine a regional budget for physician services. The regional budget for physician services cannot rise by more than the average increase in wages for all sickness fund insureds.

Sickness funds pay most of the budgeted amount for physician services to the KV, which processes claims and pays the physicians. The KVs have flexibility to distribute payments to physicians according to their own methodologies. However, physician payments must stay within budget limits, so the actual fee level depends on overall physician utilization rates. There is an explicit trade-off between volume of services and unit payments. If the number of services provided by all physicians exceeds projections, the monetary conversion factor is reduced for all physicians, to keep total payments within a global cap.

The KVs also do some economic monitoring of physician practice patterns, including reviewing the hospital referral and drug use practices of a sample of physicians. Physicians whose practice patterns differ markedly from established norms are required to meet with a committee of other doctors. The general view seems to be that this process results in few denials of payment.

Doctors have always comprised a powerful, organized, and highly respected profession in Germany. However, there is considerable unrest and growing discontent among German doctors. This change has a number of causes, including a serious surfeit of physicians. Germany currently has the highest ratio of physicians per capita of any industrialized country (3.1 per 1,000 population, compared to 2.3 in the United States). The German constitution guarantees all qualified students the opportunity for a state-subsidized education to pursue the occupation of their choice if they pass the necessary examinations. However, the government has begun to take a series of steps, including limiting the size of medical school classes, imposing retirement age limits on doctors, and restricting the licensing of new physicians in regions that have excess capacity. Sixty percent of regions are closed to new ambulatory doctors. One physician representative estimates that almost 9 percent of physicians in the old *Länder* are unemployed, as are 17 percent of physicians in the new *Länder*. As part of the 1992 reform law, sickness funds and physicians must jointly determine the need for additional physicians in an area before new physicians are allowed to practice there. When this new law was passed, the number of ambulatory physicians increased by almost 10 percent as thousands of hospital-based physicians switched into office-based practice during the grace period before the new restrictions became effective.

The excess supply of physicians, combined with the global budgets for physician services, have resulted in a widespread perception, at least among physicians, that they are working harder and making less money. Although physicians are among the highest-paid professionals in Germany, their relative incomes compared to other workers have declined in the last decade. Physicians view themselves as being on a "hamster wheel" *(Hamsterrad)*, according to one physician representative. "A physician has to provide more and more services because if he does not, but other physicians do, his payments and income will go down." One physician agreed, "A physician who practices carefully and conservatively in Germany cannot survive financially anymore. . . . My income went down 20 percent last year even though I worked 40 percent harder." He added, "The competition among doctors is wasting so much money and resulting in poor quality. . . . Doctors are afraid to talk to each other or to send patients to each other because they think they will not get the patients back. So they send the patients to the hospital for tests and services that could be performed more cheaply in physicians' offices because they know that way they will get the patients back."

Hospitals

Germany's hospital sector is among the largest in the world relative to its population. The country has twice as many hospital beds per capita as the United States. Admission rates are high and lengths of stay are very long. (Average length of stay in 1994 was 12.7 days.) As a result, occupancy is higher than in most other countries. However, hospital costs are relatively low compared to other countries, the result of less intensive case mix and less intensive care. The division between the ambulatory and hospital sectors results in the hospitalization of many patients who could be treated as outpatients. In addition, Germany has few nursing home beds, and sickness funds do not pay for long-term care, so many individuals are hospitalized for social rather than medical reasons. Most hospitals are publicly owned or nonprofit community institutions. Hospitals have dual sources of revenue: they negotiate with sickness funds over payment for operating expenses and receive payments from the government for capital expenses.

Until recently, hospitals were paid on a per diem basis. Each hospital negotiated a budget with the regional association of sickness funds, which resulted in an all-inclusive per diem that was paid by the funds for each day of care. Some services, such as ICU, often had separate per diem rates, and some expensive procedures were paid on a fixed case or DRG-type basis. The per diems were uniform for all patients of a given hospital. Although sickness funds are permitted to cancel or refuse to renew contracts with hospitals that demonstrate chronic inefficiency and waste, few sickness funds have attempted to do so. Hospitals had a legal right to receive rates that enabled them to cover all operating costs. The system essentially operated as a cost-based payment system.

Not surprisingly, this per diem cost-based payment system and lack of coordination between office-based and hospital physicians contributed to rising hospital costs. In addition, although patients are theoretically required to consult an office-based doctor before seeking hospital care except in an emergency, as many as 40 percent of non-emergency hospital admissions are patients who come directly to the hospital. In an attempt to control rising costs, as part of the 1992 reform law increases in hospital budgets for 1993–1995 were limited to the rate of increase in the wages and salaries of sickness fund members (with some allowances for additional spending in certain categories of cost). Beginning in 1996, hospitals moved to a DRG-type payment for a substantial percentage of all hospital services.

Drugs

Some of Germany's most aggressive cost containment actions have been taken in the area of prescription drugs, where utilization rates and costs have historically been very high. For instance, the number of prescriptions per capita is three times as high as in the United States. Twenty percent of sickness fund expenditures are for drugs, approximately two to two and a half times the percentage spent in the United States. High use and costs are attributed to a number of factors, including high prices, the surplus of physicians, and insensitivity to costs by both physicians and patients because of comprehensive coverage with minimal cost-sharing.

Drugs in Germany can only be dispensed by free-standing pharmacies. There are no drug chains because pharmacists cannot legally own more than one store. Physicians have the freedom to decide what drugs to prescribe and to provide needed care, with little or no coordination or communication between physicians and pharmacies. Pharmacists are not permitted to make drug substitutions. Drug prices are the same at pharmacies across the country. Mail order pharmacy is illegal.

Germany has enacted a range of cost-containment measures in recent years, including reference pricing (or maximum allowable reimbursement levels for the sickness funds), the adoption of a "negative list" of therapeutically questionable drugs, consumer copayments, and global drug budgets. As part of the 1992 reform law, physicians are held collectively liable for spending in excess of the drug budget negotiated by the KVs and the sickness funds, up to certain limits (approximately 1–2 percent above the budget). Individual physicians can also be penalized financially if their prescribing patterns fall significantly outside established norms. (Although the number of prescriptions fell dramatically as a result of this change, it appears that actual savings were minimal because of a significant increase in the use of drugs dispensed by hospital-based pharmacies, which are not included in the physician drug budget.) The KVs and sickness funds are also working to develop therapeutic recommendations and other types of quality management and outcomes-oriented guidelines for drug use. Despite much debate about implementing a national drug formulary, this action has not been taken.

INCREASED COMPETITION AMONG SICKNESS FUNDS

In 1992, Germany adopted a policy of promoting increased competition among sickness funds, including experimentation with "managed care elements," as a means of containing costs and improving quality of care. This policy has been somewhat controversial, with a concern about the extent to which market-driven incentives and structures can be put in place without endangering the principles of solidarity and equal access to medical care. However, so far German policymakers appear to be viewing increased competition and the introduction of managed care as tools to be used within a system that remains deeply committed to universal coverage, equal access to care, and a continuing strong role for governmental planning and regulation.

THE 1992 REFORM LAW

Over the past fifteen to twenty years, Germany enacted numerous reforms intended to contain the growth of health care costs and stabilize sickness fund contribution rates. Although these reforms were generally somewhat successful, the average contribution rate for the statutory system continued to increase. In 1992 Germany enacted a reform law, *Gesundheitsstrukturgesetz* (GSG), or the Law on the Stabilization and Structural Reform of the Statutory Health Insurance System. This law went into effect on January 1, 1993. Besides the cost containment measures described in the preceding sections, the GSG introduced a number of far-reaching structural changes into the statutory insurance system that are designed to move the system toward more competition and to permit experimentation with managed care.

The move toward competition comprises three major elements: a risk compensation scheme designed to reduce differences in sickness fund contribution rates caused by differences in the risk of members, expanded choice of sickness funds for most members of the statutory system, and the creation of pilot managed care programs.

Risk Compensation Scheme

The implementation of a risk adjustment mechanism was viewed as a necessary precondition to increased competition among the sickness funds. In recent years, the disparity between the lowest and highest sickness fund contribution rates has been growing, with an especially wide gap between the local and substitute funds. It was generally acknowledged that this disparity was, in large part, the result of risk selection caused by a number of factors, including a shift in the German labor force toward more white-collar workers, who have a greater choice of sickness funds; higher rates of unemployment and hence a lower income base, especially among the largely blue-collar membership of the local and craft funds; and efforts by the substitute and company funds to attract and retain lower-risk members.

The goal of the risk compensation scheme (RCS) is to reduce risk segmentation, more equitably distribute health care costs among sickness funds, and promote competition among funds based on efficiency, quality, and service rather than selection of risk. The principle underlying the scheme is that no fund should be advantaged or disadvantaged financially because of the risk of its members, and that differences in the contribution rates of the funds should reflect differences in performance, not risk structure. Under the scheme, the financial strength and ability to pay of each fund is assessed, based on the total income of sickness fund members subject to the contribution rate. This amount is compared with an estimate of the fund's expected standardized expenses, based on its demographics and average national expenditures for each demographic group (that is, age, sex, disability status). Funds whose members are relatively younger, richer, or more likely to be male or single or less disabled contribute money to the compensation scheme. Funds whose members are relatively older, poorer, female, or more likely to be receiving disability pensions, or that have higher proportions of large families, receive compensation from the scheme.

Each sickness fund is still self-supporting and must set its contribution rate at a level adequate to cover its costs, taking into account expected payments to or from the RCS. Funds continue to have an incentive to keep their costs below the average for sickness funds, since the risk adjustment scheme is calculated based on average national standardized expenditures. Regional differences among funds will still persist because regional variations in costs are not taken into account in the formula. This works to the disadvantage of local funds, which have regional contribution rates, compared to substitute funds, which set their contribution rates on a national basis. The question of requiring residents of high-cost regions to bear those costs has roused considerable controversy, but the final structure of the RCS was explicitly designed to use differences in contribution rates as an incentive to reduce regional costs and overcapacity and to penalize regions with above-average consumption of medical resources.

The RCS calculations were done for the first time for active employees in 1994; retirees were added in 1995. There appears to be widespread agreement that the risk adjustment scheme has somewhat narrowed the gap in contribution rates among funds, although the amounts that were redistributed were relatively small (approximately 1.5–2 percent of sickness fund revenues in total). The local and craft funds were the big recipients from risk adjustment, while the substitute and employer sickness funds were net contributors.

Competition Among Sickness Funds

Beginning in 1996, Germans have increased freedom to choose among sickness funds. Individuals can register their intent to switch funds during 1996, with the change of funds to become effective at the beginning of 1997. The degree of competition and openness varies among the categories of sickness funds. The substitute and local funds must be open to all sickness fund members, although a local fund can restrict membership to individuals who live in the fund's region. Employer and craft funds can choose whether to have open membership; if they choose to be open, they are required to take any sickness fund member who wishes to join. The special purpose funds will not be open, and their members will have no choice of funds.

Prior to this change, approximately half of sickness fund members had a choice of sickness fund. It is estimated that more than 80 percent of sickness funds members now have a choice as a result of the reform law.

It is unclear how sickness fund members will respond to their expanded choice of sickness funds. Although many members have historically had a choice of fund, most observers believe the competition among sickness funds has been quite limited. According to one observer, "Most of the competition has been around risk selection, with funds offering health promotion and wellness programs as a way to compete . . . but a study by the Federal Ministry of Health showed that these programs were not really health promoting because they were used only by people who would have engaged in such behavior anyway." However, with uniform benefits, many funds plan to offer additional benefits, including health promotion and prevention programs, to attract new members. Funds are also beginning to focus more attention on improving service and quality of care. "Sickness fund employees have been like civil servants," according to one sickness fund manager. "They need to be trained to be courteous and to be given more discretion and not trained to automatically say no. . . . A fund could pay nine times out of ten, but the member will only remember the time you said no."

Research indicates that quality is one of the most important considerations for consumers, and that Germans are willing to pay more for health care rather than sacrifice quality of care. Many believe that the substitute funds will benefit from a belief among many Germans that they are higher-quality funds, a perception that grew out of the higher payments that the substitute funds historically made to physicians, which created an impression of better access and quality of care (although these impressions have no data to substantiate them). In addition, the substitute funds may benefit competitively from the "cachet of exclusivity," since they were previously open primarily to white-collar workers. However, the substitute funds have had to make significant contributions to the RCS, which has reduced their capacity to make higher payments to physicians. According to one physician representative: "Substitute funds will not be the darlings of the system anymore because of the risk compensation scheme. They will not have as much money to spend. . . . They will have to offer something other than higher payment to doctors to maintain their competitive position."

Although studies show that most Germans have little knowledge of actual contribution rates for statutory sickness insurance and are not highly sensitive to price differences among funds, many observers believe that with uniform benefits, the contribution rate will emerge as one of the most important factors in choice of fund. It is unclear whether lower contribution rates will be an inducement to join or taken as an indicator of possible poor quality of care.

Employers have been particularly supportive of the move to a more competitive system. According to one employer representative:

> Our goal is to first stabilize and then lower the employer's contribution rate. . . . We would like a private insurance system, but because of the U.S. experience, there are concerns that a totally private system would be too costly and the unions have been able to oppose it. . . . So we will have to have an evolution, not a revolution. Regulation has not worked very well, so deregulation and competition should be tried. . . . Individuals need to assume more responsibility. For instance, drugs are used too much because the drug copayment is too low. And we should pay only for medically needed and essential services. . . . For example, eyeglasses are not a necessary service because people will still get them if there is no coverage. Employers should not have to pay for extras, for employee preferences, but only for 50 percent of the cost of medically needed services. . . . Competition and managed care may not work. . . . It's always a question of hopes and beliefs and whomever has the better argument will get a try. But we have seen that competition works in other parts of the economy.

But many policymakers and providers are cautious about moves to promote competition among funds. They worry that competition will increase administrative costs, which are now very low, approximately 5 percent of sickness fund revenues, and much lower than the 12–13 percent administrative cost ratio of private insurers in Germany.

(Administrative costs are less than 10 percent if the costs of the sickness funds and the regional provider associations are included.) Because of these concerns, the Federal Ministry of Health froze the administrative costs of sickness funds for 1993–1995.

Observers also express concern that the risk compensation scheme is not adequate to eliminate undesirable competition among funds, particularly cream skimming. Although funds must take all comers, many observers believe funds will engage in selective marketing practices, through sales methods or product design. For example, one pointed to criticism that the AOKs, the local funds, have used much of their payments from the risk compensation scheme for advertising rather than to reduce the contribution rate for members. Others worry that employers and other purchasers (such as the local welfare offices that pay for coverage of welfare recipients) will pressure sickness fund members to join the lowest-cost sickness funds, even though this type of behavior is not permissible under federal law. In particular, critics note that competition among insurers in the United States has not been shown to be effective either at reducing costs in the long run or at improving health. Even proponents of the competitive approach are quick to note that, in the words of one sickness fund manager, "We do not want to Americanize our system."

Managed Care Pilot Programs

The 1992 reform law allowed sickness funds to develop managed care pilot programs and implement them beginning in 1996. The interest in experimenting with managed care appears to have developed as much, if not more, out of concerns about quality than out of cost concerns. Among the quality concerns frequently mentioned by observers are the lack of communication and coordination between ambulatory and hospital-based physicians, unnecessary referrals to specialists, underuse of ambulatory surgery and mid-level practitioners, long hospital stays, excess high-tech capacity (particularly in physicians' offices), financial incentives for overprovision of physician services, the frequency of overprescribing and adverse drug interactions, and a historic lack of an organized focus on improving quality of care and health outcomes.

There seems to be widespread agreement that changing physician behavior should be a primary goal of the managed care pilots. In the words of one sickness fund representative,

We are stuck with fixed budgets for medical care, and more specifically for physician services. The goal has to be to get better quality for the same money. . . . At the moment, we do not reward the right things. Physicians are forced to do more of the things they are paid for and less of the things they aren't paid for. . . . We have set up a system that economically drives physicians to bad medicine and protects bad doctors. We need to get physicians off the treadmill and reward doctors for providing the best medicine they can within the resources available. . . . Now, performing more services is the only way doctors can stay even or increase their incomes.

Another observer gave a concrete example of how the current physician payment system adversely affects quality of care: "Seventy-five percent of pregnancies in Germany are categorized as 'high-risk' by physicians because that designation is necessary for the doctor to receive payment for office ultrasound. However, this is terrible quality, not only because there are many unnecessary ultrasounds but because it unnecessarily frightens so many patients."

Even physicians and their representatives agree that changes are needed: "The present cannot be allowed to be the future," said one. "Competition and managed care presents many risks as well as opportunities. But since we are limited on the income side, we must limit costs. We must change the structures because we will not get out of our financial problems. . . . We have to create incentives for physicians to stop competing, get into group practices, and to stop the medical arms race."

Managed care is often viewed as a means to improve quality of care. Many observers commented on a lack of attention to quality improvement or health outcomes in Germany. One sickness fund representative remarked:

Health measurement, health promotion, and disease prevention programs are not well developed in Germany. We have very limited research in health services, epidemiology, and health economics. The public does not talk about the deficits in quality in the current system, although there is growing suspicions about physician self-interest and perverse financial incentives. . . . The movement to seek alternative care, which is strong, is one sign of disaffection with the traditional system. I think there is lots of interest among consumers in more and better information but we don't have it.

A physician agreed: "Patient suspicions are making the system even more costly. . . . Patients are doubtful and so they go for other opinions and more tests. . . . There used to be an assumption of quality. Now that is not the case." He added wryly, "But I think the focus of all parties is changing for the better. For example, in the past the sickness funds hired economists and lawyers to work on health policy. Now they are beginning to hire physicians."

The development of managed care approaches has been advocated mainly by sickness funds and employers. "We want to combine medical decision making and financial responsibility as much as possible, to eliminate the organizational segregation of the different health sectors and establish a more integrated system of care and financing," said one sickness fund representative. Managed care is also seen by the sickness funds as a way to empower sickness funds and limit the power of physicians' associations. "One of the major goals of the sickness funds with managed care is to modify our contractual relationships with providers," noted a sickness fund employee. "We want to break the physician monopoly. If sickness funds will now compete, physicians have got to as well."

The move to managed care has been greeted more cautiously by some providers, who worry that it will impede their autonomy and power, and will also be an administrative burden. At least in part to deal with these concerns, Germany has adopted a cautious, incremental approach to managed care. Although sickness funds are frustrated about not being allowed greater flexibility in developing managed care pilots, particularly in the areas of benefit design, product pricing, and provider contracting, there seems to be widespread agreement that a pilot program approach makes sense. According to one employer, "We support managed care and competition, but we think model projects are a good approach. . . . We want an evolution not a revolution. . . . We should do this carefully and evaluate the results before we decide how useful managed care will be." A representative of the Ministry of Health described the federal government's approach to managed care: "We are experimenting with managed care for a limited time. We are cutting down some old trees to plant some new ones. . . . But there is no competitive or managed care strategy, just room for some managed care and competitive elements."

Although some observers worry that managed care will only exacerbate the undesirable aspects of competition, particularly risk selection, this does not seem to be a focus of the sickness funds.

According to one sickness fund spokesperson:

> Sickness funds should compete on efficiency, not benefits or risk selection. We want to make service provision more efficient, not cut costs by reducing benefits or offering benefits that would only attract better risk members. We cannot save money on healthy people. We need and want sick ones to enroll in the program so that we can manage their care. That is how we will improve quality and contain costs. In fact, we believe that there will be a windfall to other sickness funds from our managed care activities. If we change physician behavior and infrastructure it will also benefit other sickness funds.

Although some worry that competition and managed care will undermine the principle of solidarity, many others believe that managed care may be best way to preserve comprehensive, universal coverage. One managed care advocate said, "We need to contain costs without reducing quality, and, in fact, hopefully improving it. The liberals are old-fashioned and isolated. They have simplistic notions about competition. . . . They think the best way to cut costs is to cut benefits. . . . [Some professionals, including physicians and lawyers] want to keep their incomes high and continue to have clinical autonomy. . . . Their alternative solutions [to managed care] are to cut benefits, increase cost-sharing, and move to more of a private insurance model. . . . I think this undermines solidarity principles and would not improve quality." A union representative agreed: "We need to work to establish new interfaces between consumers and providers. Managed care is one way to do this. If we do nothing, if we do not participate in making positive changes, other regressive measures will be adopted, like cuts in benefits and increased cost-sharing."

Another physician summarized his hopes for managed care in discussing his reasons for wanting to participate in the managed care pilot designed by one of the sickness funds:

> I want to have more pleasure in my work and patients who are happy. German patients are not happy. People do not like being in the hospital when it is not necessary; they want to be home in their own beds. . . . Doctors don't speak to their patients; they keep them at a distance emotionally because if they come close it is too scary. It is much easier to give them a prescription. Physicians are afraid to take care of patients so they send them to the hospital to be safe. Doctors want to be king of their own patients. . . . Half of them are afraid to work with

other doctors because they are afraid their colleagues will see their mistakes. But I am not afraid, I can only learn more. It is not possible to know everything. We also need to change the mindset of German patients. People do not always need to go to doctors. They need to be trained early to take care of themselves, before they come to expect drugs or to be sent to the hospital. The sickness funds used to be seen by the doctors as the enemy, as the ones having all the money. But now there is one big pot and there is a lid on top; there is no more money. The only way to save money is to come together and work toward the same end. . . . It cannot go on this way. There is so much money to be saved, if there are supports for doctors. We must do it."

THE BKKS' MANAGED CARE PROPOSAL: *PRAXISNETZ*

The BKKs selected Berlin as the site for their managed care pilot program. Berlin, a city of 3.5 million people, has a number of attractive characteristics, including high medical costs (particularly for hospital services as a result of the city's eighty hospitals and three medical schools) and, perhaps more important, a local KV that is willing to work with the BKKs to develop the program. Although the BKKs' share of the Berlin population is only 10 percent, they believe the city offers considerable opportunity to use elements of managed care to contain costs and improve quality of care for their members, despite the significant program design constraints they face under the 1992 reform law.

Working with the Berlin KV, the BKKs have developed a new managed care program called *Praxisnetz,* or Practice Network. The program has three major goals:

- To develop a new basis for coordination and cooperation among physicians
- To eliminate the adverse financial incentives and effects resulting from the current structure of separate budgets for ambulatory services, hospital care, and prescription drugs
- To improve quality of care

The program will attempt to achieve these goals by reconfiguring the structure and financial system in which ambulatory physicians operate. The delivery system will be altered by creating a network of ambulatory physicians in certain regions of Berlin to provide care to members of the BKKs who choose to participate in the program. The members of any company-based sickness fund in Berlin will be eligible to join *Praxisnetz* or to remain in the BKKs' traditional plans. A member who selects *Praxisnetz* will be required to remain in the program for at least three months. Although members will be strongly encouraged to use *Praxisnetz* providers, the BKKs cannot legally prohibit members from going out of the network for any service. The benefits covered by the program will be the same as in the BKKs' traditional plans.

Physicians are required to apply to participate in the program by responding to an "invitation to tender," or RFP, developed and issued by the BKK and KV. To be eligible for the network, physicians have to meet a number of objective criteria:

- Have a practice with a minimum concentration of members of the BKK (that is, at least 12 percent of the physician's patients must be members of the BKK)
- Have the capability to submit claims electronically
- Be willing to participate in a variety of new utilization review and quality management programs
- Agree to have longer office hours for *Praxisnetz* members
- Meet various credentialing standards, including requirements regarding postgraduate education and experience with quality improvement activities

Praxisnetz providers must also agree to belong to the network for at least two years.

Based on an analysis of physician practices in Berlin, the BKKs believe that approximately six hundred ambulatory physicians have a large enough percentage of BKK members to be eligible for the network, and they estimate that half of these doctors have the required information systems capability. The BKKs hope to enlist two hundred physicians in the program.

Praxisnetz is designed to change financial incentives for physicians by creating a prospective "global communicating budget" for the program, which will operate within Germany's overall structure of separate global budgets for ambulatory physician, hospital, and drug services. The budget will be based on the standard expenditure profiles from the German risk compensation scheme, adjusted for costs in Berlin and the age and sex composition of *Praxisnetz*'s enrollment. This budget will be designed to cover all physician, hospital, and drug services, with the exception of care for certain catastrophic conditions (for example, AIDS, kidney failure requiring hemodialysis, hemophilia). Ninety-seven percent of this budget will be allocated to the physicians, and 3 percent will be allocated to the BKKs for the costs of administering the program.

The budget does not change the overall systems for paying ambulatory physicians or hospitals, although physicians will receive additional payments for providing care during evening hours and for certain utilization management and care coordination activities. However, the budget will provide the financial structure for attempting to change practice patterns and for evaluating the performance of *Praxisnetz* physicians. Every three months, there will be a comparison of actual and budgeted expenditures. The upside financial potential for the physicians and the BKKs is that network doctors and the BKKs collectively will each receive one-third of any budget surplus (the amount by which actual costs for *Praxisnetz* members are lower than the budget); the other one-third will be used to improve the network (for example, paying for new health promotion services, making investments in the development of quality improvement programs). Although physicians are not at direct financial risk for budget overruns, any program deficits will be carried over into the budget for the next period. Because of data limitations, the initial budgets include only hospital and physician services; budgets for drugs and devices will be added to the program as soon as reliable data are available. The BKKs have instituted a variety of mechanisms to ensure that the financial results of the program can be monitored carefully on an ongoing basis in order to give timely information to *Praxisnetz* physicians and to detect any serious budget trouble.

Perhaps the most important components of *Praxisnetz* are a variety of new utilization management and quality improvement programs. Participating physicians must agree to communicate with one another and with hospital-based physicians about *Praxisnetz* members. (Since the BKKs are not permitted to contract with hospital-based physicians, they cannot include hospital-based doctors in the *Praxisnetz* program. However, the program will attempt to influence both hospitals and hospital-based physicians indirectly.) *Praxisnetz* physicians will also be required to take part in a range of new activities, including a mandatory second surgical opinion program for selected procedures, periodic case conferences, quality circles, and adherence to clinical protocols and a drug formulary. In the future, the BKKs also intend to develop provider networks for certain targeted specialty services, including diabetes and mental health. *Praxisnetz* physicians will be encouraged to use these networks. All of the utilization management and quality management programs are being developed in close collaboration with the KV in Berlin. The BKKs are developing a variety of new information collection and reporting capabilities, so that they can monitor the program overall, as well as be able to provide detailed reports to individual *Praxisnetz* physicians on their utilization and cost performance.

Although the BKKs are excited about *Praxisnetz*, they are uncertain how consumers will receive the program. "We know from focus groups with consumers that the attractiveness of the program will depend, in part, on which doctors join," said a BKK staff member who has worked on designing *Praxisnetz*. "But we think that consumers should be attracted by the focus in the program on quality of care and service. We need to figure out how to market *Praxisnetz*," she mused.

—∿∿— Epilogue: The Fate of *Praxisnetz*

Sabine Richard, Ph.D.
Allgemeine Ortskrankenkassen
Berlin, Germany

In July 2001 the *Praxisnetz* contract between the BKK and the Berlin KV ended. The *Praxisnetz*—one of Germany's earliest and most notable managed care models—had failed.

What had happened?

THE PHYSICIANS

The *Praxisnetz* started with about two hundred physicians of different specialties all over Berlin in 1996. They were organized in eleven regional teams of varying size. In 1998, due to the entry of another sickness fund into the contract, the *Praxisnetz* was enlarged to ensure easy access to providers for a larger number of patients. The *Praxisnetz* included almost six hundred physicians in the end. The new physicians were selected by the regional teams to assure a complete supply in the city districts. The selection had to be approved by the joint council of sickness funds, physicians, and KV and became a regular item of the agenda of its meetings. The members of the council indulged in lengthy discussions on the overall strategy.

Whereas one side pleaded for a large expansion of the number of doctors to raise the group's attractiveness for as many patients as possible in terms of choice, the other side worried that the weak internal management structure of the *Praxisnetz* would be unable to successfully integrate a large number of new members.

The loose group of physicians never transformed into a managed organization based on principles and targets shared by everyone. Physicians simply didn't modify their behavior in terms of better cooperation between primary care physicians and specialists or adherence to the guidelines developed in the network. Even the spokespersons of the regional teams, who were important collaborators, did not agree on a development strategy. Moreover, active physicians complained about the large number of colleagues in the physician network who were ignoring their duties. The sickness funds and the spokespersons tried to strengthen the management structure. One first attempt was a procedure to exclude noncompliant members. The joint council agreed on a procedure that—as a result of legal objections of the KV—did not prove to be operational and led only to very few exclusions. Therefore, additional instruments to motivate the physicians were necessary to improve the cooperation in the network.

Early in 2000, spokespersons of the *Praxisnetz* and the sickness funds negotiated management targets for the physicians. Among the agreed targets were regular participation in team meetings, reduction of waiting time, reduction of the use of controversial prescription drugs, and more effective recruitment of patients to the *Praxisnetz*. The targets were to be signed by each physician in order to emphasize personal commitment to them. The target process made it entirely evident that a management structure had not evolved. Several of the spokespersons of the regional teams did not motivate their teams to sign the targets; in other teams the spokespersons could not convince their colleagues. Finally, the sickness funds proposed to end the contract.

THE MEMBERS

By the time *Praxisnetz* ended, enrollment had risen to about twenty-five thousand members of eighteen different sickness funds. From the beginning, the recruitment of patients to a managed care model entailing certain rules for the members proved to be one of the biggest challenges. The sickness funds had no experience to market managed care models and the patients were used to using the health system without being restricted to certain providers. The partners of the *Praxisnetz* emphasized the advantages of better cooperation and systematic quality management, and some sickness funds offered modest financial incentives (when these became legally permissible in the late 1990s). But apart from colorful marketing brochures and chip cards the *Praxisnetz* hardly materialized because the physicians did not alter their practice behavior, and so the patients did not see many differences compared to the care process outside the *Praxisnetz*.

Analyses by the sickness funds showed that *Praxisnetz* patients did not restrict their practice visits to the *Praxisnetz* physicians. Therefore, the physicians in the network complained that they were not able to control the entire process of care of the enrolled patients.

THE BUDGET

The financial framework distinguished the *Praxisnetz* in Berlin from other managed care models in Germany. The *Praxisnetz* received a capitation that covered the physicians' remuneration, the cost for hospital care, and prescription drugs. The capitation was risk-adjusted for age, sex, and disability status and reflected the high level of expenditures in the city of Berlin. Additionally, high risks were excluded from the budget: patients with yearly costs above a certain limit were shifted back into the financial responsibility of the sickness funds. The stop loss limit increased over the years with growing membership. When the first balance was presented, it became obvious that the budget mechanism was poorly understood by most of the physicians.

Budgets were calculated in 1998, 1999, and 2000. In 1998 and 2000, the *Praxisnetz* generated a surplus, whereas in 1999 a loss resulted. It was very difficult to analyze the budget results for critical factors of the *Praxisnetz*, considering the fact that the *Praxisnetz* had little impact on the decisions of the participating physicians. Analysis of the financial results for the different sickness funds participating in *Praxisnetz* showed no systematic patterns: for some sickness funds deficits were caused by the cost of prescription drugs, while for others the cause of deficits was hospital care. Some speculated that the results primarily reflected the activities of the sickness funds (such as case management), which included *Praxisnetz* members. There was no evidence of adverse risk selection.

THE ENVIRONMENT

During the operation of the *Praxisnetz* the legal framework was changed to facilitate the introduction of managed care models. The new law allows sickness funds to contract directly with groups of providers including physicians, challenging the central position of the KV. The government had hoped that the reform of the contract law would generate a rapid boom of managed care models in Germany. But the last year has shown that many obstacles still prevent selective contracts.

Although the monopoly position of the KV has been challenged, its influence is still considerable because the remuneration a sickness fund is willing to pay for the services of a network is to be deducted from the budget of the KV to avoid double payments. The KV has to agree to the deducted sum.

Physicians in private practice have not developed satisfactory organizational models to manage care processes beyond their premises. Moreover, no investors have volunteered to support the development of managed care entities. Although many physicians are dissatisfied with their current financial situation, they are not interested in participating in innovative forms of care. Many physicians are afraid to be closely monitored and to lose their clinical autonomy to the managers of the sickness funds. Therefore, sickness funds are rarely offered contracts with established groups of providers.

For the sickness funds, the operation of models like the *Praxisnetz* consumes a lot of time and resources without clear prospects for success.

References

Confederation of German Employers' Associations. *Social Provision in Germany: The Welfare State at the Crossroads.* (Trans. A. Jackson.) Cologne: Confederation of German Employers' Associations, Oct. 1994.

Federal Ministry of Health. *Health Care in Germany: The Health Care System in the Federal Republic of Germany.* Bonn: Bundesministerium für Gesund, Feb. 1994.

Schönbach, K. H., and Richard, S. "German Sickness Funds: Under Fixed Budgets." In F. W. Schwartz and others (eds.), *Fixing Health Budgets: Experience in Europe and North America.* New York: Wiley, 1996.

CHAPTER SEVEN

Disease Management at Harvard Pilgrim Health Care

If You Build It, Will They Come?

—⁓— "Itt's never easy to do disease management, but the challenges are even greater when you're talking about a loose, fragmented delivery system rather than a staff or group model HMO," observed one of the associate medical directors in the Massachusetts region of Harvard Pilgrim Health Care Inc. (referred to here as "Harvard Pilgrim" or "the Plan"). This associate medical director, and other staff in Harvard Pilgrim's corporate Office of the Medical Director, had some ambitious goals for disease management programs in the next year. Harvard Pilgrim had implemented several strong disease management programs in the staff and group model parts of its delivery system, as well as some more limited efforts in the network part of the Plan. Now they wanted to broaden these efforts in several ways, both by increasing access to the programs for members enrolled through the network part of its delivery system and by increasing the number of members with targeted diseases who participated in the programs. But they realized that the approaches that had been

This case was originally written by the authors in 1998. Funding was provided by Astra USA.

successful in the more tightly structured and integrated parts of the Harvard Pilgrim provider system would not work in the network part of the Plan.

BACKGROUND ON HARVARD PILGRIM HEALTH CARE

Harvard Pilgrim is a 1.3 million-member health plan based in Massachusetts and licensed in Maine, Massachusetts, New Hampshire, Rhode Island, and Vermont. (The Rhode Island, Vermont, and New Hampshire affiliates do business as Harvard Pilgrim Health Care of New England.) Harvard Pilgrim offers HMO, point-of-service, and preferred provider plans to more than eight thousand employers, and also serves the individual, Medicaid, and Medicare markets. It is widely regarded as a national leader among managed care plans, particularly in quality measurement and improvement. In 1997, the Plan received its second three-year full accreditation from the National Committee for Quality Assurance (NCQA). Harvard Pilgrim has been consistently ranked as one of the top plans in the country in a variety of national and regional reports.

Harvard Pilgrim is the largest HMO in Massachusetts. Its main competitors are Tufts Health Plan, HMO Blue (a subsidiary of Blue Cross Blue Shield of Massachusetts), and Fallon Community Health Plan. These four HMOs account for more than 85 percent of all HMO members in the state. Massachusetts is one of the most heavily penetrated states in terms of managed care, with more than 50 percent of the population enrolled in an HMO—almost 70 percent of insured people. Approximately one-quarter of Massachusetts Medicare beneficiaries are enrolled in HMOs. (See Table 7.1.)

Harvard Pilgrim was created by a merger of two of the state's largest HMOs, Harvard Community Health Plan and Pilgrim Health Care. Harvard Community Health Plan (HCHP), which began in 1969 as a staff model HMO, merged in 1988 with a large group model HMO, MultiGroup. In 1991, HCHP acquired Rhode Island Group Health Association, a staff model plan. Pilgrim Health Care, an IPA model HMO, was formed in the early 1980s, and grew rapidly, acquiring Family Health Plan, a direct contract HMO, in 1989. In a "merger of equals," HCHP and Pilgrim combined in 1994. In early 1998, Harvard Pilgrim affiliated with Neighborhood Health Plan, a 50,000-member Boston-based HMO owned by the community health

HMO	Total Members
Harvard Pilgrim Health Care	972,000
HMO Blue	699,000
Tufts Health Plan	441,000
Fallon Community Health Plan	178,000
Others (12 plans)	410,000
Total Massachusetts HMO Membership	2,700,000

Table 7.1.   HMO Membership in Massachusetts: Four
Largest HMOs as of Year-End 1996.

centers in Massachusetts and serving a primarily Medicaid popula-
tion. The Plan has also entered into a partnership with Baystate Health
Systems, the largest health delivery system in western Massachusetts.
As part of the partnership, Harvard Pilgrim assumed partial owner-
ship of Health New England, a regional managed care company.
Harvard Pilgrim also operates a number of other companies, includ-
ing Harvard Pilgrim Insurance Company and Harvard Pilgrim
Medical Practice Corporation. (See Figure 7.1 and Figure 7.2.)

Another significant change occurred in January 1998, when
Harvard Pilgrim's health center division, the original HCHP staff
model HMO, reorganized as a separate, nonprofit multi-specialty and
multi-site medical group called Harvard Vanguard Medical Associates. Harvard Vanguard, which is governed jointly by Harvard Pilgrim
and clinicians of Harvard Vanguard, has a contractual relationship
with Harvard Pilgrim to provide or arrange for comprehensive care
to Plan members who select primary care physicians at Harvard
Vanguard practices. (Harvard Pilgrim still owns the actual health center sites and leases them to Harvard Vanguard.) At present, Harvard
Pilgrim is the only HMO with which Harvard Vanguard contracts,
although the group provides care to patients with other types of health
coverage.

Harvard Pilgrim is structured as four regions:

• The Massachusetts Region, with approximately 725,000 members

• Harvard Vanguard, with approximately 300,000 members

• The Southern New England region (Rhode Island), with approximately 150,000 members

• The Northern New England region (Maine, New Hampshire
and Vermont), with 56,000 members

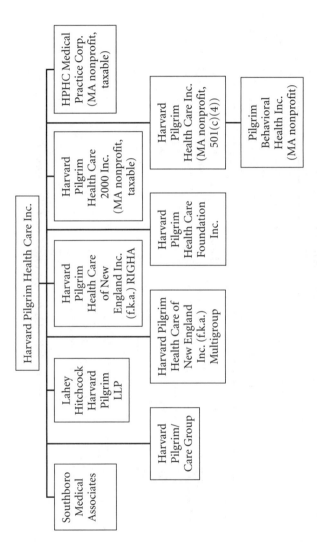

Figure 7.1. Organizational Chart (Nonprofit).

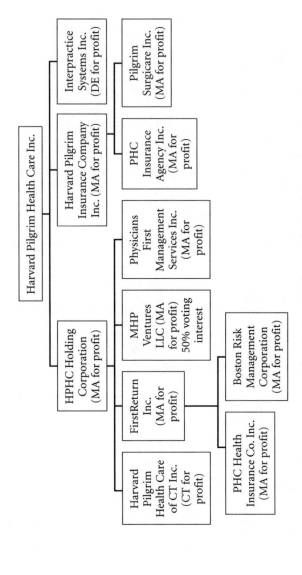

Figure 7.2. Organizational Chart (For-Profit).

Harvard Pilgrim's provider networks include more than 22,000 physicians and 140 hospitals. Physicians practice in many different settings, including multi-specialty group practices and health centers, small groups, community health centers, and individual practices.

HARVARD PILGRIM'S DELIVERY SYSTEM IN MASSACHUSETTS

Harvard Pilgrim members in Massachusetts are generally enrolled through one of four different types of physician delivery sites:

- *Harvard Vanguard,* which has fourteen different practice sites in the greater Boston region.
- *The Medical Groups* (which evolved from the former Multi-Group delivery system), with approximately 220,000 members. These eleven groups are tightly structured practices, mostly multi-specialty groups, which are closely aligned contractually and financially with Harvard Pilgrim. While Harvard Pilgrim is a dominant payer, the groups contract with other HMO and non-HMO payers as well.
- *Joint Ventures* (JVs), which have approximately 415,000 members. There are between seventy and eighty JVs, which can be structured as physician-only or physician-hospital organizations. Some JVs are highly structured, tightly integrated organizations, while others are individual doctors who have joined together for contracting purposes but have no other formal relationship or managed care infrastructure. Harvard Pilgrim membership per JV ranges from 1,000 to more than 13,000 members.
- *Pilgrim IPA (PIPA),* which includes the 7,000 physicians who contract with Harvard Pilgrim to serve 165,000 Harvard Pilgrim members with the Plan. PIPA is mainly a contracting entity; it has very little managed care infrastructure and provides few services to its member physicians. The physicians belonging to PIPA also contract with other HMO and non-HMO payers.

Harvard Pilgrim also has a fairly small number of members who are enrolled through primary care networks (PCNs). PCNs range in structure from primary care group practices to community health centers. Their financial relationship with Harvard Pilgrim varies, but generally involves a limited degree of financial risk, often only for primary care services.

The Medical Groups, JVs, and PIPA members located in Massachusetts collectively make up the Massachusetts Region of Harvard Pilgrim. (See Figure 7.3.) The term *network* refers to PIPA and the JVs.

Table 7.2 describes the predominant payment method used by Harvard Pilgrim for each of the four types of physician delivery sites.

DISEASE MANAGEMENT

Disease management (DM) is a term used to describe programs that provide a comprehensive longitudinal continuum of care and other interventions to help manage patients with (or at risk for) a specific chronic disease. The goal of disease management is to identify at-risk patients and coordinate and manage their care throughout the course of their disease. "The aim of DM is to look at all the barriers to care for a patient with a particular disease and figure out how to break them down," according to one Harvard Pilgrim clinician.

The DM approach differs from case management in that it goes beyond intensive management of a given patient who is already in the hospital with an acute exacerbation of a condition; it is designed to manage the condition across all settings of care, placing a heavy emphasis on prevention and maintenance. While DM programs focus on the care of individual patients, they also generally try to maintain a population-based, longitudinal perspective. "We want to provide a systematic approach to improving outcomes and quality of life by improving quality of care and coordination of resources for all patients with a targeted disease," the clinician reports. Identifying the population of patients at risk of developing a chronic condition or having an acute episode related to the chronic condition makes it possible to target prevention activities effectively.

DM programs have grown explosively in the last decade for several reasons. One factor has been the so-called 80/20 rule: 80 percent of health care costs tend to come from 20 percent of patients. "Given this fact, we should focus our attention on those 20 percent when we can, particularly for diseases where there is wide variation in how people with a particular disease are treated," said one medical director at Harvard Pilgrim. "Which," she added wryly, "is practically every one." The rise of "evidence-based medicine" has also fueled the growth

Planwide

Regional

**Model
Type**

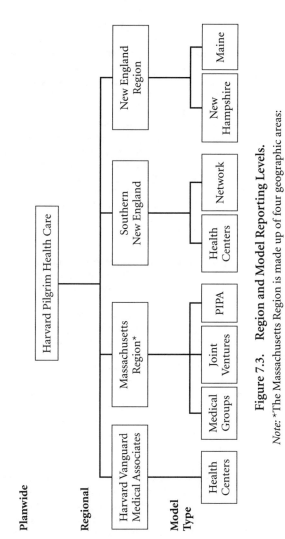

Figure 7.3. Region and Model Reporting Levels.

Note: *The Massachusetts Region is made up of four geographic areas:
Southern, Northeast, Central, and West.

Delivery System	Predominant Method of Physician Payment
Harvard Vanguard Medical Associates	Harvard Pilgrim pays HVMA on a global capitation basis, with a year-end settlement of budgeted versus actual costs. Most HVMA physicians are paid a salary. A portion of the salary, 10 percent, is withheld and at risk for performance against the budget. If performance is better than the budget, HVMA keeps the surplus above the amount withheld. If performance is worse than the budget, HVMA is at risk up to the full amount withheld. Any distribution of surplus is also dependent upon HVMA meeting certain clinical and customer service performance targets.
Medical Groups	The medical groups are paid on a per member per month or percentage of premium capitation basis, depending on the line of business (for example, the usual arrangement for Medicare risk members is percentage of premium). The range of capitated services varies somewhat from group to group, but generally includes substantially all covered services. Groups are also eligible for bonus payments if they meet certain clinical and administrative performance targets.
Joint Ventures	JVs are paid on percentage of premium capitation basis. The JVs are at risk for all services except mental health and substance abuse. JV providers are subject to a withhold of 10 percent for office-based services and 20 percent for hospital and obstetric services. There is a year-end settlement of actual JV performance compared to a budget. If actual performance is worse than the budget, the JV is at risk for the amount of the withhold. If actual performance is better than budget, the JV keeps any surplus up to the amount of the withhold, and any additional surplus is shared between Harvard Pilgrim and the JV according to a formula that varies by JV. JVs are also eligible for bonus payments if they meet certain clinical and performance targets.
Pilgrim Independent Practice Association	Physicians are compensated on a fee-for-service basis (based on a fee schedule), subject to a withholding of 20 percent of hospital-based services and 10 percent of office-based and obstetric services. The physician withhold is at risk for performance against a budget. If performance is worse than the budget, PIPA is at risk for up to the full withholding amount. If performance is better than budget, PIPA receives up to the full withholding amount. Any surplus beyond the withhold is retained by Harvard Pilgrim.

Table 7.2.   Physician Payment Methods.

of DM programs by emphasizing both how much of accepted clinical practice has never been shown to be effective in rigorous trials and how widely clinical practice varies. Another impetus for DM is the fact that a substantial number of hospital admissions in most plans involve patients with chronic disease being rehospitalized for emergency treatment of their conditions. "We started to figure out that these patients often wind up in the hospital because they are often treated only episodically and lack continuity of care," said one Harvard Pilgrim staffer. "The hope is that if we devote more resources to preventing admissions and readmissions instead of focusing only on reducing lengths of stay and increasing the use of step-down facilities, it will be a much more cost-effective approach, and one which will improve quality of care."

The increasing cost and prevalence of chronic diseases has also prompted the DM approach, as have the aging of the population and the booming market for Medicare HMO programs. "We can't change the demographics of our members," said one Harvard Pilgrim clinician, "so the best way to deal with the tide ahead is to try to keep more people from getting chronic diseases and to make treatment of chronic disease less expensive." Many observers point to the correlation between NCQA's requirement that managed care plans have outcomes data and the growth of disease management programs.

Both the focus and structure of DM programs vary widely. Among the most commonly targeted diseases are asthma, hypertension, AIDS, diabetes, congestive heart failure, and coronary artery disease. "The biggest bang for the buck comes from managing patients with conditions that are common, expensive, and treatable," said one staffer.

DM programs generally have a number of common elements:

- Patient identification, most commonly by referrals from physicians or from analysis of hospital admissions and ER visits
- Referral to the DM program, generally by the patient's physician
- Patient screening and assessment
- Active disease management, generally involving a variety of interventions—physician education, care management based on clinical guidelines, and patient education and support to improve compliance with care plans (particularly drug regimens and lifestyle changes)
- Outcomes measurement, including clinical outcomes and patient satisfaction

Harvard Pilgrim has been a leader among health plans in the development of disease management programs. One of its major DM initiatives has been targeted at asthma.

Asthma: The Disease and Its Care

Asthma affects more than 14 million people in the United States. Harvard Pilgrim estimates its planwide asthma prevalence at 4–5 percent, or approximately forty-five thousand members. During an acute episode of asthma, the muscles surrounding the airtubes (bronchial tubes) of the lungs go into spasm. (*Asthma* is the Greek word for panting.) However, asthma is actually a chronic condition that inflames the lining of the small airways of the lungs; the mucous lining swells, and secretions build up, reducing the overall air exchange capacity of the lung. Acute episodes are more likely to occur if the chronic inflammation is not controlled.

Asthma generally develops in childhood but can also begin later in life. Many children outgrow asthma as they get older but will still be at risk in adulthood. Many things can trigger acute episodes, including allergens such as house dust mites, cockroaches, pollen, mold, and animal dander. Other common triggers are exercise, cold air, pollution, cigarette smoke, colds or the flu, and analgesics (especially aspirin). Asthma cannot be cured, but most asthmatics can control their asthma by avoiding triggers and using medications to minimize the chronic inflammation. Many people with asthma have acute episodes only occasionally, but others struggle every day. Asthma that is not treated adequately can be disabling and even life threatening. Many acute episodes result in emergency room visits and even hospitalization.

Two types of medication are commonly prescribed for asthma:

- *Preventive anti-inflammatory medications:* These help reduce or prevent the chronic swelling of the bronchial tubes and subsequent secretion buildup. The two types of anti-inflammatory medication are steroid inhalers and nonsteroid inhalers. Recent research suggests that steroid inhalers provide the best long-term benefits without serious side effects.

- *Rescue medicines (bronchodilators and beta-agonists):* These are medications that open up the bronchial tubes when an asthmatic is having difficulty breathing or shortness of breath (an acute episode).

"In many ways, asthma is an easy disease to target for a disease management program," said one Harvard Pilgrim nurse. "There are care guidelines that are well accepted by physicians and well known, so you don't have to argue over standards of care. It just requires patient and provider education. But the hard part is that asthma is a disease of denial. Asthma attacks are episodic and people feel better quickly. Many people pretend that their attacks come from nowhere, but that's not the case—there are always warning signs. But patients often want to pretend that they don't have a chronic disease that needs to be managed. And often physicians do not want to label people as asthmatics because they are afraid it will have negative consequences at school or in the job market."

HARVARD PILGRIM'S ASTHMA MANAGEMENT PROGRAMS. Harvard Pilgrim is a national leader among managed care plans in asthma care. "There has been a lot of internal pressure from clinicians and external pressure from purchasers and organizations like NCQA and the state Medicaid program to focus on asthma," said a Plan employee. The Plan participates actively in a range of statewide and national asthma initiatives, including the NCQA group developing new measures for assessing health plan performance in asthma management. The Plan is also participating in a two-year AHCPR-funded project to study the cost effectiveness of a number of different asthma education interventions targeted at physicians.

Harvard Pilgrim's asthma management program (AMP) is nationally recognized. "Asthma is Harvard Pilgrim's most robust and well-developed disease management program," according to a Plan medical director. "We developed a model that clearly worked in the health centers, and there were best practices to share. There was clear buy-in from other parts of the delivery system that this was a priority. And we learned how to adapt the program from the health centers to other delivery models."

The first asthma management program was a pilot developed in the 1991 in one of the Harvard Vanguard centers, which was then in the staff model part of Harvard Community Health Plan. In 1992, based on the publication of national asthma management guidelines developed by the National Heart, Lung and Blood Institute, as well as the success of the earlier pilot, HCHP identified improving asthma care as a planwide priority. "We formed a multi-disciplinary task force to design the program," said one participant. "It took us a couple of years. The health center culture is very participatory and consensus-driven, so it's slow. But we do eventually get from here to there." An AMP was implemented in all the Harvard Vanguard centers in 1993. The Harvard Vanguard program has several goals:

• Improving the quality of life for asthmatics by increasing their control over acute episodes

• Increasing the use of anti-inflammatory medications, home peak flow meters, and written home treatment plans by moderate and severe asthmatics

• Improving ER and hospital utilization trends and reducing associated costs

• Improving patient satisfaction with care received for asthma

The AMP program uses clinical practice guidelines based on the National Heart Lung and Blood Institute guidelines (revised in 1997), which emphasize use of effective therapies and monitoring, along with an approach to asthma care based on disease severity. Patients are referred to the AMP either as a result of an ER visit or inpatient admission for asthma, or by their physician. The Harvard Vanguard program uses specialized asthma management nurses, who are assigned to particular health centers to do outreach, one-on-one patient education, and case management of severe asthmatics and high service utilizers. Each patient has an individual treatment plan that takes into account symptoms and respiratory parameters such as peak flow. Patients learn about triggers and how to monitor their own flows and use their inhalers or nebulizers. They learn what peak flow numbers should prompt a call to their physician or other intervention. A key component of the program is ongoing clinician education focusing on clinical guidelines implementation and effective techniques to coach patients in asthma management skills.

"The structure and culture of the health centers make it much easier in most ways to do disease management," observed one clinician. "The doctors are all in one place, so you can do centralized education, and the chiefs can require people to attend. The asthma nurses are on site, so they get to know the nurses and the case managers, and it becomes second nature to refer patients to the program. . . . And although the doctors have no financial incentive to be innovative, because they are salaried, there is peer pressure and a culture of excellence. All in all, it's easy in the health center to get people to do the right thing in terms of asthma care."

An AMP was implemented in Harvard Pilgrim's Medical Groups in 1993. The program shares most key components with the Harvard Vanguard program. According to one Harvard Pilgrim staffer, "The Medical Groups are enough like the health centers that we could implement a very similar program. There is strong medical leadership and a highly developed infrastructure. Although the practice culture is less consensus driven, the arrangement between the Plan and the groups puts the groups at financial risk for emergency room visits, so they want to avoid any unnecessary ER use."

The AMP at the Medical Groups uses asthma management nurses, either Harvard Pilgrim staff or practice nurses employed by the groups who have been trained by Harvard Pilgrim to do patient and clinician education. "One of our biggest problems was that the doctors in the groups have no time to do patient education but thought that if they didn't do it, no one else could," said a program designer. "But it's not cost-effective for physicians to do the education. So we focused on nurses as the key audience in the groups and trained the RNs and LPNs on the use of peak flow meters and spacers. Nurses are better at patient education anyway, and also better at taking the care plan and making it usable to the member." One difference between the AMP at Harvard Vanguard and the Medical Groups is that the latter added home visits as a program component in 1996. "Home visits are very useful," said one Harvard Pilgrim clinician. "They are convenient for the patient and a good way to provide support for the whole family. Plus they are the only reliable way to check the home environment for triggers and other important conditions."

By all accounts, the AMP has been very successful in Harvard Vanguard and the Medical Groups, resulting in significant improvements in processes of care and utilization, and substantial cost savings. The Plan assesses its results using claims-based data, as well as survey-based patient-reported information. The survey data show significant improvement in performance on a variety of measures, such as the percentage of asthmatics who have steroid inhalers, the percentage who have home peak flow meters and use them, and days lost from school or work (see Table 7.3).

The results of the program have been better in the pediatric population than among adults. "Asthma management elicits an emotional and passionate response from pediatricians," observed one Harvard

Measure	Pre-1996 Baseline	Adults Post-Program
Percentage of moderate and severe asthmatics with anti-inflammatory inhaler	69	78
Percentage of moderate and severe asthmatics with home peak flow meter	35	64
Percentage kept home from work or school one or more days in past four weeks	17	12
ER visits per thousand asthmatics per year	73	57
Hospital days per thousand asthmatics per year	138	106

Table 7.3.   Key Measures: Asthma Management Program, Harvard Pilgrim Health Care—Adult Population (All Pre/Post Comparisons, $p < 0.05$).
Note: Population includes Harvard Vanguard and Medical Groups.

Pilgrim clinician. "Asthma has a profound impact on kids and it's a more important cause of avoidable hospitalizations than for adults, so it gets the attention of the pediatric chiefs more than the chiefs in internal medicine, who treat lots of important diseases like chronic obstructive pulmonary disease, cancer, heart disease. The pediatric service is also smaller than internal medicine, so it's easier to change practice." It also helps that in addition to the AMP, Harvard Vanguard has a consultative service and referral center for severe pediatric asthmatics, as well as a special program for their families.

ASTHMA MANAGEMENT IN THE JVS AND PIPA. Harvard Pilgrim began developing an AMP for the JVs and PIPA in early 1996. Although Pilgrim Health Care had an asthma management program before its merger with HCHP, the program was very small. "The program was very hit or miss," according to one observer. "Physicians could refer patients with asthma to Pilgrim case managers. It helped those patients who were referred. But it was very reactive in relying exclusively on physician referrals to identify patients and never served many members."

It was clear from the outset that Harvard Pilgrim could not use the same approach to an AMP for the JVs and PIPA as had been used for Harvard Vanguard and the Medical Groups. However, the Plan believed that many of the core elements of its existing programs were transferable to the rest of the network. "The development model in disease management is shamelessly stealing from other programs that work," said one Harvard Pilgrim clinician. "In this case, we were lucky that we could steal from ourselves. We could use the same clinical practice guidelines, the same patient education material, and much of the same clinician education material. But the issues were how to engage clinicians and deliver the program to patients."

An AMP was implemented in the network in late 1996. The program has the same goals as the Harvard Vanguard and Medical Groups AMPs, and it has many common program elements, including reliance on referral of patients to the program by physicians or as the result of an ER visit or inpatient admission, and nurse managers who do patient and clinician education as well as case management of patients with severe asthma. As in the other sites, a key component of the program is to eliminate operational barriers to optimal care by providing equipment such as peak flow meters and spacers to physician offices, so that the equipment will be available to patients. "We have always covered the equipment as a benefit, but often members had to figure out how to get it," said a nurse. "When we actually put them in the supply cabinets at the doctors' offices, they are more likely to be used." Harvard Pilgrim also requires its contracting pharmacies to stock equipment so it will be easily accessible to members.

Harvard Pilgrim decided early on that home visits would be an important means of assessing and educating patients in the network. "The network is very diffuse and there are no real sites for patients to come to for classes or one-on-one sessions. We knew we would have to have a more flexible distribution system if we were going to get patients into the program," explained a program manager. As the program developed, Harvard Pilgrim decided to contract with a vendor to do home visits with asthmatic patients for whom this was deemed an appropriate intervention. The vendor employs respiratory therapists rather than nurses to do the home visits. The RTs receive didactic training from Harvard Pilgrim and then shadow Harvard Pilgrim clinicians until the Plan is comfortable that they are adequately trained in the AMP. "RTs know about asthma and are very experienced with the equipment and its proper use. Nurses generally do not have experience with asthma because it is not as much a hospital disease." After completing the home visit, the vendor sends a record to the primary care physician. The AMP then follows up with patients identified as in need of further case management. The vendor is paid on a per-visit basis.

In 1997, Harvard Pilgrim combined the AMPs in the Medical Groups and the network under one administrative structure. Although the components of each program are model-specific, the AMPs in the Medical Groups and network are under common management and have a common referral management system.

THE CHALLENGES AHEAD FOR ASTHMA MANAGEMENT. All Harvard Pilgrim members in Massachusetts now have access to an AMP, including case management, regardless of their primary care delivery site. But although access is theoretically universal, Harvard Pilgrim staff want to increase penetration of the programs (that is, the percentage of all asthmatics who have received care from an AMP), particularly in the network (JVs and PIPA) part of the Plan. "We are just beginning to develop a methodology to measure penetration," said one staffer. "Each region needs to figure out how it will determine how many members with asthma have participated in the program. But even though we do not have the data, we know that penetration is much higher in Harvard Vanguard and the Medical Groups than it is in the network."

Among the issues that must be addressed to increase access are identifying and stratifying patients at risk, increasing referrals, and increasing physician buy-in to the program.

Population Identification. The Plan's approach to patient identification and stratification is evolving. For purposes of determining the number of asthmatics in Harvard Pilgrim and for measuring program results, the Plan defines as an asthmatic any member who has had two outpatient visits or one ER visit or one hospital admission (the "2:1:1 algorithm") with a primary diagnosis of asthma in the last two years (along with related codes with a secondary diagnosis of asthma).

It is difficult to get accurate and timely data because of the Plan's multiple systems. "We have sixteen different claims information systems," said one Plan analyst. "Disease management requires comprehensive information, but the Plan has to struggle with data from a variety of nonintegrated systems—medical claims, encounter information, lab and pharmacy claims, health risk assessments, and other patient-reported outcomes. . . . Plus if members change delivery sites, until recently we gave them a brand new ID number, so we can't necessarily follow patients longitudinally."

Getting timely information is also a problem because of the lag in the availability of outpatient data for the Medical Groups and the network. "In Harvard Vanguard we have every outpatient visit in the system within forty-eight hours. It takes three to four months to get complete claims data from the network." Another problem is inaccurate diagnostic coding. For example, a recent study by NCQA found that using claims data to identify asthmatics resulted in many false positives on the East Coast compared to other parts of the country, because many cases coded as asthma turn out to be something else, like pneumonia or chronic obstructive pulmonary disease (COPD).

Patient Stratification. Asthmatics vary significantly in severity and costs, and Harvard Pilgrim would like to develop methodologies to identify and target its interventions to patients based on the severity of their asthma. It is particularly interested in determining which patients are at greatest risk of exacerbation. "We want to know who the 'ticking time bombs' are," said one clinician. So far, Harvard Pilgrim has used both inpatient and outpatient claims data as one means to identify high-risk members. It has recently begun to use an algorithm based on flagging patients with two inpatient admissions or two ER visits in two years, a group they refer to as "frequent flyers." Of the seventeen thousand asthmatics in the Massachusetts region, approximately nine hundred were identified as frequent flyers. But these nine hundred patients are spread across six hundred PCPs. "This dispersion makes it almost impossible to get the attention of the primary care physician," said one program manager. "We figure you need to have at least three or four patients in a practice before the physician focuses on the problem."

Perhaps an even greater issue is that high use in one period is not a good predictor of future use. According to Harvard Pilgrim's analysis, only 30 percent of the frequent flyers in any year could have been identified from prior claims data. The Plan is currently working with a vendor that has developed a regression model that can be used to identify as many as 70 percent of the asthmatic population at risk of high cost and use. (Harvard Pilgrim and the vendor will also work together to develop interventions to improve asthma care in the network, including physician education, patient education, and patient outreach.)

Harvard Pilgrim is also using pharmacy claims data as a means to identify high-risk patients. "It is very hard to get timely pharmacy data," said one person. "But at least it's quicker than waiting for the hospital claims. For example, we could have a member who gets too many albuterol [a beta-agonist] scripts in January, then has an ER visit or is hospitalized in February. We will know about the drugs in February or March, but not about the inpatient admission until May or later."

In an initiative in the fall of 1997, the Plan and its pharmacy vendor, PharmaCare, identified members in the Massachusetts region who had high use of beta-agonists (defined as more than 1.5 beta-agonist inhalers a month). (Beta-agonists are one type of asthma rescue medicine. Heavy use of beta-agonists can be one indicator of poor asthma care.) The list of patients was sent to the medical directors of the medical groups and Joint Ventures, as well as to individual doctors who had more than a certain number of patients on the list. Harvard Pilgrim suggested to the physicians that the patient lists be reviewed to determine the possible need for changes in medication management of these patients to use more inhaled steroids and anti-inflammatories. The letter also encouraged physicians to refer patients to the AMP. Physicians were asked to respond to the letter and indicate any follow-up action they had taken. The Plan got a response from 40 percent of the PCPs of the 753 patients identified, indicating that some action had been taken, including seventy-six referrals to the AMP. The next step will be to follow up directly with the patients of the physicians who did not respond.

In a recent follow-up initiative, Harvard Pilgrim and PharmaCare identified patients in the Massachusetts region who had received at least six beta-agonist inhalers within the prior six months. A ratio comparing beta-agonist use during the six-month period to inhaled anti-inflammatory use during the same period was calculated for each patient, and compared to the Plan's treatment goal ratio of less than 0.5:1 for beta-agonist inhalers versus anti-inflammatory inhalers per month. This information was sent to individual physicians, and to the medical directors of the Medical Groups and JVs. Also included was the patient's drug profile with a list of common prescription medications that could precipitate asthma. Physicians were asked to review the data, along with any current patient information they had, and to respond to PharmaCare if they wanted to make any medication change. If a doctor requests a different medication or dosage, the patient will receive a letter from Harvard Pilgrim announcing the change and the availability of a new prescription at the usual pharmacy. Physicians were also given the opportunity in their responses to refer patients to the AMP.

Patient Outreach and Referrals to the AMP. To date, Harvard Pilgrim has relied mainly on clinician referral of patients to the AMP, along with identifying patients who have an ER visit or inpatient admission. While clinician referral has been quite an effective outreach technique in Harvard Vanguard, Harvard Pilgrim believes it needs to do more in the Medical Groups, JVs, and PIPA, and is considering a new "direct to member" approach. The Plan would identify members with asthma, using the 2:1:1 algorithm, and provide a list of asthmatics to each primary care physician in the network. Unless the physician tells the Plan not to do so ("a regrets only" response), it will contact patients to inform them about the AMP. "Our benchmarking of other programs suggests that direct-to-member strategies work, and that physicians almost never exercise the regrets only option," said a staff member working on the program design. The direct-to-member approach has been approved by Harvard Pilgrim's Joint Clinical Quality Committee, which has representatives from all delivery systems, and is being considered for implementation starting in the fall of 1998.

Physician Support and Participation. According to one Harvard Pilgrim staffer who has been very involved in the AMP, "The $64,000 question is: What will get more physicians in the Massachusetts region to participate in the AMP and to provide better care to their patients with asthma? Direct-to-member strategies are only a partial answer. Asthma is a chronic disease, so people will eventually go to the doctor when they get sick. If the doctor is not hooked in and part of the disease management program, the doctor will undermine the HMO. We can't put patients in the middle. We have to reach the doctors. HMOs don't manage the care of patients, doctors do. But so many doctors are not doing the right thing now in terms of asthma care."

Harvard Pilgrim recently ranked physician practices in the Massachusetts region according to their degree of alignment with the Plan's asthma management activities. On a scale of 0–5, where 0 is no alignment and 5 is shared accountability with a significant Harvard Pilgrim oversight role, the most highly aligned providers (at level 4 and 5) accounted for only 7 percent of the region's asthmatic members, while over 40 percent of asthmatic members were enrolled in practices with a ranking of 0 or 1, or in practices not ranked because they were in the PIPA model. (See Table 7.4.)

The Plan sees a number of barriers to getting more of the physicians in the network to be more aligned with the AMP. "The network

Provider Rank	Member Distribution	Asthmatics	Percentage of Asthmatic Members
Rank 5 (Shared accountability: Harvard Pilgrim role oversight)	8,015	241	1
Rank 4 (Active support to existing process: Harvard Pilgrim consult, CME/CEU programs)	32,059	966	6
Rank 3 (Practice working to create process: Harvard Pilgrim actively involved)	164,302	4,951	29
Rank 2 (Medical director engaged, outreach to PCP)	120,221	3,623	22
Rank 1 (No contact to date—assess for problem areas)	36,066	1,086	6
Rank 0 (No response—outreach to member directly)	40,074	1208	7
Subtotal	400,737	12,075	
PIPA affiliated	161,288	4,721	28
Total	562,025	16,796	100

Table 7.4.   Provider Rank: Total Membership and Asthmatic Distribution for Massachusetts Region.

is very diffuse and hard to reach, with wide variations in practice," said one observer. "In Harvard Vanguard and the Medical Groups, there are systems and mechanisms in place to detect practice problems. But the network practices often have little structure, particularly clinical infrastructure, even in many of the joint ventures. Being able to contract is not the same as having processes and systems to support clinical practice. Plus our risk model is lousy—there's little or no economic incentive for most of the physicians. And there's very little clinical leadership." Another Harvard Pilgrim clinician echoed the concern about lack of medical leadership: "In the staff and groups, the medical director is empowered, has significant responsibilities, makes a definite time commitment, and is compensated for being medical director. Often in the JVs the medical director is just picked at random. The person in the position may have been stuck with the job and have little interest in changing practice."

If engaging the JVs more actively is seen as a challenge, PIPA is even more daunting. "PIPA is a difficult entity to get your arms around," said one Harvard Pilgrim clinician. "The doctors are self-selected; they are ones who did not want to join another model. As long as we pay them, the attitude of many of them is that the less they hear from us, the better. In fact, some of them think that they can just play a waiting game and managed care will go away." Added another Harvard Pilgrim staff member: "At least with the JVs we can try to get the attention of the physicians by talking about money. For example, I had one twenty-four-year-old member with asthma who is in the ER one or two times per month. His doctor is supposed to be the gatekeeper, he writes the scripts. So he needs to be more proactive to get this member to come in for office visits and to help him develop better self-management skills. I finally got the doctor's attention by sitting down with him and explaining in detail how his JV is at risk for the ER and inpatient use for this member. Now he understands that it's in his financial interest to do something different, and he's getting more active. But if that member's PCP were in PIPA, there's nothing similar I could have said."

Some Thoughts About Disease Management from a Few Physicians in the Massachusetts Region

In our interviews with a number of primary care physicians in the Massachusetts region, most (but not all) appeared to be supportive of disease management in general, and of Harvard Pilgrim's programs. The doctors did, however, raise a variety of issues and concerns. Some selected comments:

I think some of these disease management programs have been very useful and others are a complete waste of time. Harvard Pilgrim's asthma management program has done a terrific job changing the focus from managing acute episodes to managing asthma as a long-term illness. The care guidelines are good. The clinician education component has been very effective at teaching our physicians and nurses about the use of peak flow meters and spacers. It's amazing that none of us really knew basic care techniques like how to use inhalers until we were taught by the asthma program nurses. Harvard Pilgrim has made very clever use of pharmacy data, and the lists we get about beta-agonist and steroid inhaler use have been very helpful, as have the printouts on ER and hospital use by asthmatics in our practice. This information allows us to identify and work with our patients who are getting into trouble. We would never be able to do this without Harvard Pilgrim's support.

But there are often problems with the timeliness of the data we get from Harvard Pilgrim (although they are no worse than other HMOs).

The lag in claims is really a problem—I get data for 1997 in May or June of 1998, which is a bit late to intervene in many cases (like flu shots for the winter). A lot of the information we get is also wrong. For example, we got a list of our patients with congestive heart failure (CHF) from Harvard Pilgrim and it turns out that a large percentage of the patients Harvard Pilgrim identified did not have CHF at all. Using diagnosis codes for identifying patients is a weak component of all of the programs, and it creates so much work for us because we need to pull charts to verify the information. And patients move from plan to plan. If we had computerized medical records, it would be easier. But no Harvard Pilgrim practices except Harvard Vanguard have computerized records, which I think the people who develop the disease management programs sometimes forget. They need to focus more on how the network is very different from the health centers.

Some of the other disease management efforts have been less effective. For instance, Harvard Pilgrim had an initiative to increase the use of ACE inhibitors. This is an area where it's easy to tell if patients are on ACE inhibitors, so it's easy for the plan to focus on. But at least in our practice it had very little yield or value, but required a lot of effort. I worry that NCQA and HEDIS are driving what the plans focus on—they are all following each other to develop the same programs. This is producing some duplication and confusion. For example, in asthma, you need to be sure that you are using the right drug for *that* patient's HMO. Different HMOs have different formularies and it's hard to keep them all straight. And we are fortunate because most of our patients are enrolled in just three or four plans. I can't imagine what it's like for other physicians.

—*The medical director of one of the Medical Groups*
in the Massachusetts Region

To me what's called disease management by Harvard Pilgrim and other managed care plans is really nothing more than good patient management, which I already do. I don't manage diseases, I care for patients. I am not sure why I should be enthusiastic about disease management programs that I and most other physicians in the network had no input into designing. I see these programs mainly as a cost-cutting measure—utilization review packaged in a more savvy way. Their intent seems mainly to cut out care and ration physician services, particularly referrals to specialists. I also think a lot of disease management is just a way for drug companies to do detailing with the help of the HMO. The one time I referred a patient to a disease management program, I was not impressed with the case manager and the process added no value and generated a lot of paperwork for the patient and me. I haven't made any other patient referrals.

—A PIPA physician in a two-person primary care practice

Care in a nonmanaged system is often episodic and event-centered, and I support the longitudinal focus of the disease management concept. But I worry about a disease-centered approach. Many people have multiple diseases. There needs to be someone who is responsible for the overall coordination of care for these patients. Among the Massachusetts HMOs, Harvard Pilgrim has done the best job of trying to keep its disease management programs very primary care focused, and of communicating with the physicians. But some of the disease management programs offered by other plans seem like a way for specialty physicians to segregate the care of patients by disease, and cut primary care physicians out of the picture in order to recapture the patients the specialists have lost with the growth of managed care.

—A primary care physician in one of the JVs

Disease management makes sense for managed care plans, because they care for large populations of members. But physicians don't think of themselves as caring for populations—they care for individual patients. Physicians get excited about improving the quality of care, but you have to approach them with a patient-centered not population-centered approach. And the program has got to make life easier for the doctors. Adhering to practice guidelines may be easy in settings where there are computerized practice guidelines and reminders for physicians. But we are very low-tech in my practice— and it would take a huge investment to develop the necessary infrastructure. I don't hear any of the HMOs willing to help us with that investment. Instead, a lot of the information we get from them is outdated, or incomplete and not very helpful. . . . For example, I have a number of patients enrolled in Harvard Pilgrim's Medicare program, but they have the plan without prescription drug coverage. It's going to be kind of hard to do disease management for most of their conditions when the pharmacy piece is not covered, and when Harvard Pilgrim will have no pharmacy data for these patients in its system either.

It also takes time for physicians to review those patient lists, or to talk to a case manager or go over a care plan. Since I am not being compensated by Harvard Pilgrim for that time, the program has got to add value for me in some other way. It would really help to offer physicians economic incentives to participate in these programs.

—A PIPA primary care physician in a four-person practice

We are very supportive of disease management, and of all the plans, Harvard Pilgrim's efforts seem much more clinician-led than imposed externally. But overall, the HMO programs feel very fragmented and very separated from the primary care physicians and what is actually going on in the practice. For example, we got a list of our patients who had had so-called preventable admissions for asthma. When we reviewed the cases, we had usually made incredible efforts at prevention, but there was incredible family dysfunction or other situations in these homes that resulted in the hospitalization of the patients.

The key issue in disease management is whether we should be developing categorical or practice-based interventions. Should these programs be centralized or decentralized? To the degree that the solution or program comes from the HMO, it will only apply to certain patients. That approach does not get at the systems issues at the actual practices. We would prefer to build good clinical systems in the practices for all of our patients, and not put major stress on the practices by making them use the external programs of the HMOs. You can't just import a disease management program into a clinical setting. We are talking about managing all aspects of care—primary care, specialists, hospitals, ancillaries, pharmacy, not just a small subset. If you bring in a preplanned program, it disrupts twenty other systems and relationships at the practice.

It's going to be a real challenge for Harvard Pilgrim to do disease management in the network. The approach requires teamwork between primary care physicians, specialists, nurses, and other clinicians. Most doctors in solo or small practices don't know how to work in teams, and they chose those types of practices because they don't want to. Plus, operationally a practice needs computerized medical records to do this well.

—The medical director of a large group practice in the network

It's very hard to follow any one disease management program when you have patients that could have one of dozens of insurance plans. I want to have one style of practice, one that is patient-centered, not payer-specific. I get lists of my asthmatics from many different HMOs, most of which have less than ten patients. Many of the lists are wrong, the medications are wrong, and they are not timely. And none of the HMOs probably has enough information to know what's really going on in our practice.

But we do believe that Harvard Pilgrim has good disease management programs, as do a couple of the other managed care plans, and we refer patients to those programs. But let's take asthma. We have lots of asthmatics in our practice, and our management of asthma is very good. But the prevalence of asthma in our practice keeps going up. It's fine to do patient education about inhalers and spacers and peak flow meters, and we do all of that. And it's a good thing to do home visits to identify triggers. But I have patients who scrub their floors, and vacuum and do everything right in terms of self-care. But they still have acute episodes because the hallways in their housing projects are moldy and the building authority is not getting the cockroaches and rats out of their apartments. There are lots of socioeconomic factors involved in most of these diseases, and I would like to see the managed care plans more involved in public health interventions as part of their disease management programs.

—A physician who practices in a community health center in Boston that contracts with Harvard Pilgrim

~~~ Epilogue: Harvard Pilgrim Health Care Organizational Update, Fall 2002

Roberta Herman, M.D.
Senior Vice President and Chief Medical Officer
Harvard Pilgrim Health Care

In the several years since this case study was written, Harvard Pilgrim Health Care has experienced a profound financial crisis and also an extraordinary recovery, during which the Plan's commitment to, and excellent performance in, clinical quality and disease management were maintained. At this writing, Harvard Pilgrim has experienced eight consecutive positive financial quarters.

A key element of the turnaround was the outsourcing of the Plan's claims processing and information systems, where poor performance had contributed to provider dissatisfaction and to Harvard Pilgrim's inability to foresee the depth of its financial difficulties. In addition, Harvard Pilgrim withdrew from the Rhode Island market (where its losses had been especially serious), standardized and simplified its key business processes and its contracts with physicians and hospitals, and adopted a more centralized structure organized around five key functions—finance, customer service and operations, provider contracting and operations, sales and marketing, and clinical programs and quality.

Even while Harvard Pilgrim was intensely focused on its financial recovery, the Plan continued to invest in clinical quality improvement

222

and disease management. In 2000, Harvard Pilgrim launched a comprehensive and highly successful Diabetes Program. In 2001, Harvard Pilgrim became the first health plan in its market to use predictive modeling in conjunction with case management to identify and provide customized care plans for members who are at high risk for hospitalization or serious illness. Harvard Pilgrim's Quality Awards Program, Pay for Performance Contracts, and Rewards for Excellence Program are components of a comprehensive strategy to produce excellent quality network performance. (These developments are discussed in more detail in following sections.)

In the fall of 2002, the NCQA *Quality Compass 2002* report placed Harvard Pilgrim among the top fifteen NCQA-accredited health plans in the country on key measures of clinical performance. The Plan's performance in claims processing and member services have improved dramatically and Harvard Pilgrim received New England's highest scores in the NCQA report's "Rating of Health Plan" member satisfaction measure. Harvard Pilgrim also receives high satisfaction ratings from its provider network.

DIABETES PROGRAM AND RECENT CHANGES IN APPROACH TO DISEASE MANAGEMENT

Significant changes have occurred in Harvard Pilgrim's approach to disease management, as exemplified by the Diabetes Program.

Standardized Definitions for Case Identification and Outcomes Measurement

Until quite recently, Harvard Pilgrim typically developed homegrown measures for case identification and outcomes measurement. Innovative and useful as these measures were, having a unique system of measurement left Harvard Pilgrim with limited ability to compare data and assess success. For many years, NCQA has organized national measurement systems based on national health initiatives and priorities. In recent years, NCQA's HEDIS measures have expanded from a primarily preventive focus to include chronic disease components. Harvard Pilgrim's case definition for the Diabetes Program is derived from HEDIS specifications (absent HEDIS requirements for continuous enrollment) and its outcome measures are those developed by Medicare and used by NCQA in the accreditation process. These results are obtained by review of transaction (claims) records and, in some cases, a record review for missed tests and test values. Homegrown definitions prevail for the minority of programs with no available HEDIS specifications; pharmaceutical transactions continue to be a preferred data source because of their timeliness and accuracy.

Direct-to-Member Approaches

Harvard Pilgrim continues to employ all the elements previously described in its disease management programs as well as a significant emphasis on direct-to-member strategies. In the case of diabetes, all members meeting the case definition receive basic educational material and an invitation to participate in more intense education intervention. The basic materials include a wallet reminder card listing questions the member should ask the clinician at the next office visit (see Figure 7.4).

These questions were based on recommendations that emerged from the Diabetes Control and Complications Trial and the American Diabetes Association concerning optimal care for diabetics as well as the preponderance of evidence suggesting that averting macrovascular events would have the biggest impact on overall mortality for a diabetic population. The direct-to-member approach draws from a long and successful track record of direct-to-consumer marketing by the pharmaceutical industry, as well as the tenets of Ed Wagner (2001) and others that an "activated" member is key to achieving optimal chronic disease management outcomes. Borrowing from Prochaska's readiness-to-change theory (1991, 1997), enlistment in a more intense educational intervention called the Diabetes Control Network was reserved for members who actively enrolled. This intervention included sixteen monthly mailings to members on discrete topics on diabetes self-care and management, such as diabetic foot care, and was available in several languages. A total of twenty-four thousand diabetics received a wallet card and more than six thousand have enrolled to date as a result of the Plan's outreach. In addition to hospital admissions data and physician referrals, candidates for case management were identified on the basis of co-morbidity using transaction data.

Harvard Pilgrim
Health Care

Dear Harvard Pilgrim Member:

This handy card will help you remember important questions to ask your doctor about your diabetes care. Just keep it in your wallet - all you need to remember is to take it out!

To find out more about how Harvard Pilgrim can help you learn more about managing your diabetes and how to stay healthy, please call our nurses **toll free at 1-888-471-4838.**

Sincerely,

Robert Herman

Roberta Herman, MD
Medical Director, Clinical Policy & Programs

Harvard Pilgrim
Health Care

Remember to ask your health care provider:

- Is my hemoglobin A1C sugar level ok?
- Is my LDL cholesterol level ok?
- Is my blood pressure ok?
- Do I need a yearly urine test to check my kidney function?
- Do I need a yearly dilated eye exam?
- Should I be taking a daily aspirin?
- Do my feet show signs of problems related to diabetes?

Figure 7.4. Diabetes Wallet Reminder Card.

Community-Based Interventions and Innovative Partnerships

Materials for Harvard Pilgrim's Diabetes Control Network were developed as part of an unrestricted educational grant in partnership with Pfizer. The Community Care Days Program was developed in conjunction with Stop & Shop, a popular local supermarket chain, using outlets that also offer pharmacy services in seventeen locations surrounding Boston. Three-day sessions were advertised in grocery circulars and local newspapers and offered on-site nutritional counseling, blood pressure measurement, and blood tests. Additional benefits included free home glucose monitoring devices and low-cost, diabetes-appropriate prepared meals. Harvard Pilgrim physicians in relevant neighborhoods were notified and asked to solicit participation by members who might benefit.

Outstanding Results

Harvard Pilgrim Health Care (and its legacy organizations) has a long track record of clinical program innovation with excellent measurable outcomes. What distinguishes the Diabetes Program is the speed at which outstanding program results have been achieved. The rapid success of the program (shown in Figure 7.5) is largely attributed to the addition of direct-to-member outreach.

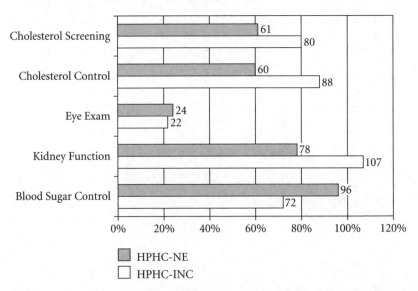

Figure 7.5.   Proven Results in Diabetes Management: Percentage Improvement over Baseline, HEDIS Comprehensive Diabetes Measures (2000–2002).

APPROACH TO QUALITY IMPROVEMENT IN THE NETWORK

The nature of Harvard Pilgrim's relationship with its network has changed significantly over the last several years. A variety of practice supports and incentives have been implemented to complement Harvard Pilgrim's disease management programs:

Network Diversity, Alignment, and Financial Models

With Harvard Vanguard Medical Associates (formerly the staff model component of Harvard Community Health Plan) becoming a self-governed, operationally separate medical practice, Harvard Pilgrim now contracts almost exclusively with independent practices. (A Plan-owned practice in Nashua, New Hampshire, is the one exception.) While the span and diversity of Harvard Pilgrim's network has been maintained, ranging from large "Integrated Delivery Systems" practices (for example, Partners) to individual practices (for example, in the IPA network), and nearly all physicians participate in Local Care Units, overall, the level of financial risk assumed by providers has decreased significantly.

Physician Involvement in Program Design and Implementation

Previously, Harvard Community Health Plan and then Harvard Pilgrim Health Care relied predominantly on employed physicians (medical directors) of the corporation to provide clinical programmatic guidance. In recent years, Harvard Pilgrim has largely adopted the approach of the legacy Pilgrim IPA. The Harvard Pilgrim Physicians Association (HPPA) and its Board (HPPA Board) are consulted regularly on matters of strategy and policy. Among the HPPA Board subcommittees are its Clinician Advisory Committees. These committees are organized by high-volume specialty (adult medicine, pediatrics and family practice, surgery, cardiology, behavioral health, and OB/GYN) and are the source of clinical input and review regarding the design and implementation of clinical programs.

Quality Improvement Supports and Tools

Harvard Pilgrim continues to sponsor educational conferences and best practice forums for network physicians in areas of high strategic importance (such as the Diabetes Workshop). Continuing medical education credits are now provided and overseen by the Department of Ambulatory Care and Prevention, a joint academic department of Harvard Pilgrim Health Care and Harvard Medical School. Case listings and defect lists continue to be used and have benefited greatly from improved data integrity; typically these now include detailed and accurate information on member demographics, recent ER or hospital usage, and drug history. Most recently, providers have been given a fax-back option to identify inaccuracies, remove individuals from the list, or enroll them in disease management programs.

Quality Awards Program

In 2000, Harvard Pilgrim Health Care launched its Quality Awards Program (QAP). This is an annual process intended to provide start-up funding to practices in the Harvard Pilgrim Network for the design and implementation of local clinical or service quality improvement initiatives. A competitive, peer-reviewed process, the QAP is overseen by the Harvard Pilgrim Quality Award Committee, which is supported by Harvard Pilgrim staff and made up of practicing primary and specialty care physicians from the community. Approximately fifty start-up grants have been awarded to date. Proposals are accepted on any topic but are expected to support Harvard Pilgrim's Quality Improvement Workplan and the corporate mission, "to improve the health of the people we serve and the health of society." As a result, many of the proposals are initiatives to address chronic diseases, and those tend to be the ones that win the best funding.

Rewards for Excellence

Beginning in late 2002, Harvard Pilgrim will also recognize and reward exemplary performance. Under this program, HEDIS scores for participating network practices are being compared to a predefined threshold, typically the national ninetieth percentile. The Plan will offer a per-member-per-month–based reward for achieving excellent levels of performance, per these defined targets. An honor roll will be posted on Harvard Pilgrim's Web site identifying practices with exemplary performance.

HARVARD PILGRIM HEALTH ADVANCE

In June 2001, Harvard Pilgrim partnered with StatusOne Health Systems to launch its *Health Advance* program in August 2001, designed to provide predictive modeling and customized care management for at-risk members. Harvard Pilgrim uses StatusOne's proprietary algorithms to identify at-risk patients based on health plan data such as diagnosis, patterns of care, place of service, failure to receive medically indicated services, and pharmacy prescriptions. In contrast to the disease-specific approach of standard disease management programs, members identified by Harvard Pilgrim Health Advance typically suffer from multiple co-morbidities (50 percent have five or more); many are also suffering from care fragmentation or psychosocial isolation. Typically, these members account for approximately 0.5 to 1 percent of the population but may account for 30–40 percent of all inpatient days and 20–30 percent of total medical expense (Lynch, Forman, Graff, and Gunby, 2000).

The Health Advance Care Management Intervention

At the program's core is nurse outreach and support. Nurse case managers work with identified members and their care providers and families to create a patient-specific care plan designed to reduce the level of illness and improve daily living. Specific goals of this voluntary, patient-centered program are to ensure the coordination of medical care, increase self-reliance, enhance daily activity and fitness, strengthen interdependence with family and friends, promote stimulation and mental challenge, and encourage community involvement and a sense of purpose. Close interaction with a member's primary care physician and relevant specialists are critically important components.

The Health Advance Care Management System

The Harvard Pilgrim Health Advance system includes a secure, Web-based care management software program focusing on the needs of the at-risk patients, a data registry of identified patients, monthly summary reports of planwide performance metrics and availability of caremanagement services. This system is in full compliance with HIPAA (The Health Insurance Portability and Accountability Act) and applicable state regulations about appropriate use of medical information.

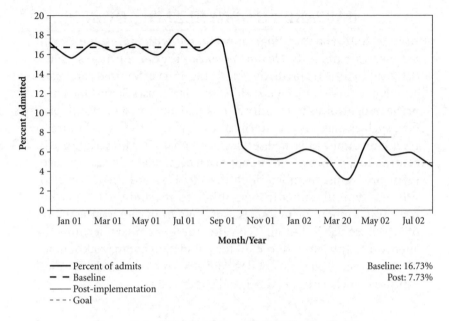

Figure 7.6.   Health Advance Hospitalization Rate.

Preliminary Results

Based on results to date, Harvard Pilgrim Health Advance holds promise to deliver significant decreases in hospital days (Figure 7.6) and a reduction in per-member–per-month costs for members participating in the program. Standard program metrics include survey-based assessment of functional status, which suggests comparably significant improvements in quality of life (Figure 7.7).

KEY CHALLENGES

During the last ten years, Harvard Pilgrim and others have become increasingly sophisticated in the design and implementation of disease management programs. Key challenges likely to continue during the next several years include developing increasingly sophisticated data mining strategies for proactive, concurrent identification and management; achieving the best balance between disease-specific and cross-population activities to leverage limited resources and optimize total population health improvement; designing programs that produce true care augmentation within a fundamentally fragmented health care

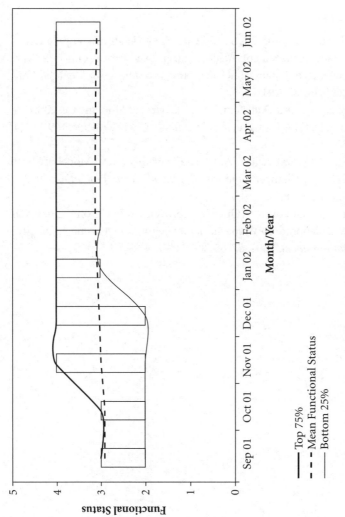

Figure 7.7. Health Advance Functional Status Improvement.

system; and demonstrating favorable combined cost and quality outcomes. Efforts directed at compliance management may be that much more important and challenging given the current trend toward insurance products that increase member financial responsibility.

References

Lynch, J., Forman, S., Graff, S., and Gunby, M. "High Risk Population Health Management: Achieving Improved Patient Outcomes and Near-Term Financial Results." *American Journal of Managed Care,* 2000, *6,* 781–791.

Prochaska, J. O., and Goldstein, M. G. "Process of Smoking Cessation: Implications for Clinicians." *Clinics in Chest Medicine,* 1991, *12*(4), 727–735.

Prochaska, J. O., and Velicer, W. F. "The Transtheoretical Model of Health Behavior Change." *American Journal of Health Promotion,* 1997, *12*(1), 38–48.

Wagner, E. H., and others. "Quality Improvement in Chronic Illness Care: A Collaborative Approach." *Joint Commission Journal on Quality Improvement,* 2001, *27,* 63–80.

CHAPTER EIGHT

Managing Care for the Dual-Eligible Population in Massachusetts

In 1996, one of the last bastions of unmanaged care in the state of Massachusetts was the *dual-eligible* population, people who are covered by both Medicare and Medicaid. The Division of Medical Assistance (DMA), the state agency that administers the Medicaid program, had been very aggressive in the preceding five years in moving most Medicaid clients into managed care programs. Now DMA had its sights set on developing a managed care approach for dual-eligible individuals.

One senior DMA official explained the situation as follows:

> We were frustrated during all the health reform discussions in the early 1990s that long-term care was not on the agenda, even though the future of health care is the services Medicaid covers. So since it looked like Medicaid was going to be eternally responsible for long-term care, we thought we should see if we could adapt some of the managed care

This case was written by the authors in 2000. Funding was provided by Astra Zeneca. The authors thank Ingrid Nembhard for her wonderful assistance with the case.

models we had used successfully for acute care to the long-term care sector. In many ways, dual-eligible people have the most to benefit from managed care approaches. They are bounced around like Ping-Pong balls in the current system. It's totally inefficient, it leads to poor quality and the ones who suffer the most are the neediest consumers. We see the dual-eligible as the next frontier for Medicaid managed care in Massachusetts. We can do much better than this.

Advocates and providers agreed with DMA that the current financing and care delivery systems did not serve dual-eligible individuals well. "There is a constant battle between Medicare and Medicaid to shift costs to one another," said one physician. "The payment rules are always changing and they have gotten so complex over the last three decades of warfare between Medicare and Medicaid that there is no logic to the system—it's a constant series of responses by both payers to the last cost shift by the other, or the last big scam or fraud by providers. So the primary rule of survival for providers has been to try to understand the complex payment rules and march to them, regardless of whether it results in optimal care." An advocate for the elderly agreed:

> Frankly, the current system could not really be much worse. The federal government spends more on Medicare because it doesn't control long-term care; nursing homes push their elderly patients unnecessarily into hospitals and other acute care providers to try to shift costs to Medicare. Meanwhile Medicaid doesn't control the acute medical care system for elders, which often practices in a way that leads to higher use of the long-term care services covered by Medicaid services. No one is in charge of the patients—doctors don't know their patients have gone into nursing homes and home care case managers don't know people have gone to the hospital. Care is incredibly fragmented and uncoordinated. The patients get bounced around with lousy results—high rates of preventable hospitalizations, unnecessary nursing home admissions, and higher costs for everyone.

Although there seemed to be nearly universal agreement on the need to improve the care of dual-eligible individuals, the road to a solution was fraught with challenges for DMA. Any new managed care approach for this population would need to be negotiated with the Health Care Financing Administration (HCFA), the federal agency that administers the Medicare program and has significant authority over state Medicaid programs as well. HCFA was notorious for being very deliberate and at times inflexible in its review of innovative proposals from state Medicaid agencies. DMA would also need the support of the Massachusetts Executive Office of Elder Affairs, the state agency that administered the Massachusetts Home Care Program, which provided a range of community-based long-term care services to lower-income elders. The state legislature would also need to give its approval to any changes proposed by DMA. State politics would play a role: the governor, who controlled DMA, was a Republican, while Democrats overwhelmingly controlled both chambers in the legislature.

But the biggest challenge was likely to be the long line of interest groups and elder advocates. Elder advocates were skeptical of managed care, and few, if any, existing managed care organizations had expertise or experience managing the care of this population. DMA had an uphill battle to convince advocates that a new managed care approach would not only reduce costs but also improve quality for the dual-eligible population. "Medicaid has been operating for years in ways that advocates and consumers don't like," said one long-time elder advocate. "So they have very little trust or good will from us. This is going to be difficult to change."

DMA was, however, undaunted by the task that lay ahead. "The current system fails everyone," said then-DMA Commissioner Bruce Bullen. "Elders don't get the services they deserve. Taxpayers pay for a system we cannot afford. A managed care program gives us a chance of reforming a dysfunctional system, helping more elders live at home where they want to be, and saving hundreds of millions of dollars. There is enough money in the system if we manage wisely. We just have to be bold and try something new."

BACKGROUND ON DUAL ELIGIBILITY

The challenge of managing dual-eligible patients is rooted in the fragmented nature of our two largest public health insurance programs.

A Brief Description of Medicare and Medicaid

Medicare is a national health insurance program for people sixty-five years of age and older, certain younger disabled people, and people with end-stage kidney disease who need dialysis or a transplant.

Eligibility is based on age, citizenship, and work history. The program has no income or asset limits. It is federally funded and administered.

Medicare pays primarily for acute and rehabilitative services. It excludes custodial care and limits coverage for care in skilled nursing facilities to about three months. Medicare Part A covers acute inpatient hospital care, skilled nursing facility and home health care for people recovering from acute hospitalization, durable medical equipment and supplies, and hospice care. Medicare Part B covers doctors, outpatient hospital care, laboratory tests, and other medical services not covered by Part A, such as the services of physical and occupational therapists. In some instances, deductibles and copayments apply. Most preventive services such as annual physical exams are not covered, nor are prescription drugs.

Medicaid is a government health care coverage program for low-income individuals. It is funded by federal and state governments and administered by the states. Eligibility is based on age, income and assets, and various "categories" of eligibility, such as being disabled or having dependent children. Eligibility criteria vary from state to state, as do covered benefits. In general, the program pays for a comprehensive range of services, including many benefits not covered by Medicare, such as nursing home care beyond one hundred days, custodial services, preventive and primary care, and prescription drugs.

The Dual-Eligibles

Approximately 6 million people are covered by both Medicare and Medicaid. Almost 90 percent of the dual-eligible population, 5.3 million people, are elderly, and the others are disabled. Nationally, the dual-eligible represent 16 percent of the Medicare population and account for 30 percent of Medicare spending. On the Medicaid side, they are 17 percent of beneficiaries and account for 35 percent of spending (original unpublished data provided to authors during interview with staff at Division of Medical Assistance).

Medicare is the *primary payer* for the dual-eligible, meaning that it pays first for any Medicare-covered services up to the extent of coverage. Medicaid acts both as the secondary payer for any Medicare services not paid in full by Medicare (for example, it pays the Medicare deductibles and coinsurance) and is also the primary payer for Medicaid services not covered by Medicare (such as prescription drugs and long-term care).

In 1997, total spending on the dual-eligible was $120 billion. The federal share was approximately $95 billion—$62 billion for Medicare and $33 billion for the federal portion of Medicaid spending. "It is vitally important to manage the dual-eligible to get Medicare spending under control," said a federal official. "Medicare spending for dual-eligibles is growing faster than spending for other types of beneficiaries, and the number of dual-eligibles is increasing as the population ages. If we can't figure out how to control these costs, the actions we will have to take will make the Balanced Budget Act look like nothing."

As is apparent from the spending figures, the dual-eligible are a very vulnerable and high-cost population. When compared to the overall Medicare population, the dual-eligible are older, more likely to be people of color, disproportionately women, more likely to live alone, and much more likely to live in an institution. Not surprisingly, given that they are eligible for Medicaid, the dual-eligible population is also much poorer on average than other Medicare beneficiaries— 80 percent have annual incomes of less than $10,000.

The Problems of the Dual-Eligible

Elders who are eligible for both Medicare and Medicaid often have enormous difficulty navigating between the two programs. Many of their difficulties result from the fact that two payers, offering distinct yet overlapping benefit packages with different sets of rules, are responsible for the same patient, yet there is no coordination between the two. One state official said, "There is constant warfare between Medicare and Medicaid as they battle to shift costs to each other. Case management for the dual-eligible becomes, 'Can you find a way for the other program to pay?' Medicare is viewed as the primary payer but Medicaid actually has most of the costs."

One of the major differences in benefit coverage between Medicare and Medicaid is that Medicare covers no more than one hundred skilled nursing facility days (and usually considerably less), while Medicaid covers unlimited nursing facility care when it is medically necessary. Because Medicare is the primary payer for dual-eligible individuals and thus pays for most hospital care, a major problem is that Medicare wants to push the patient into nursing home care while Medicaid wants to hospitalize nursing home patients whenever possible.

Medicaid officials express particular frustration that they cannot participate in acute care decisions made when Medicare is the primary payer, despite the fact that coverage for long-term care services is the financial responsibility of Medicaid. According to one Massachusetts DMA employee:

> The fact that the state has no control over what happens to dual-eligible people in the acute system is particularly troubling when you look at the comparative cost of serving frail seniors in the community versus serving seniors in nursing facilities. The Medicare per capita cost for dual-eligible seniors in nursing facilities is nearly three times *less* than that for frail dual-eligible seniors in the community. For Medicaid, however, costs are more than five times greater for seniors residing in the nursing facilities. This means that Medicare has incentives to shift patients into nursing facility services. Medicaid, as part of its mandate to remain the payer of last resort, tries to find all claims that should have been billed to Medicare. The cost-shifting by both programs doesn't consider the ramifications of such behavior on total health care spending—which is 30 percent less for frail seniors residing in the community. More important, neither program pays attention to the impact of this cost-shifting on patients and their quality of life.

Medicaid's financial eligibility rules further compound the cost-shifting problem. It is much easier for low-income elders to obtain Medicaid if they reside in a nursing facility than if they live in the community, because they generally quickly spend down their assets to eligible amounts by paying for nursing home care. Many low-income, high-risk seniors who would prefer to remain out of nursing facilities cannot afford community-based services, such as assistance with personal care, which they need to remain in the community, unless they have Medicaid coverage. But these elders cannot qualify for Medicaid because their assets are too great. Without the personal care services, they often quickly deteriorate physically, lose function, and lose the ability to live independently. Under these circumstances, a nursing facility admission often becomes the inevitable solution. Soon after admission to the nursing facility, these elders deplete their assets and become eligible for Medicaid. But by then, community-based resources may be insufficient to sustain them, and family resources needed for community living have been lost.

State officials, providers, and advocates all have their favorite anecdotes to put a human face on the problems experienced by the dual-eligible. Here are a few samples:

Vivian was diagnosed with Alzheimer's disease when she was seventy-seven. She was cared for at home by her husband and children. At age eighty-one, Vivian fell and was taken by ambulance to the hospital. After four days in the hospital, she was transferred to an intermediate rehabilitation hospital for ten days. From there, she was transferred to another floor and spent nearly two weeks in a transitional care center. She was then discharged to a skilled nursing facility, where she stayed for five days before being transferred to a rest home. A week later, she fell again and was transferred to the hospital emergency room. Agitated and violent, she was admitted to a psychiatric hospital for two weeks. Vivian was bounced around continuously for the next seven months. During this time she was evaluated by more than twenty doctors, countless direct care nurses, and fourteen discharge planners, and she was cared for in fourteen different facilities. She fell two more times, broke her hip and lost her independence. . . . With the constant movement, her dementia advanced quickly, and her husband could no longer bear the emotional strain of being with her and began to suffer from severe depression. Vivian now lives in a nursing facility. Her daughter said, "Alzheimer's disease had taken some of my mother's mind and independence, the disjointed system that moved her around like a piece of cargo has taken the rest."

—*Excerpted from testimony of Vivian's daughter before the U.S. Senate Special Committee on Aging hearing on the dual-eligible (Bullen, Perrone, and Parker, 1998)*

Mrs. Franks was an eighty-year-old woman who lived in the community. She was on Medicare, had a low income, but did not meet the asset criteria for Medicaid. She joined an HMO several years ago when her traditional medigap policy got too expensive for her. Her HMO provided only a limited drug benefit, unlike the full benefits in her old medigap plan. She could not afford all of her prescriptions so she only took some of them intermittently. She needed home health services but her HMO would not cover the services because they weren't sufficiently skilled in nature. She qualified for home care services, but these don't meet her skilled care needs and were limited because the state program can only provide services up to its budget allocation. Without drug coverage and the home health services she needed, she deteriorated in the community and had to go to a nursing home, where Medicaid picked up her tab after she spent her assets down to the limit. It would have been so much cheaper to support her in the community than to pay $60,000 a year to keep her in a nursing home. Not to mention the better life she would have had.

—*An elder advocate*

One of my elderly patients who was dual-eligible lived in a nursing home and needed a procedure that could be safely performed there. But the nursing home transferred her to the hospital for the procedure so it could get paid by Medicare when she got back to the home, because then she met the three-day prior hospitalization requirement for skilled nursing facility care and Medicare payment was more than they were getting for her from Medicaid. Medicare paid for several days of SNF care at the nursing home, then it said her care was not sufficiently skilled, so the nursing home transferred her to a new bed to free up a Medicare-certified bed so the nursing home could get the higher Medicare payment for another patient. So she ended up on the same floor but in a different room at the end of the whole saga. That's a lot of unnecessary disruption for an eighty-six-year-old woman just to get a few more bucks for the nursing home, and an unnecessary expense for the system.

—*A primary care physician*

I had a diabetic patient who had a stroke and was having great trouble giving himself insulin at home. He was deemed ineligible for home health services because his need was not acute, so he started having a cycle of emergencies and hospitalizations. After he was discharged he would qualify for home health for a few weeks, then Medicare would cut him off, and he'd go into the hospital again. He finally had a really bad incident and ended up in a nursing home and on Medicaid. Medicare gets skittish when it is confronted with the real home needs of patients, so it retreats into a medical coverage model. Everyone becomes a strict constructionist about their own benefits, never focusing on the skill needs of the patient. But this ends up being so much more expensive in the long run and tragic for the patients.

—*A nurse practitioner*

A classic example is the elderly person who enters a hospital on Medicare and is transferred to a nursing facility for a Medicare-covered skilled nursing facility stay. The elder needs to stay in the nursing home because he has inadequate supports at home. But then he discovers that Medicare covers only a limited amount of nursing home days. He can't afford the services he needs in the community so he stays in the nursing home and spends down to Medicaid. Since the Medicare beneficiary goes to the nursing home before he or she is eligible for Medicaid, Medicaid cannot avert this admission by offering preventive or alternative care not included in the Medicare benefit package. So the low-income elder gets whipsawed between the two systems because neither program is ultimately responsible for the performance of the entire system.

—A DMA official

BACKGROUND ON MASSACHUSETTS

In 1995, there were 861,000 people age sixty-five or older in Massachusetts. This represented 14.1 percent of the state's population, higher than the national average of 12.8 percent. Census trends indicate that the number of elderly persons in the state will increase dramatically over the next few decades, rising by nearly 50 percent by 2025. (See Table 8.1.) Those most at risk for long-term care services are persons seventy-five and older, and especially those over eighty-five. The proportion of elders in Massachusetts who are in the very oldest age category exceeds the national average by 21 percent and the Census Bureau estimates that by the year 2025, the population in Massachusetts who are eighty-five and above will have increased by more than 50 percent.

Who Pays for Long-Term Care in Massachusetts?

Long-term care services are paid primarily from three sources: Medicaid, Medicare, and out-of-pocket payments by individuals. In

Year	1995	2000	2005	2015	2025
Number of residents age 65+	861,000	843,000	827,000	965,000	1,252,000
Percentage of state population	14.1	13.5	13.0	14.6	18.1

Table 8.1. Elderly Population in Massachusetts.
Source: Bruce and Schulman-Green, 2000.

Massachusetts, 40 percent of payment for long-term care services comes from MassHealth (the name for Medicaid in Massachusetts). Out-of-pocket payments by individuals represent the second-greatest source of payment (32 percent) and Medicare payments are third (24 percent). These expenditures do not include the cost of care provided by informal caregivers, which has been estimated nationally to be $196 billion per year and to involve 25 million family caregivers, three-quarters of whom are women. A shift to paid care could greatly increase the expenditures for long-term care. More than 60 percent of family caregivers who provide at least twenty-one hours a week have suffered from depression; caregiver burnout, rather than any change in the patient's functional status, is often a major reason for institutionalization.

Private insurance is not a major source of financing long-term care services. The state government in Massachusetts estimates that fewer than forty thousand people had private long-term care insurance policies in 1995. Although the number of policies in force is increasing, private insurance would have to grow considerably to become a major payer. The cost of coverage is the major barrier. Several studies estimated that only 10–20 percent of the elderly could afford high-quality long-term care insurance policies.

Provider Supply

Massachusetts has a large supply of long-term care providers, particularly nursing homes. Table 8.2 presents an inventory of the current supply in most categories.

As shown in Table 8.3, the state has significantly more licensed nursing beds per thousand elderly age seventy-five and above, but a much lower ratio of residential beds and home health agencies per thousand elderly. The number of nursing facility residents in Massachusetts, at 55.6 per thousand seniors, exceeds by 25 percent the national average of 43.7 per thousand seniors. The divergence from the national average is even greater when examining the number of Medicaid nursing facility recipients per thousand elderly, with Massachusetts—at 47.3—65 percent greater than the national average of 28.6 (AARP, 1996). Nursing facility lengths of stay fell from 2.4 years in 1988 to 1.4 years in 1994 as a result of the shift by nursing homes into short-term, post-acute care (covered by Medicare).

Provider Type	Capacity	Oversight Agency
Nursing facilities	55,067 beds in 1997; 66 beds/1,000 elders	Licensed by Department of Public Health
Chronic care and rehab hospitals	19 facilities; 2,805 beds in 1998	Licensed by Department of Public Health
Rest homes	147 facilities; 4,410 beds in 1998	Licensed by Department of Public Health
Assisted living residences	89 facilities; 5,500 units	Certified by EOEA
Respite care		Offered by Respite Care Program of EOEA
Home health services	201 agencies	
Personal care and homemaker services		State Home Care Programs
Adult family care	17 providers; can arrange families for up to 650 individuals	DMA
Adult day health	103 providers; 4,800 slots	Certified by payers: DMA and EOEA
Hospice care	24 providers	DPH

Table 8.2. Inventory of Long-Term Care Providers in Massachusetts.

In Massachusetts, new and replacement nursing homes require a certificate of need from the state government. To control expenditures, the state has had a moratorium on new nursing home construction since 1989 and a moratorium on applications from existing homes for renovation and replacement. But a large number of new nursing home beds approved in 1989 have not yet been licensed, so the supply of nursing home beds is expected to increase over next decade. The increase in beds, combined with some slack in occupancy, means access to nursing home beds is not a problem generally.

The Medicaid Program in Massachusetts

Massachusetts is a high-income state with a long progressive history and tradition, and this philosophy is reflected in its social programs, including Medicaid. MassHealth is large and generous by national Medicaid standards, with broad benefits, less stringent eligibility requirements, and relatively high provider payments. Table 8.4 outlines the Medicaid eligibility rules for elders in the state.

In 1995, total Medicaid spending in Massachusetts was $5.7 billion, equivalent to $6,189 per enrollee, higher than every state except

	Licensed Nursing Facilities			Community Residential Facilities			Home Health	
	Number of Facilities	Total Beds	Beds/1,000 Residents Age 75+	Number of Facilities	Number of Beds	Beds/1,000 Residents Age 75+	Number of Agencies	Agencies/1,000 Residents Age 75+
Massachusetts	591	56,912	168.7	167	5,500	16.3	178	0.53
United States	14,246	1,781,912	133.1	44,564	707,024	52.8	13,140	0.98

Table 8.3. Long-Term Care Provider Supply in Massachusetts and United States: 1995.

Source: Weiner and Stevenson, 1998, Table 2, p. 3.

MassHealth Program	Description of Coverage	Income Requirements	Asset Limit: Individual***	Asset Limit: Couple***
MassHealth Standard:				
Individuals	*Full MassHealth (Medicaid) benefits.* Pays for MassHealth services provided by Medicaid providers, and for services also covered by Medicare if the Medicaid payment rate is higher than the amount paid by Medicare.	Less than or equal to 100 percent Federal Poverty Limit (FPL): $716/month per individual; $958/month per couple	Less than $2,000	Less than $3,000
SSI recipients*		Automatically eligible	Automatically eligible	Automatically eligible
Former SSI recipients ("Pickle Amendment"— Persons who would meet SSI standard but for Social Security cost-of-living increase)		Greater than 100 percent; less than $3,000 per couple	Less than $2,000	
Medicaid Spend Down	Within this limit, MassHealth will pay the Medicare beneficiary's cost-sharing liability, which includes paying the MC premiums, deductibles, and coinsurance for MC Part A and Part B.	Income minus medical bills must be less than or equal to $522/month per individual; $650/month per couple	Less than $2,000	Less than $3,000
MassHealth Senior Buy-In				
Qualified MC Beneficiary (QMB)	Pays for MC premiums, deductibles and coinsurance for MC Part A and Part B	Less than or equal to 100 percent FPL; $716/month per individual, $958/month per couple	$4,000 or less	$6,000 per couple living together
Specified Low-Income Beneficiaries (SLMB)	Pays the monthly MC Part B premium	Between 100 percent and 120 percent FPL, $855/month per individual; $1,145/month per couple	$4,000 or less	$6,000 per couple living together

(Table 8.4 Continued)

MassHealth Program	Description of Coverage	Income Requirements	Asset Limit: Individual***	Asset Limit: Couple***
Qualifying Individuals 1 (QI 1)**	Pays the monthly MC Part B premium	Between 120 percent and 135 percent FPL; $960/month per individual; $1,286/month per couple	$4,000 or less	$6,000 per couple living together
Qualifying Individuals 2 (QI 2)**	Pays $2.87 monthly per person toward the MC Part B premium; payments made directly to individual.	Between 135 percent and 175 percent FPL; $1,238/month per individual; $1,661/month per couple	$4,000 or less	$6,000 per couple living together

Table 8.4. MassHealth Eligibility Standards for Medicare-Related Programs.

Notes: *SSI is a cash assistance program for those who are aged, blind, or disabled. SSI recipients (present and former) whose income, assets, or both exceed the limits may become eligible by reducing their assets, meeting a deductible, or both.

**Limit on total expenditures for the Qualifying Individual Programs (QI 1 and QI 2): "If enough money is not available to provide benefits for all eligible individuals, preference is given to members who were qualified for MassHealth Buy-In or MassHealth Senior Buy-In the previous year." MassHealth Buy-In pays private health insurance premiums for persons under age sixty-five.

***Assets excluded: The home in which individual resides, certain household goods and personal belongings, one car, irrevocable burial contracts, up to $1,500 in separate burial account for an individual and his or her spouse.

New York. Medicaid is the second-largest item in the state's general fund budget, after elementary and secondary education. The program accounted for 13 percent of state general revenue spending, and 22 percent of the entire state budget (which includes funding from federal and other sources). As shown in Table 8.5, long-term care is a higher percentage of Medicaid spending in Massachusetts than nationally. The proportion of Medicaid beneficiaries in Massachusetts who are elderly is somewhat higher than the national average. (See Table 8.6.)

There were approximately 106,000 dual-eligible individuals in Massachusetts in 1996. Most dual-eligible individuals receive full Medicaid coverage. Some other low-income disabled and elderly Medicare beneficiaries have incomes too high to be eligible for full Medicaid coverage, but qualify for Medicaid's assistance with Medicare cost-sharing or payment of the Medicare Part B premium. Most of this latter group of beneficiaries count as Qualified Medicare Beneficiaries (QMB) or Specified Low Income Medicare Beneficiaries (SLMB). However, the focus of this chapter is dual-eligibles who receive full Medicaid benefits.

In calendar year 1997, the total Medicaid expense in serving the dual-eligible population was projected to be $1.44 billion. Approximately 83 percent, or $1.20 billion, of this spending went toward long-term care services, primarily nursing facilities. Medicare spending on dual-eligible seniors in 1997 in Massachusetts was projected to be $960 million.

As shown in Table 8.7, Medicaid expenditures for long-term care grew at a modest annual rate of 5.2 percent from 1990 to 1995, compared to an annual increase of 10.7 percent nationally. State officials attribute this modest growth to a variety of efforts to moderate nursing home spending, including restructuring admission criteria, freezing the supply of beds, and squeezing reimbursements. DMA reimburses nursing homes using a prospective, cost-based, resident-specific rate methodology. Care for each resident is based on one of ten rates per facility, determined by the resident's level of disability. In 1995, the average nursing home rate per day was $94.25, one of the highest in the country. The state has been very aggressive in negotiating very low increases in this rate of payment since then. DMA also attempted to raise the level of disability needed to qualify for nursing home placement, but this met resistance from the nursing home industry and elder advocates and was defeated by the legislature.

	Total Long-Term Care Spending (billion)	Long-Term Care as Percentage of Total Medicaid Spending	Spending per Elderly Beneficiary	Spending per Elderly Resident	Percentage of Long-Term Care by Type			
					Nursing Facility	Mental Health	Home Care	Other
Massachusetts	$1.3	23.3	$12,872	$1,763	92.7	1.1	4.0	2.3
United States	$30.4	19.5	$7,821	$967	84.1	3.6	10.3	2.0

Table 8.5. Medicaid Long-Term Care Expenditures: United States and Massachusetts: 1995.

Source: Weiner and Stevenson, 1998.

	Elderly Population	Elderly as Percentage of Total Population	Number of Elderly Medicaid Beneficiaries	Elderly as Percentage of Total Medicaid Beneficiaries
Massachusetts	841,000	14.1	101,000	14.0
United States	34,100,000	12.8	3,889,000	11.1

Table 8.6.   Number of Elderly and Elderly Medicaid Beneficiaries: 1996.
Source: Massachusetts Division of Medical Assistance, unpublished data provided to the authors by staff.

	LTC Expenditures (million)						Average Annual Percentage		
	1990	1991	1992	1993	1994	1995	1990–1995	1990–1993	1993–1995
Total	$1,010	$1,061	$1,087	$957	$1,136	$1,302	5.2	−1.8	16.7
Nursing home	$950	$1,006	$1,027	$900	$1,065	$1,208	4.9	−1.8	15.8
Other	$21	$18	$20	$16	$15	$29	7.0	−7.9	33.9
Mental health	$2	$1	$5	$7	$9	$14	43.2	41.7	45.6
Home care	$38	$37	$36	$34	$46	$52	6.9	−3.3	24.1

Table 8.7.   Massachusetts Medicaid Long-Term Care Expenditures.
Source: Weiner and Stevenson, 1998.

DMA also funds a range of home and community-based services as one strategy to divert people from inappropriate and expensive nursing home care. Medicaid also covers a variety of home and community services, including home health care, adult day health care, adult foster care, group adult foster care, hospice care, case management, private duty nursing, and personal care services. As with other Medicaid benefits, home and community-based services are offered as open-ended benefits, without cost-sharing or benefit maximums. To control payment for these services, DMA imposes strict medical necessity criteria and prior approval requirements. "We do not pay for services if they are not medically necessary," said a DMA clinician. "We don't cover respite care or social supports. That is not the purpose of the program."

In addition to the long-term care benefits covered for regular MassHealth members, the state also operates a Home and Community-Based Services Waiver Program targeted to low-income, frail elders who are eligible for institutional care but want to remain in the community. It offers a range of services not otherwise covered by Medicaid, including homemaking services, residential support, and respite care. Eligible elders have access to all MassHealth services. Approximately 3,700 elders were in the program in 1997.

Medicaid has pursued an aggressive strategy of billing Medicare whenever possible for nursing facility and home health services. "Medicaid should be the payer of last resort, and we have been tough on Medicare, tough on consumers trying to qualify for Medicaid by transferring assets, and vigilant in recovering payments from estates when beneficiaries die," said one DMA official. "We also killed a proposal for a private-public partnership to promote long-term care insurance developed under Dukakis [the previous Democratic governor] because it would have made Medicaid easier to get for the middle class."

The state has also been aggressive on the revenue side, engaging in active efforts to maximize the amount of federal matching funds for MassHealth (called FFP, for federal financial participation). For example, the state has passed some of the appropriation for the Departments of Mental Retardation and Mental Health through the Medicaid budget so that this spending will technically qualify as state Medicaid spending and be eligible for federal matching funds.

The Massachusetts Home Care Program and ASAPs

In addition to Medicaid expenditures, the state also spent $120 million on state-funded home and community-based care for the elderly through the state's Home Care Program. This program, administered by the Executive Office of Elder Affairs (EOEA), provides home care services to eligible low-income elders. Financial eligibility criteria are separate from those for MassHealth and are based on income rather than assets. The criteria vary from year to year. In 1996, elders with incomes below approximately $18,000 for an individual and $25,000 for a two-person household were eligible. In general, elders must have a care need other than assistance in managing activities of daily living to qualify for services. The Home Care Program is subject to a limited appropriation rather than being an open-ended entitlement. This means that the program limits the amount of services provided to otherwise eligible elders if demand exceeds the amount budgeted by the state legislature.

EOEA provides services through a system of Aging Services Access Points (ASAPs), formerly known as home care corporations. The twenty-seven ASAPs are local, private nonprofit agencies designed to provide one-stop shopping for community-based long-term care, and generally also serve as the federal Area Agency on Aging for their geographical areas. ASAPs are geographically based and provide services in specific, nonoverlapping regions. Under the Home Care Program, ASAP case managers arrange community-based services (personal care, homemaker services, home-delivered meals) to enable local elders to live in the community safely and independently for as long as possible. Some ASAPs also provide care management services to private, paying clients who do not meet the income eligibility criteria for the Home Care Program.

ASAPs also administer two relatively small EOEA programs for high-risk elders. The Managed Care in Housing Program provides personal care and after-hours support to high-risk elders in housing complexes. It provides twenty-four-hour emergency response, as well as a range of individualized services such as adult day health, adult foster care, and in-home services.

The Enhanced Community Options program provides similar community-based services to elders who live in their own homes.

The ASAPs also perform certain functions for the state Medicaid program, including preadmission screening for all Medicaid clients seeking nursing home care, with the goal of diverting these individuals to the community if possible.

THE MASSACHUSETTS APPROACH TO THE DUAL-ELIGIBLE

For several years Massachusetts had worked with the other New England states and HCFA (now CMS) to develop a regional approach to integrated care for dual-eligibles. But this regional effort faltered, and Massachusetts had decided to go it alone and design a new program to manage care for the dual-eligible. As one advocate told us, "It was apparent that all of the New England states are different. Some are rural, some have much higher numbers of uninsured, some have no managed care penetration, and some have very little agency infrastructure to support this type of program. The politics in the other states are all different too. Only one of the states other than Massachusetts had a chance of actually doing a program for the dual-eligible. The nursing home industry there gave a big donation to the governor and he killed the initiative."

One of the major challenges to the planning process in Massachusetts was to obtain data on the dual-eligible population from Medicare and Medicaid. With the cooperation of HCFA, DMA undertook a complicated process to merge claims data files from Medicare and Medicaid. The results provided much more detailed information on dual-eligible individuals than was ever available before. Some of the results of DMA's analysis of state and national data on the dual-eligible are outlined here:

Of the 136,000 dual-eligible individuals in Massachusetts, 92,000— or two-thirds—were elderly, and one-third were disabled under age sixty-five. One-third of dual-eligible elders were institutionalized.

Based on national data, compared to other Medicare beneficiaries, dual-eligibles are more likely to have one or more chronic conditions. A significant proportion are cognitively impaired. They are much more likely to need help with activities of daily living, and almost one-fifth need help with four or more of these ADLs, which is total dependency. Dual-eligible individuals are much heavier users of acute care and long-term care services.

As noted earlier, dual-eligibles account for a disproportionate share of Medicare and Medicaid spending. In Massachusetts, Medicaid spending per beneficiary on the dual-eligible was more than seven times the spending on individuals enrolled through the Transitional Assistance to Needy Families (TANF) program, $14,097 and $1,857 respectively.

The data confirmed the cost-shifting incentives under the two systems. The average overall costs for frail elders in the community were significantly less than for frail elders living in institutions ($2,380 versus $3,310 per member per month, respectively). But the distribution of costs between Medicare and Medicaid was much different. Medicare costs were nearly three times as high for elders receiving care in the community compared to institutionalized elders, while Medicaid costs were much lower for elders receiving community-based care.

According to national data, dual-eligibles were more than twice as likely as other Medicare beneficiaries to be hospitalized for preventable conditions.

DMA's belief that a managed care approach could improve care and reduce costs for dual-eligibles comes, at least in part, from the state's experience with managed care for other groups covered by Medicaid.

"We have gotten excellent value from our managed care programs," said a DMA staffer. "The same benefits of care coordination and management oversight could be brought to bear successfully for dual-eligibles. The purchasing expertise and infrastructure already in place would be directly applicable to a new program for dual-eligibles."

Massachusetts instituted statewide mandatory enrollment in managed care for most Medicaid clients in 1992. Of approximately 650,000 Medicaid beneficiaries, 378,000 are subject to mandatory managed care enrollment for most care. Beneficiaries age sixty-five or older form the major group not required to enroll in one of the state's managed care programs.

Medicaid managed care members had a choice of several managed care plans. About 75 percent of Medicaid managed care members selected the Primary Care Clinician Program, a fee-for-service gatekeeper model plan administered by DMA. The other quarter of Medicaid managed care members were enrolled in one of several HMOs that contract with DMA. Although DMA would like to move more Medicaid members into HMOs, enrollment in HMOs has been flat since 1993. Some of the contracting HMOs did business with Medicaid only so they could have access to contracts for state employees and retirees, which the state offered only to HMOs with Medicaid contracts. In particular, many HMOs expressed frustration over the low rates of payment they received from DMA, as well as the significant oversight by DMA. "The rates are far too low and the administrative costs of dealing with DMA are incredible," said one HMO official. "There is not another purchaser that exercises such micromanagement over us. If we didn't think we'd get bad publicity, we'd cancel our DMA contract."

Possible Approaches

DMA would like to develop an approach to integrate payment and service delivery for dual-eligibles. The new program would combine funding from Medicare and Medicaid, administered by the state on behalf of both programs. DMA would use this funding to provide the full Medicare and Medicaid benefit package while instituting new managed care approaches to reduce the use of institutional services (hospital and nursing home) and make the programs work together instead of against each other.

The state was aware that dual-eligibles have not shown great enthusiasm thus far for managed care on a voluntary basis. Less than

5 percent of dual-eligibles in the United States have enrolled in traditional Medicare HMO plans, less than one-third the rate of other Medicare beneficiaries. In Massachusetts, the proportion is no higher, even though Medicare HMO penetration in the state is nearly double the national average. DMA officials were not surprised or discouraged by these figures. "Medicare HMOs provide little of value to dual-eligibles," said a senior DMA official, who continued,

> The plans only manage Medicare benefits, so they don't address the lack of coordination between Medicare and Medicaid, or the problems integrating long-term care, acute care, and social services. Dual-eligibles have absolutely no financial incentive to enroll in Medicare HMOs because of their Medicaid coverage. All of the cost-sharing in Medicare is picked up by the state, and they get all these additional benefits as well. Plus they keep complete freedom of choice of provider. Most dual-eligibles never had employer-sponsored health insurance so they also have no experience with managed care. Would you join a Medicare HMO if you were dual-eligible? I sure wouldn't!

PACE-TYPE PLANS. Rather than look at the poor record of Medicare HMOs in serving dual-eligibles, DMA was inspired by another managed care program for frail elders called the Program of All-Inclusive Care for Elders (PACE). PACE was instituted by HCFA in 1990 as a demonstration program, with funding from HCFA and the Robert Wood Johnson Foundation, to allow the development of a series of pilot managed care plans for frail elders, using pooled capitation. (The 1997 federal Balanced Budget Act changed PACE into a permanent program.) PACE was modeled on the On-Lok program in San Francisco, which had been successfully operating since 1971. As of 1996, there were twenty-four PACE sites across the country, including five in Massachusetts.

PACE programs are designed to help frail elders remain as healthy and independent as possible, while staying in the community as long as possible. Individuals must be certified as nursing home eligible to enroll in a PACE program. (The certification is done by the local ASAP in Massachusetts.) The program provides all services covered by Medicare and Medicaid, including acute and long-term care services, in return for a capitation payment from Medicare and Medicaid. Medicare pays 2.39 times the adjusted average per capita cost (AAPCC) for each member. The AAPCC is the methodology used by

Medicare to pay Medicare HMOs. Payment varies depending on certain member characteristics, such as age, sex, county of residence, institutionalization, disability, and Medicaid status. On average, Medicaid pays 88 percent of the estimated Medicaid costs in the fee-for-service system for a similar population.

PACE programs then use these capitation payments to create integrated models of care. Most PACE programs include two central features. They have *interdisciplinary geriatric teams,* consisting of a physician, nurse practitioner, social worker, nutritionist, home health aide, rehabilitation specialist, and home care coordinator. This team provides or arranges for all care of participants, and is available twenty-four hours a day. Participants must use the PACE doctor as their primary care physician. In addition, they offer an *adult day health center,* which provides a range of services on site, including podiatry, rehabilitation therapy, social services (for example, personal support, assistance with financial aid), prescription pickup, hot meals, and recreational activities. Participants are generally required to come to the adult day health center at least two or three time per week, both for services and so that they can be evaluated by the care team. The program arranges transportation for all participants.

PACE programs across the country have been shown to improve quality and reduce overall costs by 20–40 percent, mainly by keeping participants out of hospitals and nursing homes. This track record impressed DMA. "We looked at the PACE experience and saw significantly better quality measures, very high patient and family satisfaction, and much lower costs," one DMA executive said. "This showed us that it's possible to redesign care if you combine the funding streams from Medicare and Medicaid."

Despite these impressive results, only six thousand frail elders were enrolled in PACE programs nationwide. Marketing has been a major challenge for most sites. A major obstacle has been the requirement that participants must change their primary care provider to one of the limited number affiliated with PACE. Frail elders who are not poor enough to be eligible for Medicaid can buy into PACE programs, provided they have Medicare coverage and have been certified as nursing home eligible. But the cost is generally at least $2,000 per month, and few of these elders can afford PACE until they spend down their assets to qualify for Medicaid. Those who could afford the personal contribution, middle- and upper-income individuals, are among the least likely to give up their existing primary care physician relationship.

OTHER OPTIONS. DMA was considering a number of possible approaches to better manage care for some or all dual-eligibles. Among the most notable were the following:

- An intensive case management program for frail elders in the community and for nursing home residents to better coordinate acute care and long-term care services. The state could create its own program, as it had done with the Primary Care Clinician program, or contract with an outside entity to provide case management services on a fee-for-service or capitation basis.

- Carving out long-term care services from the rest of the Medicaid benefit package and contracting on a full-risk or partial-risk basis to a third party that would provide or manage these services (similar to the approach DMA had adopted for behavioral health services).

- Develop programs for targeted groups of dual-eligibles (for example, individuals with Alzheimer's disease or other cognitive impairments). DMA had used this approach successfully in the under-sixty-five population for individuals with HIV and severe physical disabilities.

- A state-supported expansion of the PACE program, to make start-up funds and technical assistance support available to qualified entities interested in setting up PACE programs.

- Expanding the PACE model to include groups of dual-eligibles other than those who were already nursing home eligible. Under this approach, DMA would contract with managed care plans, provider systems, and other entities to provide all Medicare and Medicaid covered services to dual-eligibles on a capitated basis.

DMA did not see these approaches as mutually exclusive.

The Political Lay of the Land

The state's approach to this problem would require the support and approval of numerous other organizations. Among the key players were HCFA, elder advocates, and the provider community.

No new approach to the dual-eligible could be adopted without the approval of HCFA. In general, the federal government supported the policy goal of improving care and reducing costs for the dual-eligible population. But any approach would be subject to a number of requirements, including a demonstration that it was budget neutral (that is, did not increase the cost for the federal government). This meant that the state government would ultimately bear the financial risk of any new approach. While DMA had a good and productive relationship with HCFA, it knew that the process, personalities, and politics of the federal review and approval process would be brutal. According to one senior DMA official:

> HCFA is completely dominated by Medicare staff. The agency has only a small Medicaid outpost. There is also no rational organizational structure in the agency, and it is constantly reorganizing. This uncertainty results in a lot of unproductive politicking and positioning. The HCFA staff are suspicious, alarmist, and distrustful of states. You cannot trust them. And they are threatened by state proposals. They don't understand that health care is a local issue and it needs a light touch—not a command-and-control model. It takes years of lobbying and meetings to get anything done. The Medicaid director's group is taking up the issue of the dual-eligible as a test case to see whether states can actually do something. But that was also a struggle. Long-term care politics are brutal for Medicaid directors because of the political power of nursing homes and the power of seniors. So it is just easier for state Medicaid directors to stay away from long-term care.

When Massachusetts first began working with the other New England states to attempt to develop a regional approach to the dual-eligible, the advocacy community began to organize. Over a dozen community groups formed the Senior Health Care Coalition (the Coalition), with the goals of helping "shape the future of the health and long-term care system for elders in Massachusetts" and "to ensure that any new program contains adequate protections for consumers." The membership of the Coalition was diverse, and included the largest and most powerful consumer and elder organizations in the state (for example, Massachusetts Senior Action, AARP, Health Care for All, and the Older Women's League), as well as some providers, most notably Massachusetts Home Care, which represented the ASAPs.

The Coalition supported DMA's overall goals. "We think it is vital to alleviate fragmentation in the delivery system and to coordinate acute and long-term care," said one Coalition member. "We should not allow the financing scheme to be the determining factor in what services elders get. The system is Byzantine and fragmented, and you need a Ph.D. in health care to get it. In fact, even a Ph.D. is not enough."

But at the same time, advocates had numerous concerns. They were wary of managed care in general and particularly concerned about any proposal that included capitation to managed care plans or providers. "We think capitation would provide a great opportunity for managed care plans to profit by underserving frail and vulnerable elders," said a member of the Coalition. "There is almost no expertise anywhere in managing care of frail elders. Certainly most of the managed care plans have no experience with this population. Managed care will become a vehicle for rationed care."

Long-term care providers had a variety of other concerns. The ASAPs believed that the state might undermine their unique role helping elders navigate through the long-term care system. According to one ASAP executive, "We worked for years to create a coordinated, geographically based system for providing home and community services. The system will be destroyed if DMA carves out services or lets managed care plans take control. Neither of them knows the community services. We need to build on the resources that exist, not just go around them." But other observers believed the ASAPs' interests were really self-serving. "The home cares are just concerned that they may not all do as well if they have to contract through a third party," said one provider. "Now they have their nice geographic monopolies and they don't have to compete."

The nursing home industry felt the DMA initiative as a direct attack. An industry member said,

> We're afraid this initiative will just be a cost-savings measure, disguised in improving-care clothing. Nursing homes have been chronically underfunded by Medicaid for years. The first goal DMA announced was to prevent or delay institutionalization. Well, that was a problem for us. We support preventing inappropriate nursing home stays, but we don't support postponing appropriate ones. We think DMA will try to keep people out of nursing homes, even if that is the best place for them to be. And they won't provide enough other services to maintain people decently at home. It would be the long-term care equivalent of deinstitutionalization of the mentally ill in the 1970s. That would be even worse than our current system.

Observers of the nursing home industry noted, however, that the industry did not necessarily have a united front. "Nursing homes are concerned about any change that would allow selective contracting," said one person. "There is a real mix of nursing homes in Massachusetts and excess capacity. The nonprofits and family-owned facilities are worried that the for-profit chains will strike good deals and put them out of business."

Advocates and providers were also concerned that a managed care initiative might be used by DMA as a means to tighten the clinical standards for nursing home care and other services, attempts they had thwarted in the past. Eligibility for Medicaid-covered nursing facility care was currently based on the so-called Score 3 criterion, which meant that the individual had to meet a clinical standard of three care needs, one of which was a nursing need and two of which could be the need for ADL (Activities of Daily Living) assistance (Score 3). Advocates and providers were adamant that Score 3 continue to be the maximum threshold.

The Choices Confronting DMA

As DMA moved forward to design its managed care approach for dual-eligibles, it needed to decide which programmatic approaches it would adopt. It also needed to make a number of other key decisions:

• *Which elderly dual-eligibles to include?* DMA had definitely decided to focus its initiative on elderly dual-eligibles. But within this group it could target elders residing in nursing facilities, for whom Medicaid was by far the dominant payer, or elders in the community, whose costs were borne more by Medicare, or both.

Some DMA staff were also urging the inclusion of an "early enrollment option," which would allow frail elders of modest income who were not yet eligible for Medicaid to buy into the Medicaid program so their care could be managed before they became eligible for Medicaid, most likely after they entered a nursing home. The goal of this option would be to provide case management, Medicaid services, and social supports to these elders to prevent, or at least delay, nursing home admission.

• *Should the program be mandatory or voluntary?* Providers and advocates were united in their position that any new managed care initiative should be voluntary for dual-eligible individuals. The Coalition's position was clear: "One of the criteria used to evaluate any new program should be whether people will join it." The group also opposed the use of any penalties to encourage elders to enroll in a managed care program. According to one advocate, "We oppose any negative incentives to force elders out of the traditional Medicaid program. Our position is: no increased copayments, no reduction in benefits, no narrower provider networks, no tighter clinical criteria, no financial requirements in terms of assets or income if people want to stay in the regular program." They also insisted that elders have the freedom to enroll and disenroll from any managed care program at any time and return to the traditional Medicaid program. "People need a meaningful choice of providers, particularly nursing homes. Some people have religious, specialty, or ethnic reasons for wanting to be in a particular nursing home. DMA must accommodate these preferences in any new program, otherwise elders could end up in nursing homes far away from their families and have no recourse."

But DMA was not yet persuaded that a voluntary program would achieve its goals. It had successfully mandated managed care for most of its other populations. It was particularly concerned that if the program was voluntary, there were few positive incentives it could incorporate to make enrollment attractive. The PACE program was having marketing problems and it provided a range of additional benefits to elders. DMA also knew that providers and advocates had the political power to oppose the use of negative incentives.

• *Should the initiative be designed as a pilot or as a statewide program?* The Coalition favored implementing any new approach on a pilot basis. "We think a full-blown program would be a bad idea," said a Coalition member. "It would be better for DMA to encourage a limited demonstration, perhaps of a number of new ideas, and then evaluate those approaches before moving forward with a statewide program. You cannot make the most frail and vulnerable join a managed care program until you know it works." But DMA was interested in a big and bold new initiative. "The tendency of the providers and advocates is to fear change more than the status quo because they are risk averse," said one government official. "If we are that timid, nothing will ever change. If you want to have a major effect on a system that's badly broken, you can't rely on aspirin and Band-Aids."

Many observers agreed with DMA that the current system needed major reform. But they were somewhat less sanguine about the prospects for achieving it. "No one likes to talk about this, but much of the publicly funded long-term care system is poor women taking care of even poorer women," said one long-term care consultant. "They are not empowered advocates for themselves. So change comes about based on the political power of other interest groups. The current medical and long-term care systems have lots of vested interests.

As much as people really do want a better system, every group will hang onto their piece of the pie come hell or high water. In the final analysis, people might just care more about turf and money than about designing a better system."

FOUR YEARS LATER . . . JULY 2000

Since 1996, the DMA has made considerable progress on developing its managed care initiative for dual-eligible individuals. As DMA anticipated, the process was slow and complex, and involved significant negotiation with the federal HCFA, providers, and advocates for the elderly.

The new program is called MassHealth Senior Care Options. Through this program DMA and HCFA will offer dual-eligible elders the option of joining comprehensive, integrated managed care programs, to be called Senior Care Organizations (SCOs). SCOs do not exist at the time of this writing, but it is DMA's hope that they will be created by a variety of entities, including managed care plans, provider systems, and community-based organizations. DMA and HCFA will contract with SCOs to provide or arrange for the delivery of all Medicare and Medicaid covered services, including primary, acute, and specialty care; institutional and community-based long-term care; and mental health and substance abuse services. SCOs will receive separate monthly prepaid capitation payments from DMA and HCFA, resulting in an integration of Medicare and Medicaid funding at the SCO level. DMA hopes SCOs will become operational in early 2001. (See the Epilogue to this chapter for developments through early 2003.)

DMA filed its application for the Senior Care Options program with HCFA in June 1997. The application was amended in October 1998, to address concerns raised by HCFA and to reflect the fact that the passage of the 1997 federal Balanced Budget Act eliminated the need for DMA to seek a federal waiver for the Medicaid portion of the proposal. HCFA approved the proposal in principle in March 1999, with the Medicare portion of the program approved as a five-year demonstration project. DMA and HCFA subsequently negotiated a memorandum of understanding that will govern the procurement, financing, and administration of the project.

Before and during the HCFA review process, DMA undertook a range of activities to involve interested parties in the Senior Care Options Initiative. Three public advisory groups—one each for consumers (Medicaid recipients), advocates, and providers—were formed and met regularly, as did workgroups on integrated care delivery and outreach and education approaches. DMA circulated a draft of its application to HCFA, and a draft of SCO purchasing specifications to the public for review and comment. DMA also held a series of technical assistance workshops to assist provider networks considering bidding to become a SCO.

DMA viewed this public development process as, in the words of one senior official, "by far the most input we have ever gotten from the public on any subject," but the views of advocates and providers were somewhat mixed. "Their process initially was nonexistent," said one advocate. "DMA's attitude was, 'OK, now we have gotten all the younger recipients into managed care, it's time to do the elderly.' But they learned fast and they came to work well with elder advocacy groups." Another advocate agreed, "DMA worked hard over the last four years to develop good will, and we got lots of what we wanted. Although we still aren't excited by the SCO idea, we have decided it's time to get off the dime and hold our breath and try. We will suffer less harm by trying something new and seeing if it works than by not doing anything."

But others are critical of the SCO development process. "Providers have been viewed as the enemy since the beginning of the process," said one hospital representative, "DMA never involved us in any meaningful way. We were invited to the so-called consultative sessions and then lectured at all day. No one really wants to hear our opinions. All the decisions had already been made—they were a fait accompli. DMA just told us what they were going to do." An elder advocate echoed this view: "We got access from DMA. They would listen, nod their heads, and then never change anything. They went to HCFA for approval before they had a plan that was acceptable to all parties. Now they are trying to shove a bill through the legislature at the last minute to get the state approvals needed to go forward with the SCO initiative. DMA did not want to get the legislature involved until HCFA was already approved. So the legislature has become the final battleground. We want to get all the key features of the program we care about into statute so DMA will have no discretion to change them."

A bill to authorize the Senior Care Options Program is pending in the state legislature. One of the key bones of contention is the clinical criteria that may be used by SCOs to determine eligibility for home care services. The Aging Services Access Points (ASAPs) are arguing that SCOs should be required to provide home care benefits if a member has at least two ADL impairments. DMA and most other interested parties support a tougher standard of two ADL impairments and one skilled care need, arguing that the more lenient standard supported by the ASAPs would make a much higher portion of dual-eligibles in the community eligible for home care services than under the current Medicaid program, thereby greatly increasing the cost of the program. "It's an unfunded mandate," said one advocate. "I think it would be great to provide unlimited home care to everyone who might benefit from it, but that's living in fiscal la-la land."

Although most observers believe the state legislature will pass a SCO bill, its content is unclear. But even with federal and state government approvals, the road ahead for the Senior Care Options program still looks somewhat rocky.

Key Features of the SCO Program

The key objectives of the Senior Care Options initiative, as articulated by DMA, are as follows:

- To improve the quality and coordination of care provided to dual-eligible and MassHealth-only seniors (that is, those who qualify for MassHealth but are not eligible for Medicare, usually because they haven't worked enough quarters to qualify for Social Security)
- To expand their access to covered services
- To maximize their satisfaction with services provided
- To increase the cost-effectiveness of care

Among the key aspects of the SCO program are the following:

- Dual-eligible elders and elders covered only by Medicaid (MassHealth-only seniors) will be eligible to join a SCO. Assuming qualified bidders present themselves in every area of the state, DMA intends to implement the Senior Care Options Program on a statewide basis.
- Enrollment in SCOs will be voluntary, and members will be able to disenroll from a SCO and return to the traditional Medicaid program at any time.
- DMA and HCFA will jointly select qualified SCOs through a selective contracting process. DMA has developed a draft of

detailed "Purchasing Specifications" that will govern the process of SCO contracting and contract management. (DMA uses this same type of contracting approach in its contracts with other managed care plans.) A copy of excerpts from the draft purchasing specifications is included as Exhibit 8.1, just before the Epilogue, to put the discussion in this chapter in context.

- An independent third-party enrollment broker, hired by DMA, will conduct all SCO enrollments to explain enrollment options to elders in a clear and objective manner.

- SCOs will be required to contract with ASAPs, which will employ geriatric support services coordinators to manage community long-term care services for SCO members. The state EOEA will assist DMA in implementing this provision of the initiative, as well as provide other support, as outlined in a formal letter of agreement between DMA and EOEA.

- DMA and HCFA will each make a separate capitation payment to SCOs for each member, permitting an integration of payment streams and an elimination of the incentive for cost-shifting between Medicare and Medicaid.

The Medicare capitation will be based on the AAPCC payment methodology used by HCFA for Medicare HMOs (now called Medicare+Choice plans), with a different risk adjustment factor for frail elders living in the community. (HCFA agreed to incorporate this risk adjuster after DMA's analysis of the linked Medicare and Medicaid claims data demonstrated that the standard AAPCC payment methodology would result in significant underpayments by Medicare for individuals living in the community who meet nursing home eligibility criteria.)

The Medicaid capitation will be based on a standard methodology called the Upper Payment Limit, which ensures that Medicaid payments for SCO members will not exceed the cost of providing Medicaid-covered services to an actuarially equivalent population. (This limit on Medicaid payments was required by HCFA to ensure that the Senior Care Options program will be budget neutral in terms of the federal government's share of Medicaid costs for the program.) Separate Medicaid rating categories will be developed for each of four populations of dual-eligibles: nursing home residents, with three rate subcategories based on patient acuity (expected need for medical and daily living services), using Medicaid's case mix categories for nursing home patients; community frail (who meet the state's nursing facility eligibility criteria); community residents with a diagnosis of Alzheimer's disease, dementia, or chronic mental illness; and all other community-dwelling elders. There will be two separate rates for each category of community-based elders, one for residents in certain towns in the greater Boston area and another for individuals living elsewhere in the state. (Table 8.8 shows sample capitation rates developed by DMA.)

The final form of the Senior Care Options program is different in some respects from DMA's original design. According to one health policy observer,

> HCFA was a major reason for the delay in getting this program off the ground. They are overwhelmed as an agency with all the things they have to do and it takes them forever to review everything. The feds would not agree to a mandatory program—it had to be voluntary for beneficiaries. They would not approve the early enrollment option because they said it did not meet the budget neutrality test. They would not agree to a single payment methodology but insisted on having separate Medicaid and Medicare capitations. They would not agree to have the program managed solely by DMA with delegated authority from HCFA. One of our biggest fears, and that of many potential bidders, is that HCFA and DMA will continue to be tangled up in their own arguments once the program gets going. The big question is going to be: How much will Medicare interfere? Medicare tries to turn everything into fee for service.

Concerns About the Draft Purchasing Specifications

Many of the entities that participated in the SCO development process express reservations about major aspects of the initiative, and about whether the timing is favorable for the project. The most common concerns about the program itself fall into several categories:

THE PAYMENT METHODOLOGY. Many worry that the proposed payment methodologies will produce inadequate capitation payments. A hospital expressed the common view: "The financing is just too risky. No one is making money now on the Medicare+Choice plans, which are

Female, Age 78, Living in Boston

Status	Community Resident: Alzheimer's Disease or Chronic Mental Illness	Community Resident: Nursing Home Certifiable	Community Resident: Other	Nursing Home Resident: Tier I (lowest acuity)
Medicare Rate	$847	$1,628	$847	$1,088
Medicaid Rate	$230	$1,585	$130	$2,200
Total Rate	$1,077	$3,213	$977	$3,288

Male, Age 67, Living in Framingham (western suburb of Boston)

Status	Community Resident: Alzheimer's Disease or Chronic Mental Illness	Community Resident: Nursing Home Certifiable	Community Resident: Other	Nursing Home Resident: Tier I (lowest acuity)
Medicare Rate	$608	$1,638	$608	$1,018
Medicaid Rate	$215	$1,490	$120	$2,200
Total Rate	$823	$3,128	$728	$3,218

Female, Age 87, Living in Worcester (central Massachusetts)

Status	Community Resident: Alzheimer's Disease or Chronic Mental Illness	Community Resident: Nursing Home Certifiable	Community Resident: Other	Nursing Home Resident: Tier I (lowest acuity)
Medicare Rate	$842	$1,346	$842	$1,092
Medicaid Rate	$215	$1,490	$120	$2,200
Total Rate	$1,057	$2,836	$962	$3,292

Table 8.8.   SCO Draft Monthly Rates: Calendar Year 2000.

Source: Massachusetts Division of Medical Assistance, 1999b.

paid using the same methodology. And SCOs will serve a much riskier population. We think the risk adjustment for the community frail is too low. Plus, SCOs will assume full financial risk, with no risk sharing by DMA or HCFA and no help with reinsurance. So you take a money-losing capitation and all of the new requirements in the purchasing specs, and this program sinks under its own weight." A PACE program manager noted, "The PACE rating methodology is hard to figure out for a couple hundred people. The SCO methodology is much more complex—more people and more rate cells. It is going to boggle the mind to project revenues accurately and then to reconcile payments. . . . Plus the state is offering no help with start-up costs, which PACE sites got. I find it very ironic that the DMA has asked for $10 million for its own start-up costs but no money for the SCOs."

MARKETING AND ENROLLMENT. Potential bidders worry that enrollment in SCOs will be small, particularly when SCOs will be unable to enroll elders directly but will be required to make referrals to the third-party enrollment broker. "The population of dual-eligibles is quite small, particularly in the suburbs," said one provider. "With a voluntary program, the likely number of enrollees will not support the costs of the program. We know this from the experience of the PACE programs." A colleague added, "You cannot spend time trying to market this program to elders in crisis and their families, and then make them take twenty steps back to talk to an enrollment broker who will show them all the options again. DMA and HCFA are so concerned that there are all these shady marketing practices out there but there's no evidence that's true for the dual-eligible population. Believe me, no one is going to make money off the Medicaid capitation."

THE MANDATED RELATIONSHIP WITH THE ASAPs. The requirement that SCOs contract with ASAPs is viewed as extremely problematic by many observers. "So the payment is low, the enrollment numbers don't look so hot, but maybe you think you can perform a miracle on the program side and really manage the hell out of the program," said one provider. "The only breath of hope here is case management—it is *the* vital service. But for purely political reasons, SCOs are required to use the ASAPs. So the case management function has been taken out of the SCO's control and turned over to an employee of another organization that has no ownership in or risk for the success of the SCO."

Another observer added, "The discussion about the role of the ASAPs was one of the more difficult parts of the process. The ASAPs are not part of the new reality of health care. They don't want to be competitive, they just want to provide services. So EOEA and DMA had a real tough time agreeing on the approach. Finally, one of the top state government people had to be brought in to broker a deal between the two agencies. The result is pure politics."

OTHER CONCERNS. Some of the other provisions of the draft purchasing specifications cause particular concern to potential bidders:

• *Care management and integration* (section 2 of the purchasing specifications): "These requirements are understandable but they will be hard to administer," said one long-term care provider. "They're drawn from a PACE model, where the individual comes in person to the adult day health at least three times per week and there's an interdisciplinary team on site, meeting every day, and they know all the patients very well. SCOs will be much more far-flung enterprises. There will be lots of doctors, most of whom will have only a few SCO members. You cannot expect the same level of case management, particularly when we have to use a geriatric care manager from the community who is not part of our organization and probably won't have any medical background.

• *Centralized enrollee record* (sections 2.7–2.9 of the purchasing specifications): "A good idea but not easy even for those of us with sophisticated systems," said one provider. "It will be a killer for others."

• *The program initiatives* (section 3 of the purchasing specifications): "All of these initiatives make sense, in an ideal world," said a managed care manager. "But in my world of limited resources, we don't adopt new clinical programs unless we can demonstrate that they produce savings. I don't think the scope of these initiatives is realistic for most entities that might want to become SCOs."

• *The financial stability requirements* (section 6 of the purchasing specifications): "We think these requirements favor large, capitalized vendors like nursing homes and hospital chains," complained one elder advocate. "Community-based agencies don't have $1.5 million in net worth, so they'll never be able to bid." But another advocate disagreed, "This is a financially risky proposition and shouldn't be undertaken by thinly capitalized entities. . . . The recent insolvency of Harvard Pilgrim Health Care [the state's largest HMO] taught us all a lesson about the need for tougher solvency requirements."

• *The reporting requirements* (section 7 of the purchasing specifications): "You can tell these requirements were thought up by someone who knows little about the information systems in most provider organizations," said one executive of a large delivery system. "Our system is really good and even we would never be able to produce all of this data. Even if we could, I don't understand what DMA would do with all of it."

Will Anyone Come to the SCO Party?

At this point, it is unclear how many potential SCOs might develop in response to the Senior Care Options initiative. Many observers believe the timing is not good. "Time has been a real player here," said one hospital executive. "Through no fault of DMA's, SCOs may just be a good idea at the wrong time." "I cannot think of a worse time to launch such an initiative," said a manager from a home care agency. "The HMOs are in terrible shape, the LTC companies are in terrible shape, and the hospital systems are in terrible shape. Who will take the risk? SCOs will be expensive, they have high fixed costs and start-up costs, and they will need capital." The view from another community provider was the same: "Five years ago, provider systems were supportive of vertical integration and interested in risk. As they have lost money, they are reducing investments and experimentation. The specialists are doing fine again and they are the major source of income for the hospitals. Nursing homes are less interested in initiatives like this—they are hurting and the level of service is dropping since the BBA hit. Home health is the worst—they are focused on survival. As each piece of the system is worried about its own bottom line, the interest in working together is evaporating. People are much less willing to experiment—they don't want to lose money."

Not everyone is worried about having only a few SCOs. "Many of us wanted this to be a demonstration all along so if there are only a few bidders and that's what we get by default, that's good," said one elder advocate. But other advocates are more concerned. "We still fear that the forces of evil will prevail," said another advocate. "There will be bidders. But they will be for-profit companies with deep pockets and strategic reasons for wanting a greater presence in the state. The irony may be that many of the things the advocates pushed for have guaranteed that they will get what they did not want most: big for-profit chains dominating the SCO landscape."

If You Build Them, Will They Come?

Even if SCOs do develop, the question of how many elders will join them remains open. "It's a good plan conceptually," said one nursing home person. "But it's flawed because it's voluntary and there are no new services. Why would you be willing to have your choice of provider limited for no new services? If PACE has problems marketing, how will

SCOs get many people to join? Elders don't want to be in nursing homes, so some might join a SCO to try to stay out as long as possible. But then if they need to go into a nursing home, they won't get to go where they want, so they will just disenroll and go back to fee for service. So there will be no real savings." A primary care doctor agreed, "In a way the Medicaid population will be the hardest to sell this program to. They already have the best insurance. The privately insured face more restrictions, more copays, less choice of providers. It would be an easier sell to them." He also noted, "People who are frail have constructed their own systems of care, and these would rarely correspond to whatever networks are put together by SCOs."

Other advocates expressed similar views. "There is no carrot now in the SCO program," said one. "SCOs can provide certain discretionary benefits if they want, but there won't be enough money in the capitations for that. So better care management is the only incentive. That's not going to be much of an advantage to the elders. These programs are very hard to understand. You won't realize what they provide until you get into them and need services. It's like the long-term care system generally. Plus most of the public thinks Medicare covers long-term care."

DMA believes that the promise of better coordination of care in the SCOs will be attractive to elders, along with other advantages like reduction in paperwork associated with Medicare, screening and risk assessment, and one-stop shopping for people using a range of services. "I would pitch the SCO concept to an elder based on the ability to build a system around your needs and not what the system pays for," said one DMA staffer. "There are many effective messengers for this notion, particularly physicians and other individuals who are already plugged in to the elders, like home health aides and meals on wheels. If SCOs can work with organizations that are already known and trusted in the communities, these connections can be made." A hospital executive thought the challenge would be great: "The current system is sheer confusion—where to go, who to see. Having a care manager is very attractive, someone who will put the services together. The caliber of support is the appeal to dual-eligibles. The message needs to be that we will help you stay out of a nursing home. But elders at highest risk are exactly the ones who want to preserve their rights to choose a nursing home and other providers."

Another factor working against the SCOs could be the recent track record of Medicare managed care plans. "Elders in many parts of the state have been left holding the bag when HMOs did their disappearing act the past couple of years," said one elder advocate, with good reason. In 1999, forty-five managed care organizations nationwide did not renew their contracts with Medicare, and fifty-four others reduced their service areas. These changes affected 407,000 beneficiaries nationwide, 51,000 of whom had no other managed care option. The disruption for Medicare enrollees continued in 2000, with forty-one withdrawals and fifty-eight service area reductions, affecting 327,000 people, 79,000 of whom had no other Medicare managed care plan available to them. More withdrawals have been announced for 2001. Managed care plans say the major problem is inadequate payment; federal officials discount these claims, saying Medicare managed care plans are overpaid as a result of positive selection. Managed care plans also criticize the amount of new regulation imposed on them by HCFA, which is complex and very costly to implement. The advocate adds, "The HMOs cried financial loss but they sure weren't complaining when they were making millions of dollars in recent years. Elders don't trust HMOs, and they will be very skeptical of any new managed care entities like SCOs."

But some DMA officials do not expect traditional managed care plans to be at the forefront of the SCO movement. "Managed care plans are not the best entities to lead the way on SCOs," according to one DMA executive. "Managed care plans are used to an insurance model, not a care management model. SCOs will have to overcome real cultural issues, particularly finding the right management team to shift the focus away from acute care. Long-term care managers are much better suited to playing the lead role—they understand the dynamics of continuum of care in a way that managed care folks and acute care providers do not."

What kind of impact SCOs can have on addressing the problems of the dual-eligible remains to be seen. As is usual in Massachusetts, skeptics are not hard to find. "I am afraid that changing the financing model will not completely change the system infrastructure and practice patterns," sighed one long-time observer of the system who has worked in the acute and long-term care sectors. "Deeply entrenched interests will not be swayed by this little managed care model, however pretty and well-intentioned. The hospitals in particular are entrenched into a 'feed and protect the beds mentality.' To get the waste out we would need to completely restructure the system. SCOs will not restructure the system." See Exhibit 8.1 for excerpts from the DMA SCO specifications.

Exhibit 8.1.   Excerpts from the DMA SCO Specifications.

INTRODUCTION

The Massachusetts Division of Medical Assistance (DMA) and the federal Health Care Financing Administration (HCFA) are establishing a comprehensive, integrated and coordinated program, entitled Senior Care Options, to deliver health care and related social support services for MassHealth members aged 65 years and over. All services currently covered by Medicare and Medicaid will be incorporated into the program, including primary, acute and specialty care; institutional and community-based long term care; mental health and substance abuse service. Qualified Senior Care Organizations (SCOs) shall each be responsible for the entire continuum of care for its Enrollees. Enrollment in a SCO will be voluntary for eligible individuals. SCOs will be required to contract for Geriatric Support Service Coordinators, on a selective contracting basis, with one or more Aging Services Access Points (ASAPs) designated by the Massachusetts Executive Office of Elder Affairs (EOEA), in order to assure effective collaboration between the medical and aging networks. State home care services, not funded by Medicaid, will continue to be available through the ASAPs according to current rules and regulations.

These Purchasing Specifications for a Senior Care Organization (SCO) are based on the concepts of a geriatric model of managed care. Medicare and Medicaid funding will be combined at the SCO level, with reimbursement to be prepaid and based on risk-adjusted capitation. DMA will work in partnership with HCFA to implement and monitor the SCO program.

Each SCO shall be responsible for the provision of all Covered Services in a manner consistent with the following objectives:

- To enhance the quality of life and autonomy of Enrollees;
- To maximize dignity and respect of Enrollees;
- To enable Enrollees to live in their homes and in the community as long as medically and socially feasible;
- To preserve and support the Enrollee's family unit; and,
- To coordinate primary, acute, specialty, mental health/substance abuse, and long term care services.

These Purchasing Specifications set forth the requirements that SCOs will be required to fulfill in order to qualify for contracts with DMA and HCFA. Information reported to DMA and HCFA in accordance with these specifications will be used to establish benchmarks and standards by which quality of care will be measured. Where applicable the requirements of the federal Quality Improvement System for Managed Care (QISMC) will apply.

DMA and HCFA will conduct a procurement to select and contract with qualified SCOs. DMA and HCFA will utilize a stringent contract management process to assure that the standards in these Purchasing Specifications are met. Failure to meet performance standards or any other contractual requirement will generate corrective action plans or other intermediate sanctions, and if unresolved, may result in termination of the SCO contract.

SECTION I: DEFINITIONS

1.1 **Advance Directives:** Written instructions, such as a living will or durable power of attorney for health care, recognized under state law, and relating to the provision of such care when the individual is incapacitated.

1.2 **Aging Services Access Point (ASAP):** Agency organized under section 4B under Chapter 19 MGL, under contract to the Executive Office of Elder Affairs to manage the state-funded home care program, and which serves as the Division's agent to perform screening and authorization activities for certain MassHealth long term care services.

1.3 **Centralized Enrollee Record:** Centralized and comprehensive documentation, containing information relevant to maintaining and promoting each Enrollee's general health and well-being, as well as clinical information concerning illnesses and chronic medical conditions. (See *Purchasing Specifications 2.6, 2.7, 2.8.*)

1.4 **Complex Care Needs:** Any condition or situation that demonstrates the Enrollee's need for expert coordination of multiple Senior Care Organization (SCO) services (see *Purchasing Specification 2.3*) including, but not limited to: eligibility for institutional long term care; medical or psychiatric illness or cognitive impairment which requires skilled nursing to manage essential unskilled services and care.

(Continued)

Exhibit 8.1.   Excerpts from the DMA SCO Specifications. (*Continued*)

1.5 Consumer: A MassHealth member, aged 65 or older, or the spouse, sibling, child, or unpaid primary caregiver of a MassHealth member who is aged 65 or older.

1.6 Covered Services: Those services listed in APPENDIX A [not included with this exhibit] delivered in accordance with these specifications.

1.7 Emergency Condition: A medical condition that manifests itself by acute symptoms of sufficient severity (including severe pain) such that a prudent lay person, who possesses an average knowledge of health and medicine, could reasonably expect the absence of immediate medical attention to result in: (1) placing the health of the individual in serious jeopardy; (2) serious impairment to bodily functions; or (3) serious dysfunction of any bodily organ or part.

1.8 Enrollee: A MassHealth member aged 65 or over, who is eligible for and who has voluntarily enrolled in a SCO.

1.9 Enrollee Services Representative (ESR): An employee of the Contractor who assists Enrollees with questions and concerns in accordance with *Purchasing Specification 4.14.*

1.10 Enrollment Broker: An agent under contract with DMA and HCFA who will perform outreach activities to educate potential Enrollees regarding all MassHealth enrollment options, and if a senior chooses a SCO will perform the operational enrollment process.

1.11 External Ombudsman: An entity designated by DMA and the Executive Office of Elder Affairs (EOEA) to assist the Enrollee with issues which have not been resolved by the Contractor to the satisfaction of the Enrollee.

1.12 Geriatric Support Services Coordinator: An employee of an Aging Services Access Point (ASAP) who meets the qualifications listed in *Purchasing Specification 5.4c* and performs the following:

  a. as a member of the Primary Care Team (PCT), participating in comprehensive assessments and reassessments of health and functional status, including determinations of appropriateness for institutional long term care services and developing community-based care plans and related service packages necessary to improve or maintain enrollee functional and health status.

b. arranging, and with the agreement of the PCT, coordinating and authorizing the provision of appropriate community long term care and social support services, such as assistance with the Activities of Daily Living (ADLs) and Instrumental Activities of Daily Living (IADLs), housing, home delivered meals and/or transportation; and, under specific conditions or circumstances established by the Contractor, authorizing a range and/or amount of community based services.

c. monitoring the appropriate provision and functional outcomes of community long term care services, according to the Enrollee's service plan, and making periodic adjustments to the service plan as deemed appropriate by the Primary Care Team.

d. tracking Enrollee transfers from one setting to another (e.g., hospital to home, nursing home to adult day health, etc.) and adjusting the service plan as deemed appropriate by the Primary Care Team.

1.13 Health Care Proxy: A document delineating to an agent the authority to make health care decisions in accordance with state and federal law, when a person is unable to make such decisions independently.

1.14 Informed Consent: A process in which an Enrollee has voluntarily agreed to a proposed procedure or treatment, or has voluntarily agreed to forego a proposed procedure or treatment, after the provider has disclosed to the Enrollee in a reasonable manner (i) all significant medical information that the provider possesses that is material to an intelligent decision by the Enrollee whether to undergo, or forgo, the proposed procedure of treatment, and (ii) any information required by applicable law.

1.15 Initial Assessment: An evaluation of clinical status, functional status, nutritional status, the medical history of the Enrollee and relevant family members and physical well-being, illnesses; screenings for mental health status, and tobacco, alcohol and drug use; and an assessment of the Enrollee's need for long term care services including the availability of informal support. For Enrollees who are able to self-report, the assessment shall include administration of the Health Outcomes Survey in accordance with HEDIS Reporting Set 3.0 requirements. In addition, the assessment shall include specific functional elements of the Minimum Data Set (MDS).

(Continued)

Exhibit 8.1.   Excerpts from the DMA SCO Specifications. (*Continued*)

1.16 MassHealth: The health coverage program provided by the Massachusetts Division of Medical Assistance.

1.17 Medical Necessity (Medically Necessary, adj.): Those services (1) which are reasonably calculated to prevent, diagnose, prevent the worsening of, alleviate, correct, or cure conditions in the Enrollee that endanger life, cause suffering or pain, cause physical deformity or malfunction, threaten to cause or to aggravate a disability, or result in illness or infirmity; and (2) for which there is no comparable medical service or site of service available or suitable for the Enrollee requesting the service that is more conservative or less costly; and (3) are of a quality that meets generally accepted standards of health care.

1.18 Minimum Data Set (MDS): A clinical assessment tool for frail elders and persons with disabilities, which includes key functional status indicators, and which is currently required by federal regulation in all nursing facilities.

1.19 Ongoing Assessment: A reevaluation of an Enrollee's health status conducted in accordance with *Purchasing Specification 2.10.*

1.20 Primary Care Physician (PCP). A licensed physician who is able and willing to meet all of the PCP requirements in these specifications. (See *Purchasing Specifications 2.13 and 2.14* for PCP responsibilities, and 5.4 for qualifications.)

1.21 Primary Care Team (PCT): A team consisting of a Primary Care Physician (PCP) working in conjunction with a Nurse Practitioner (NP) or Registered Nurse (RN) or Physician's Assistant (PA) and a Geriatric Support Services Coordinator (GSSC), all of whom shall have experience in geriatric practice. In order to assure effective coordination and delivery of care, the PCT may be enlarged at the discretion of the PCP to include other professional and support disciplines, when the Enrollee belongs to special high risk populations and/or requires additional expertise to assure adequate, safe care. (See *Purchasing Specification 5.15* for Primary Care Team qualifications).

1.22 Provider Network: PCPs, PCTs, mental health/substance abuse providers, community-based and institutional long term care providers, and all other providers employed by or under subcontract with the Contractor. A provider is any entity or individual, whether direct employee or subcontractor, delivering one or more of the Covered Services listed in APPENDIX A [not included with this exhibit].

1.23 Urgent Care: Medical services required promptly to prevent impairment of health due to symptoms that a prudent lay person would believe require immediate attention, but are not life-threatening and do not pose a high risk of permanent damage to an individual's health. Urgent care is appropriately provided in a clinic, physician's office, or in a hospital emergency department if a clinic or physician's office is inaccessible. Urgent care does not include services provided to treat an Emergency Condition nor does it include primary care services.

SECTION II: CARE MANAGEMENT AND INTEGRATION
A. General

Goal: DMA and HCFA believe the needs of the elderly population can best be met by the implementation of a geriatric model of care which incorporates an interdisciplinary approach to provide assessment, prevention, treatment, and other interventions which minimize disability, promote positive health behaviors, and maintain health status and function for each senior Enrollee. To achieve these objectives, the Senior Care Organization (SCO) Contractor must provide, integrate, and coordinate care across all service areas for its Enrollees.

Service Delivery: The Contractor must provide all Medically Necessary Covered Services, or their equivalent, to Enrollees. (See APPENDIX A [not included with this exhibit].)

2.1 Primary Care Physician (PCP) Selection: Contractor shall assure that each new Enrollee selects a PCP upon enrollment.

2.2 Initial Triage: The Contractor must have a mechanism for making an initial clinical determination of emergency, urgent, or routine Enrollee status, and must provide for the transition of existing services, equipment and other resources to assure safe, efficient continuity of care at enrollment.

2.3 Assessment and Determination of Complex Care Needs: Upon enrollment, and as appropriate thereafter, the Contractor shall perform an Initial and Ongoing Assessment, using an assessment tool approved by DMA. This process will identify all the Enrollee's needs, and, in particular, the presence of Complex Care Needs. The

(Continued)

Exhibit 8.1.   Excerpts from the DMA SCO Specifications. (*Continued*)

presence of Complex Care Needs shall trigger a comprehensive evaluation process to be performed by a Primary Care Team (PCT), which will include an in-home component. Enrollees with Complex Care Needs will have their care managed by a PCT. (See *Purchasing Specifications 1.4, 1.15 and 1.19* for definitions of Complex Care Needs and Initial and Ongoing Assessment.)

2.4 PCP Responsibility: When no Complex Care Needs exist, the Contractor shall assure that the PCP is responsible for overall clinical direction and serves as a central point of integration and coordination of Covered Services listed in APPENDIX A [not included with this exhibit]. For individuals with Complex Care Needs, the PCP shall create a PCT, and participate as needed.

2.5 Integration Plan: The Contractor shall assure that clinical linkages exist among all providers, including subcontractors (i.e., acute, specialty, mental health/substance abuse, and long term care). The PCP or the PCT will be accountable for integration and coordination of services. The Contractor must demonstrate effective linkages of clinical and management information systems among all providers in the Provider Network.

Integration and coordination of services will include, but not be limited to, the following:

a. an individualized care plan for each Enrollee, developed by the PCP, or if applicable, the PCT, and the periodic review and modification of this treatment plan by the PCP or PCT;

b. protocols for generating or receiving referrals, and for recording and tracking the results of referrals;

c. protocols for sharing clinical and care plan information, including management of medications;

d. protocols for determining conditions and circumstances under which specialty services shall be provided appropriately and without undue delay to Enrollees without established Complex Care Needs (for example, Geriatric Support and specialty physician services).

e. protocols for tracking Enrollee transfers from one setting to another (i.e. hospital to home, nursing home to adult day health, etc.) and assuring continued provision of necessary services;

f. protocols for obtaining consent from Enrollees to share individual medical and care planning information among the Enrollee's caregivers in the Provider Network, and with DMA and HCFA for quality management purposes; and, a provider training curriculum, flow charts, correspondence or brochures created to assure coordination and linkage.

2.6 Coordination and Access to Emergency and Urgent Care Services: Procedures concerning access to Emergency and Urgent Services must be included in Enrollee education materials and be part of Enrollee orientation curriculum. The Contractor will ensure linkages among the PCP, the PCT and any appropriate acute, long term care and mental health/substance abuse providers to keep all parties informed regarding Emergency and Urgent Service utilization.

2.7 Centralized Enrollee Record: To facilitate coordination of care, the Contractor must maintain a single, centralized, comprehensive record which documents the Enrollee's medical, functional, and social status. The Contractor must ensure that the PCP and all members of the PCT as well as any other appropriate providers, including subcontracted providers, make appropriate and timely entries regarding care provided, diagnoses determined, medications prescribed and treatment plans developed. The organization and documentation included in the Centralized Enrollee Record shall meet all applicable professional requirements. The Centralized Enrollee Record must contain the following:

a. Enrollee identifying information;

b. documentation of all services provided, including who provided the services and how they may be contacted;

c. multidisciplinary assessments, including diagnoses, prognoses, reassessments, plans of care, treatment and progress notes, signed and dated;

d. laboratory reports;

e. prescribed medications, including dosages and any known drug contraindications;

f. reports regarding the involvement of community agencies who are not part of the provider network, including any services provided;

(Continued)

Exhibit 8.1.   Excerpts from the DMA SCO Specifications. (*Continued*)

   g. documentation of contacts with family members and/or persons giving informal support;

   h. physician orders;

   i. disenrollment agreement, if applicable;

   j. enrollee's individual Advance Directives and Health Care Proxy, recorded and maintained in a prominent place;

   k. plan for emergency and urgent situations, including identifying information on emergency contact person(s); and

   l. allergies and special dietary needs.

2.8 Coordination of Enrollee Record Information: Systems must be implemented to ensure that the Centralized Enrollee Record:

   a. is updated in a timely manner by each provider of care; and

   b. is available and accessible, either in its entirety or in a current summary of key clinical information, to triage and acute care providers for emergency and urgent situations; and

   c. is available and accessible to specialty, long term care, and MH/SA providers.

2.9 Confidentiality of Enrollee Record Information: The Contractor must develop policies to ensure the confidentiality of Enrollee record information. Such policies shall include the following:

   a. at a minimum, compliance with all state and federal legal requirements as they pertain to confidentiality of Enrollee records including without limitation M.G.L. c.66A and, if applicable, M.G.L. c. 123 §36 104 CMR 15.03 (4), 104 CMR 2.07–08, and 104 CMR 3.19.

   b. informing Enrollees upon enrollment how their Centralized Enrollee Record will be used and who will have access to it;

   c. informing Enrollees how to obtain a copy of their Centralized Enrollee Record, upon written request;

   d. requiring all subcontractors to abide by the confidentiality protections established by the Contractor;

   e. assuring that documentation of MHSA treatment in the Centralized Enrollee Record shall include only documentation of MHSA assessment, diagnosis, treatment plan, therapeutic outcome/disposition, and any medications prescribed. Psychotherapeutic session notes shall not be recorded in the Centralized Enrollee Record; and

f. providing records at DMA and/or HCFA's request for monitoring the quality of care provided by the Contractor in accordance with federal law (e.g. 42 USC 1396a (a)(30)), and conducting performance evaluation activities.

2.10 **Ongoing Assessments:** Assessment of the needs of Enrollees must be performed at least once every 6 months, and for Enrollees with Complex Care Needs, shall be performed a least quarterly. Additional assessments must be performed when the Enrollee experiences a major change that is not temporary, impacts on more than one area of health status and requires interdisciplinary review or revision of the care plan. At least annually, the HEDIS Health Outcomes Survey shall be administered to Enrollees who can self-report. Results of all assessments shall be recorded in the centralized Enrollee recon and communicated to the Enrollee's Provider Network in a timely manner.

2.11 **Process to Coordinate Services with Community Agencies:** The Contractor shall implement a systematic process for coordinating care and creating linkages for service with organizations not providing Covered Services, including, but not limited to:

a. state agencies (e.g., Executive Office of Elder Affairs, Department of Public Health, Department of Mental Retardation, Department of Mental Health);

b. social service agencies (such as Councils on Aging) and services (e.g., housing, food delivery, non-medical transportation); and,

c. consumer, civic, and religious organizations.

The systematic process and associated linkages must provide for: sharing information, generating, receiving, and tracking referrals, obtaining consent from Enrollees to share individual Enrollee medical information where necessary; and ongoing coordination efforts (e.g., regularly scheduled meetings, newsletters, joint community based projects, etc.).

2.12 **Community Involvement and Representation:** The Contractor shall obtain Consumer and community input on issues of program

(Continued)

Exhibit 8.1.   Excerpts from the DMA SCO Specifications. (*Continued*)

management and participant care. Consumer representation must be achieved both through Consumer participation on its governing board and through establishment of Consumer advisory committees.

B. PRIMARY, ACUTE AND PREVENTIVE CARE

Goal: The Senior Care Organization (SCO) Contractor shall ensure that a qualified PCP, and when necessary a PCT, will provide primary, acute and preventive care, as well as clinical expertise, and integration and coordination of care for all Covered Services listed in APPENDIX A [not included with this exhibit]. The PCP or PCT shall have both care provider responsibilities and care manager responsibilities, as specified below. In addition, the PCP or PCT will be responsible for ensuring that the Enrollee and/or his/her designated representative is involved in his/her own care planning and decisions regarding medical treatment. In order to assure access to Emergency medical and mental health/substance abuse services, certain services shall not require any referral or prior authorization (see APPENDIX B [not included with this exhibit]).

2.13 **PCP Responsibilities:** As a care provider, the PCP shall be accountable for the following but may delegate specified tasks in accordance with state law:

   a. initial and ongoing assessments as defined in *Purchasing Specifications 1.15, 1.19, and 2.7;*

   b. primary medical services, including acute and preventive care;

   c. referral of the Enrollee to specialty, long term care and/or mental health/substance abuse providers, as medically necessary;

   d. when Complex Care Needs exist, establishment of a PCT;

2.14 **Care Management Responsibilities:** As the manager of care, the PCP or the PCT shall:

   a. with the Enrollee and/or his/her designated representative, develop a care plan, including treatment goals (medical, functional and/or social), and track measures for assessing progress in reaching those goals;

   b. consult with and advise acute, specialty, long term care, and mental health/substance abuse providers regarding care plans and clinically appropriate interventions on an ongoing basis;

   c. assure that ongoing assessments are conducted appropriately, and that care plans are adjusted as necessary and communicated to the Enrollee's providers in timely manner;

   d. utilize the Geriatric Support Services Coordinator to assure that, to the greatest extent possible, independent functioning of the Enrollee is promoted, and services are provided in the most appropriate, least restrictive environment;

   e. document and comply with Advance Directives concerning the Enrollee's wishes regarding future treatment and health care decisions, and assist in the designation of a Health Care Proxy, should the Enrollee desire one;

   f. maintain the Centralized Enrollee Record, including, but not limited to making appropriate and timely entries regarding care provided, diagnoses determined, medications prescribed and treatment plans developed, and designating the physical location of the. record for each Enrollee (see *Purchasing Specifications 2.7–2.9*); and

   g. communicate with Enrollee, family members, and significant caregivers regarding the Enrollee's medical, social, and psychological needs.

2.15 Enrollee Participation in Care Planning and Medical Decision-Making: The Contractor, through its PCPs and PCTs, shall be responsible for ensuring that the Enrollee or his/her designated representative is included in the development of an individualized care plan, participates in Informed Consent, and is involved in medical decision making. The Contractor shall:

   a. demonstrate the participation of the Enrollee or his/her designated representative in the development of an individualized care plan by having the Enrollee or his/her designated representative participate in initial and ongoing assessments (see *Purchasing Specification 1.14)* and sign a copy of the care plan;

   b. include questions in the annual Enrollee satisfaction survey regarding how included and involved the Enrollee or his/her designated representative felt in developing the care plan and in medical decision-making; and,

   c. provide information to the Enrollee regarding Advance Directives (at a minimum those required in 42 CFR 489.000),

(Continued)

Exhibit 8.1.   Excerpts from the DMA SCO Specifications. (*Continued*)

designating a Health Care Proxy and other mechanisms for ensuring future medical decisions are made according to the desires of the Enrollee.

C. LONG TERM CARE

2.16 Long Term Care Delivery System: In delivering the long term care services referenced in APPENDIX A [not included with this exhibit], the Contractor must demonstrate the capacity to provide coordination of care and expert care management through the PCT. The Contractor shall assure the following:

a. The PCT will be responsible for monitoring the provision of long term care services on an ongoing basis.

b. The Geriatric Support Services Coordinator provided under contract with the Aging Services Access Points (ASAPs) will participate in determinations of appropriateness for institutional and community long term care services and shall identify and recommend to the PCP Enrollees for whom a PCT may be appropriate.

c. The measurement of the functional status of Enrollees will be performed at Initial and Ongoing Assessment (See *Purchasing Specifications 1.15 and 1.19*) applying components of the Minimum Data Set (MDS) as required by DMA. Reports will be produced in accordance with *Purchasing Specification 7.9*.

2.17 Continuum of Long Term Care: The Contractor shall provide:

a. community long term care service alternatives to nursing facility care (see APPENDIX A [not included with this exhibit]);

b. other transitional, respite, and residential support services to maintain Enrollees safely in the community, based on assessment by the Contractor of functional status and cost effectiveness;

c. nursing facility services for Enrollees who are medically eligible (in accordance with 130 CMR Chapter 456) and for whom the Contractor has no noninstitutional service package appropriate and available to meet the Enrollee's medical needs. (See *Purchasing Specification 7.8* for reporting requirements);

d. other institutional services as medically necessary.

2.18 PASARR Evaluation: The Contractor shall comply with federal regulations requiring referral of nursing facility eligible Enrollees, as appropriate, to the State's agent for Pre-Admission Screening and Annual Resident Review (PASARR) evaluation for mental illness/mental retardation treatment pursuant to OBRA '87.

D. MENTAL HEALTH/SUBSTANCE ABUSE (MH/SA)

2.19 Continuum of MH/SA Care: The Contractor shall offer a continuum of MH/SA care which shall be coordinated with PCPs or the PCTs, and include, but not be limited to:

a. a range of services from acute inpatient treatment to intermittent professional and supportive care for delivering MH/SA Services to Enrollees residing in the community or in nursing facilities; and,

b. a comprehensive alternative service system that allows for diversion from acute inpatient hospital services. (See APPENDIX A [not included with this exhibit]).

2.20 MH/SA Responsibilities: The Contractor will manage the provision of all MH/SA services. When Emergency services are needed, the Enrollee may self-refer to a qualified MH/SA provider. The care management protocol for Enrollees must encourage appropriate access to MH/SA care in all settings. For Enrollees who require MH/SA services as part of the coordinated Provider Network, the MH/SA provider shall:

a. with the Enrollee and/or his/her designated representative, develop the MH/SA portion of the care plan for each Enrollee which is consistent with established clinical criteria and protocols;

b. with the input, as appropriate, of the PCP or PCT, determine clinically appropriate interventions on an ongoing basis. Such interventions shall, to the greatest extent possible, promote the independent functioning of the patient and be provided in the least restrictive environment;

c. make appropriate and timely entries into the Centralized Enrollee Record regarding MH/SA assessment/diagnosis determined, medications prescribed, if any, and care, plans developed. As stated in *Purchasing Specification 2.9,* psychotherapeutic

(Continued)

Exhibit 8.1.   Excerpts from the DMA SCO Specifications. (*Continued*)

session notes shall not be recorded in the Centralized Enrollee Record; and

d. obtain authorization from the PCP or PCT for any non-Emergency services.

2.21 Coordination of Medication: Prescriptions for any psychotropic medications must be evaluated for interactions with the medications already prescribed for the Enrollee. To support this, the Contractor must comply with DMA's Pharmacy Online Processing System (POPS). (See *Purchasing Specification 7.12*)

2.22 MH/SA Needs Management Programming: The Contractor shall maintain a structured process for identifying and addressing complex MH/SA needs at all levels of care and in all residential settings. Qualified MH/SA providers shall pro-actively coordinate and follow Enrollee progress through the continuum of care until optimum stability in life functions is achieved.

2.23 Systematic Early Identification and Intervention for MH/SA Services: MH/SA problems shall be systematically identified and addressed by the Enrollee's PCP or PCT at the Initial and Ongoing Assessment (*Purchasing Specifications 1.15 and 1.19*) through the use of mental health screening tools and other mechanisms approved by DMA and HCFA. When appropriate, the Contractor must assure that referrals for specialty MH/SA services will be generated.

2.24 Services for Enrollees with Serious and Persistent Mental Illness: The Contractor shall assure that Enrollees with serious and persistent mental illness have access to ongoing medications review and monitoring, day treatment, and other milieu alternatives to conventional therapy, and that the PCT coordinates services with additional support services as appropriate. For such Enrollees, a qualified MH/SA clinician (See *Purchasing Specification 5.2d*) must be part of the PCT. Such Enrollees must have access to all medically necessary covered services, including inpatient hospitalization for crisis situations. As necessary, interface with the Department of Mental Health must be provided.

SECTION III: PROGRAM INITIATIVES [Excerpts]

Goal: The Contractor shall implement specific initiatives through the development of protocols approved by DMA and HCFA. Initiatives shall incorporate the geriatric model of care and shall be based on the principles of Continuous Quality Improvement (CQI) as described in *Purchasing Specification 5.1.*

3.1 Initiative to Reduce Preventable Hospital Admissions: Monitoring and risk assessment mechanisms, processes linking assessment to service delivery, timely information to providers.

3.2 Discharge Planning Initiative: Interdisciplinary planning at the point of admission to hospital or nursing home.

3.3 Preventive Immunization: Protocols and implementation processes for providing pneumococcal and influenza vaccines.

3.4 Screening for Early Identification of Cancer: Protocols and implementation processes, including testing and patient/caregiver education, for key cancer prevention services.

3.5 Disease Management: Protocols for managing congestive heart failure, COPD, diabetes, and depression.

3.6 Management of Dementia: Protocols and implementation processes.

3.7 Assuring Appropriate Nursing Facility Institutionalization: Protocols and implementation processes.

3.8 Alcohol Abuse Prevention and Treatment Initiative: Protocols and implementation processes.

3.9 Abuse and Neglect Identification Initiative: Mandates that Contractor be a mandated reporter of elder abuse under state law.

SECTION IV: ACCESS AND ENROLLEE SERVICES [Excerpts]

Goal: The Contractor shall demonstrate its ability to meet the needs of Enrollees competently and promptly. The Contractor shall offer adequate choice and availability of PCPs and PCTs, if required, as well as MH/SA and long-term care providers. The Contractor shall provide adequate access to Covered Services (listed in APPENDIX A [not included with this exhibit]) including physical and geographic access, as well as access to TTY and translation services. Such access shall be designed to accommodate the needs of Enrollees who are disabled and/or non-English speaking. Responsible areas listed below:

4.1 Training in Access and Services: Provided to provider network.

4.2 Linkage with Enrollment Broker: Daily communication system with Enrollee Broker to assure accurate Enrollee eligibility information.

4.3 Communication with Enrollees: Must be made available in a manner that Enrollees can understand.

(Continued)

Exhibit 8.1.   Excerpts from the DMA SCO Specifications. (*Continued*)

4.4 Enrollee Rights

4.5 Disenrollments

4.6 PCP Selection and Initial Assessment: Information and guidance to Enrollee.

4.7 24-Hour Coverage: 24/7 toll-free access to skilled professional who has access to Centralized Enrollee Record.

4.8 Triage System: Emergency and urgent care.

4.9 Access to Services for Emergency Conditions and Urgent Care: Processes and information systems in place to assure access.

4.10 Proximity Requirements: Each enrollee should have a choice of at least 2 PCPs and 2 MH/SA providers within 15 miles/30 minutes of their residence.

4.11 Non-Symptomatic Office Visits: Available within 30 days.

4.12 Urgent Care, Symptomatic Office Visits: Available within 48 hours.

4.13 Choice of Long Term and Hospital Providers: Enrollees should have a choice among providers.

4.14 Enrollee Service: Enrollee Service Representatives must be available to Enrollees during business hours.

4.15 Enrollee Orientation: Within 30 days of enrollment, written and nonwritten form.

4.16 Health Promotion/Wellness Activities: Information and seminars on health promotion/wellness activities.

4.17 Linguistic Competency: Telephone access to linguistically competent providers or interpreters with appropriate knowledge of care.

4.18 Access for Enrollees with Disabilities

4.19 Access to Home and Community-Based Services

4.20 Closing Enrollment: Prohibited without approval of DMA and HCFA.

4.21 Procedures for Enrollees' Complaints and Appeals: 3-1/2 pages of due process requirements.

SECTION V: QUALITY

Goal: The Contractor shall ensure the delivery of quality care through a planned, systematic quality management approach which constantly evaluates and improves clinical and non-clinical processes and outcomes. The Contractor's performance shall be evaluated by DMA, HCFA and the Contractor, through the application of Continuous Quality Improvement (CQI)/Total Quality Management (TQM) in all aspects of its organization and service delivery system.

5.1 **CQI/TQM Philosophy**: All clinical and non-clinical aspects of Contractor management shall be based on principles of CQI/TQM. The quality management program shall:

a. recognize that opportunities for improvement are unlimited;

b. be data driven;

c. rely heavily on Enrollee input;

d. rely heavily on input from all employees of the Contractor and subcontractors;

e. require continual measurement of clinical and non-clinical effectiveness and programmatic improvements of clinical and non-clinical processes driven by such measurement; and

f. require re-measurement of effectiveness, and continuing development and implementation of improvements as appropriate.

5.2 **Quality Management Resources**: Assure sufficient skilled staff and resources to implement quality management program, including a Quality Management Director, Medical Director, Geriatrician, and N41VSA specialist.

5.3 **Provider Qualifications and Performance**: Protocols for credentialing, continuing education, and provider profiling, and corrective action processes.

5.4 **Primary Care Qualifications**: PCP, RN, Geriatric Support Coordinator from ASAP.

[5.5] **Subcontracting Requirements**

5.6 **Assessment of New Medical Technology**: Maintain procedures for evaluation of new technologies and new uses of established technologies.

5.7 **Enrollee Satisfaction Survey**: Annual survey covering non-English speaking Enrollees, physically disabled Enrollees, minority Enrollees, and family members.

5.8 **Enrollee Orientation Performance**: Annually evaluate Enrollee orientation activities.

(Continued)

Exhibit 8.1.   Excerpts from the DMA SCO Specifications. (*Continued*)

5.9 Health Promotion/Wellness Activities Performance: Annually evaluate effectiveness of activities.

5.10 Ethics Committee: Written policies and procedures to assist decision making and including End-of-Life and Patient Self-Determination.

5.11 Annual Quality Management Goals: Specific goals in primary care, LTC, MH/SA areas; report on progress annually to DMA and HCFA.

SECTION VI: FINANCIAL STABILITY AND SOLVENCY STANDARDS; GENERAL BUSINESS REQUIREMENTS

Goal: The following specifications are to ensure:
- initial and continuing financial stability of the Contractor for the provision of health care benefits; and

- corrective action measures are taken to address and resolve any identified financial problems.

6.1 Minimum Net Worth: The Contractor shall demonstrate and maintain minimum net worth as specified below. Minimum net worth shall be defined as assets minus liabilities.

   a. The Contractor shall demonstrate a minimum net worth of $1,500,000 at the time of application to become a SCO, subject to the following conditions:

   1. HCFA and DMA may jointly reduce this amount to $1,000,000, when HCFA and DMA determine that a reduction in the minimum net worth requirement is necessary to increase access to underserved areas or that such a reduction is otherwise in the public interest;

   2. a minimum of $750,000 of this requirement must be in cash;

   3. the Contractor may include 100% of the book value (the depreciated value according to generally accepted accounting principles or GAAP) of tangible Health Care Delivery Assets (HCDA) carried on its balance sheet;

   4. if at least $ 1,000,000 of the minimum net worth requirement is met by cash, then the GAAP value of intangible assets up to 20% of the minimum net worth required will be allowed;

   5. if less than $1,000,000 of the minimum net worth requirement is met by cash, then the GAAP value of intangible assets

    up to 10% of the minimum net worth required will be allowed.

  b. From the date of signing a contract to operate as a SCO onward, the Contractor shall maintain a minimum net worth of $1,000,000, subject to the conditions in *Purchasing Specifications 6.1(a) 2–5.*

6.2 Working Capital Requirements: The Contractor shall maintain a positive balance of working capital at all times. (Working capital is defined as current assets minus current liabilities.) In its quarterly reports, the Contractor shall demonstrate that it meets this requirement (see APPENDIX C—Section VII.C [not included with this exhibit]). The Contractor shall provide a quarterly report within 15 days of the end of each quarter that provides detailed documentation of the balance of working capital. If a Contractor's working capital falls below zero, the Contractor shall submit a written plan to reestablish a positive working capital balance for approval by HCFA and DMA. HCFA and DMA may take action they deem appropriate, including termination of the Contract, if the Contractor:

  a. does not propose a plan to reestablish a positive working capital balance within a reasonable period of time;

  b. violates a corrective plan approved by HCFA and DMA; or

  c. HCFA and DMA determines that negative working capital cannot be corrected within a reasonable time, as determined by HCFA and DMA.

6.3 Performance Bond or Insolvency Deposit: In the event that the Contractor must be rehabilitated or liquidated, it will be necessary for the Contractor to have liquid assets on deposit. The Contractor may meet this requirement with either one of the following:

  a. a Performance Bond in the amount of $500,000 with an agent, and under terms, acceptable to HCFA and the Division. The use of funds guaranteed by the Performance Bond must be solely for insuring the provision of services to Enrollees at the time of impending or actual insolvency of the Contractor, as agreed to by HCFA and DMA; or

  b. an Insolvency Deposit of $100,000 in an escrow account with an agent and under terms acceptable to HCFA and DMA. This

(Continued)

Exhibit 8.1.   Excerpts from the DMA SCO Specifications. (*Continued*)

deposit may be considered to count toward fulfillment of the Minimum Net Worth requirement, but not the $750,000 cash requirement.

6.4 Insolvency Protection Plan: The Contractor must have an Insolvency Protection Plan approved by HCFA and DMA. Any changes to the Insolvency Protection Plan must be approved in advance by HCFA and DMA. The Insolvency Protection Plan must include the following:

a. proof of financial arrangements, satisfactory to HCFA and DMA, for the continued provision of Covered Services to Enrollees for a period of at least 45 days from the date of the Contractor's insolvency, and until Coverage for all SCO Enrollees (e.g. enrollment with another managed care organization, or Medicare fee-for-service and Medicaid fee-for-service) has been re-established, including referrals to primary care and other providers.

b. guarantees to insure that Enrollees, HCFA and DMA do not incur liability for payment of any expense which is the legal obligation of the Contractor, or any of its subcontractors or other entities which have provided services to Enrollees at the direction of the Contractor or its subcontractors. Neither Enrollees, nor HCFA, nor DMA will incur any liability for any expense which is the legal obligation of the Contractor or any subcontractor.

c. The detailed specification of the Contractor's insolvency protection arrangements, including the underwriting organization and amount of protection, as applicable, which may include, but not be limited to the following:

  1. reinsurance or insolvency insurance (which may not count as a credit against the minimum net worth requirement);

  2. hold harmless arrangement;

  3. continuation of benefits provisions;

  4. letters of credit;

  5. guarantees; and

  6. net worth.

d. timely, written notice to HCFA and DMA as soon as the Contractor has reason to be considering insolvency or otherwise has reason to believe it or any subcontractor is other than financially sound and stable.

6.5 General Business Requirements: Upon application, upon signing the initial contract, and upon contract renewal, the Contractor shall represent and warrant that the Contractor is in sound financial condition.

6.6 Risk Arrangements: The Contractor may maintain, subject to approval by DMA and HCFA, provider risk arrangements which shall improve cost-effectiveness without compromising the quality of care provided.

6.7 New Organizations: For new organizations, the Contractor must demonstrate the financial feasibility to meet the requirements specified in these Purchasing Specifications, and that adequate funding for the start-up period has been obtained. The Contractor must provide DMA and HCFA with information regarding any loans or other funds received and any prospectus materials developed.

6.8 Financial Reports: The Contractor shall report performance to DMA and to HCFA with financial statements and ratios as listed in APPENDIX C [not included with this exhibit] that measure liquidity, efficiency, composition, capitalization and profitability of the Contractor and all subcontractors, in accordance with generally accepted accounting principles (GAAP).

6.9 Right to Audit and Inspect Books and Records: The Contractor shall grant DMA and HCFA the right to audit and inspect its books and records.

SECTION VII: REPORTING [EXCERPTS]

Goal: The Contractor shall collect and report specified financial, clinical, and outcome data to DMA and HCFA. The Contractor shall also collect and report encounter data as noted in this Section. Such data shall provide meaningful management information for the Contractor to use in improving the health care management of Enrollees and for DMA and HCCFA to use to monitor the quality of the Contractor's performance.

7.1 Experience Review & Profit/Loss Report

7.2 Reports on Capacity

(Continued)

Exhibit 8.1.   Excerpts from the DMA SCO Specifications. (*Continued*)

7.3 Clinical Indicator Data: Including appropriate HEDIS 3.0 measures.

   a. Preventive Medicine: influenza and pneumococcal vaccination rates, mammography and fecal occult blood testing rates, eye, hearing, alcohol abuse testing rates.

   b. Acute and Chronic Disease

   1. Diabetes Mellitus (DM): number and rates of compliance with key tests/procedures.

   2. Chronic obstructive pulmonary disease (COPD): number and rates of compliance.

   3. Congestive Heart Failure (CHF): number and rates of compliance.

   4. Depression: number and rates of compliance.

   5. Dementia: number and percentage receiving specific services.

7.4 Appeals and Complaints

7.5 Disenrollment Rate

7.6 Institutional Utilization Data

   a. Rate of acute hospital admissions

   b. Rate of preventable hospital admissions (Pneumonia, COPD, CHF, dehydration and urinary tract infection)

   c. Rate of nursing facility admissions

   d. Various characteristics of nursing home residents

7.7 Community Health Service Utilization

7.8 Enrollees Medically Eligible for Nursing Facility Services

7.9 MH/SA Utilization Data

7.10 Functional Data: Activities of daily living—rates of need/1000 Enrollees.

7.11 Mortality Data: Deaths by site of care.

7.12 Medications: Participation in DMA's Pharmacy On Line Processing System.

—⁓— Epilogue: 2002—A SCO Odyssey

Diane Flanders and Kate K. Willrich Nordahl
Massachusetts Division of Medical Assistance

It has been almost five years since DMA filed its initial federal Medicaid waiver request to create a new health care delivery option to improve services and outcomes for dually eligible seniors. During this time, the state has faced unprecedented challenges on two fronts: it has attempted to develop consensus within the state among providers, advocates, and consumers and, at the same time, to negotiate and finalize first-in-the-nation agreements with the federal government to obtain Medicare payment rates that would be adequate to implement Senior Care Options. DMA has made many changes and important compromises in response to the input of the various stakeholders along the way. Yet, as of drafting this update (in March 2002), the Senior Care Options plan is not yet operational, and MassHealth seniors are still not receiving the coordinated health care they need and deserve.

THE STATE LEGISLATIVE PROCESS

One major issue has been the challenging evolution of state legislative authorization for SCO. For a number of years, the state budget included language that was supportive of DMA's efforts to seek a waiver and develop SCO. However, this language also required DMA to obtain legislative authorization prior to implementation. During state fiscal year 2000, Senator Richard Moore, chair of the Joint Committee on Health Care, had proposed legislation authorizing the SCO program. Certain issues surfaced at that time, largely connected with other broad-scale managed care reforms the state was pursuing. The SCO Bill passed the House, but did not pass the Senate. Instead, the FY 2001 budget directed a legislative task force, led by Senator Moore, to develop detailed recommendations for the implementation of Senior Care Options. The key advocacy organizations and provider trade associations, all of whom had participated in various advisory groups during DMA's planning phase, were named as members of the SCO Task Force, along with representatives from cabinet-level state agencies, the Executive Office of Elder Affairs and the Executive Office of Health and Human Services.

The SCO task force met eight times between September and December 2000. Senator Moore and his staff made a tremendous effort to achieve agreement on the legislative language. Some task force members attempted to use the task force meetings as opportunities to bring in issues unrelated to the SCO demonstration, which sidetracked the discussion, so the ideal of full consensus was never reached. However, major areas of agreement were approved by almost all of the SCO Task Force, who supported—in writing—new legislative language, which was filed by Senator Moore in May 2001.

Here are some of the key areas that were processed in the task force and included in the legislation:

- Definitions of "complex care" that would qualify enrollees for higher community rating category payments
- Creation of a Consumer Advisory Council and inclusion of consumer protections
- Performance measurement and report cards
- Definition of the role of elder service agencies (ASAPs)
- Creation of a special commission to report back to the legislature

Nonetheless, the legislation (Senate Bill 527), while it was reported out favorably from the Joint Committee on Health Care, still has not reached the full legislature. The budget for State Fiscal Year 2002 took nearly all available legislative attention well past the budget deadline of July 1, 2001. In fact, with the events of September 11 and the declining state revenues, the legislature did not pass an FY 2002 budget until late November, being the last state in the Union to do so. The SCO bill remains in the Senate Ways and Means Committee, and DMA continues to urge its passage with the legislature.

THE TIME FOR SCO IS NOW

In spite of these difficulties and delays, the DMA—in a remarkable partnership that has evolved with both the central and regional offices of the Centers for Medicare & Medicaid Services (CMS, formerly HCFA)—has been proceeding with the critical tasks necessary to make Senior Care Options a reality. A SCO Steering Committee initiated in November 2000, including representation from CMS and EOEA, has established subcommittees that have successfully completed design and documentation for procurement, outreach, enrollment, finance, and operational systems.

The commitment of CMS to this project is demonstrated not only by active participation in these workgroups but also by their initiation of a national effort to continue to focus on issues associated with dual eligibility. The central office leadership of CMS in Baltimore has recently established a Technical Advisory Group exclusively devoted to working with states on Medicare and Medicaid integration issues. DMA Commissioner Wendy Warring is the chair of the new group. Commissioner Warring is very concerned about the delays with Senior Care Options, and has worked very hard to move the project ahead.

The question of whether or not any providers will come to the SCO party remains a critical one. Approximately six to eight provider networks continue to express interest in bidding to be Senior Care Organizations, when and if the program becomes official. But timing now is surfacing as a critical issue. Maintaining interest and support for the project, especially in the provider and advocacy communities, requires action in the near future.

Nationally, the urgency of achieving basic quality of care in the health care system for seniors is more visible every day. In that regard, Massachusetts was one of the first states to work with CMS to link the Medicare and Medicaid databases. For the first time, the diagnostic and acute care information from Medicare has been combined with the pharmacy and long-term care information from Medicaid to produce a full picture of the services individuals receive over time. This data demonstrates that the fee-for-service system results in poor care. For example, low percentages of individuals with heart failure receive the proper medication; low percentages of individuals with diabetes receive the proper blood tests. When chronic diseases such as these are not managed, hospitalizations and institutional placements are inevitable. And hospitalization for frail elders, in particular, can be a devastating event resulting in further decline in functioning.

For Massachusetts, there are also financial implications. For example, in 2000, DMA was awarded a significant grant from the Robert Wood Johnson Foundation's Medicare/Medicaid Integration Project, making $600,000 available specifically to support SCO start-up in Massachusetts. These funds must be returned to the Foundation in August of this year if they are not spent. It would be wasteful to lose this resource.

In addition, the federal government has agreed to a favorable Medicare rate structure for SCO enrollees. The capitation payment level for the chronically ill residing in the community is more than twice the payment for a similar population enrolled in a Medicare+Choice plan. Under Senior Care Options, Medicare will bring substantial new capitation funding to SCO providers, which, in combination with the Medicaid payments, will enable them to provide flexible, personalized, integrated care far beyond what can be done in the current fee-for-service environment.

It is essential to begin accessing this funding, so that dual-eligible seniors can finally begin to reap the benefits of high-quality preventive and geriatric care. Otherwise, the problems eloquently described in the first section of the chapter will not be resolved. Vulnerable seniors will continue to receive uncoordinated and sometimes inappropriate care because the system of fee-for-service payments is not designed to allow for, much less promote, comprehensive care for the chronically ill. Despite their wishes to remain in their communities, the institutional bias in the existing Medicare and Medicaid systems will drive them increasingly into hospitals and nursing homes.

Given the state's budget crisis and the impending aging of the baby boomers in coming decades, we must develop and refine a workable infrastructure now to integrate care and align provider incentives for these members. Change is inevitable, and the SCO program presents the opportunity to proceed with a gradual, voluntary enrollment, which will allow DMA and CMS to monitor and adjust the model as needed. Senior Care Options has the ability to greatly improve quality of care and to promote cost-effective use of government funds. We are ready to carefully implement this program now!

Editors' Note: The Massachusetts Legislature finally approved legislation authorizing the SCO initiative in the fall of 2002. DMA issued a request for proposals to potential bidders in early 2003 and expects to contract with several SCOs for enrollment of members in fall 2003.

References

AARP. *Across the States: Profiles of Long-Term Care Systems.* Washington, D.C.: AARP, 1996.

Bruce, E., and Schulman-Green, D. "Background Paper on Long-Term Care in Massachusetts: Prepared for the Vision 2020 Task Force." Gerontology Institute, University of Massachusetts, Apr. 2000, p. 13. (Table 1)

Bullen B., Perrone, C., and Parker, P. "Saving Medicare: Why Medicaid Must Be Part of the Solution." *Policy and Practice of Public Health Services,* Dec. 1998. Published by the American Public Health Services Association. www.aphsa.org.

Massachusetts Division of Medical Assistance. "Purchasing Specifications for a Senior Care Organization," Aug. 1999a.

Massachusetts Division of Medical Assistance, "SCO Draft Monthly Rates: Calendar Year 2000." Unpublished data provided to the authors by staff at the Division of Medical Assistance, 1999b.

Weiner, J. M., and Stevenson, D. G. *Long-Term Care for the Elderly: Profiles of Thirteen States.* Occasional Paper #12, Assessing the New Federalism Project. Washington, D.C.: Urban Institute, Aug. 1998.

PART THREE

Managing Health

CHAPTER NINE

Threat to the Public's Health or Leaders in Public Health?

Managed Care in the Twin Cities

Minnesota is a state that cares about you more than you do.

—Public health adage in Minnesota

I hope we are not at the high water mark in community health improvement in Minneapolis.

—George Isham, Chief Health Officer, HealthPartners

"The heart of our mission is health improvement," says Ray Ahrens, past board chair of HealthPartners, the second-largest managed care health plan in Minnesota. "We believe we are doing more than any other health plan in the country to improve the health of our members and our community—in innovative, effective, and measurable ways." Indeed, the mission statement of HealthPartners is simple and clear: *"The mission of HealthPartners is to improve the health of our members and our community."*

This chapter was originally written by the authors in 1999. Funding was provided by Astra Pharmaceuticals, L.P. The authors thank the staff of Health-Partners, especially George Isham and Maureen Peterson, for their interest and assistance in preparing the case.

"Our involvement in community health is central to our mission," notes George Halvorson, president and chief executive officer of HealthPartners. "We are blessed to have the mission, resources, and talents to do this work, and we enjoy being catalytic. Our goal is to create health improvement concepts and develop them to the point where purchasers will not only accept them but demand them. If buyers' expectations change, the plans will comply."

Although HealthPartners is widely regarded as the leading health plan in the Minneapolis/St. Paul area (the Twin Cities) in terms of community health improvement work, other plans are also involved in a wide range of community health improvement efforts, both individually and in collaboration with both public and private partners. Some observers see a critical link between the maturity of the overall managed care market in the Twin Cities and the growing focus of managed care plans on population health initiatives. "The managed care market in Minneapolis is so mature that community health improvement is the only tool left that will move the needle on health care costs," one observer noted. While most health industry observers applaud the efforts of the managed care plans, a few question the motivation of the initiatives undertaken by the plans. "The efforts of the HMOs are small and blown out of proportion," said one consumer activist. "All this talk about community health improvement is just health plan propaganda to fool policymakers into thinking that managed care plans can provide salvation from the serious problems in our health care system and to prevent any real and meaningful reform."

Regardless of motivation, a wide range of community health improvement initiatives are under way. In many respects, the preconditions for effective community health efforts by managed care plans are better in the Twin Cities than in other parts of the United States: high managed care penetration, a small number of health plans, significant consolidation among delivery systems, the country's highest proportion of physicians in group practice, a history of collaboration between the public and private sectors, and a state requirement that all managed care plans in Minnesota be nonprofit. Thus the experience in the Twin Cities should be instructive about the appropriate role, as well as the long-term prospects, for relying on competitive managed care plans as an important force for community health improvement.

BUT WHAT IS COMMUNITY HEALTH IMPROVEMENT?

Both public and private organizations in the Twin Cities often use the terms *community health, public health,* and *population-based health* interchangeably. The definition of "population-based public health services" developed by the Minnesota Department of Health seems to incorporate most of the types of initiatives that are being referred to:

> Interventions aimed at disease prevention and health promotion that shape a community's overall profile . . . and improve the health status of the entire identified population. . . . They may be directed at the individual, community, or systems level, depending on how the problem may best be addressed. . . . Systems-focused interventions focus on creating change in organizations, policies, laws, and structures . . . community-focused interventions create changes in community norms, attitudes, awareness, standards or practices . . . individual-focused interventions focus on creating changes in knowledge, attitudes, belief, skills, practices, and behaviors in individuals, either single or in families, classes or groups. . . . They are person to person interventions that focus on a population at risk. . . . The most powerful public health interventions often are combinations of intervention strategies at all three levels [Minnesota Department of Health, 1997, pp. 7–8].

BACKGROUND ON MINNESOTA AND THE TWIN CITIES

As a state, Minnesota has an enviable record on health care compared to most other parts of the country. Its health care expenses per capita are 10 percent lower than the national average. The state's rate of uninsurance is 7–8 percent, compared to the national average of 15 percent. Minnesota is consistently rated in the top bracket, if not as the top state, in terms of a variety of health status measures. However, these impressive results mask significant disparities in health in certain populations, including people of color, low-income individuals, and children. For example, while the 1995 pregnancy rate for white adolescents in Minnesota, at 47 births per 1,000 females aged fifteen to nineteen, was the third-lowest among all states, the pregnancy rate for black adolescents, at 215, was the highest in the country.

Health Plan Name	Membership*	1998 Net Gain/(Loss)	Months of Expense in Reserve
Medica Health Plans	1,058,300	$14.3 million	1.8
HealthPartners	789,300	($5.7 million)	1.5
Blue Plus	526,000	($8.7 million)	1.1
UCare Minnesota	61,900	$0.3 million	1.9
Preferred One (HMO)	44,900	($0.5 million)	1.5
Metropolitan Health	27,500	($6.4 million)	1.3
First Plan	13,900	$0.4 million	2.0
Mayo Health Plan	5,700	$0.2 million	2.2
Altru Health Plan	1,900	$0.0 million	3.9
Total/average	2,528,200	$6.1 million	1.5

Table 9.1.   Enrollment and Financial Results for Minnesota HMOs (1998).
Source: Minnesota Council of Health Plans, press release dated Apr. 1, 1999.
Note: *Including self-insured accounts

The Minneapolis/St. Paul region covers seven counties and includes about 2.4 million people, more than half of the state's population. Its health care system is regarded as one of the most advanced in the country. Over 80 percent of individuals in the Twin Cities are enrolled in managed care plans. Three health plans, HealthPartners, Medica, and Blue Cross Blue Shield, have more than 80 percent of the managed care membership in the metropolitan area (see Table 9.1).

Consolidation has been significant at the provider level, with a small number of care systems dominating the delivery system. Many of the delivery systems also operate health plans. These are the major provider systems:

• HealthPartners, which includes the 325-bed Regions Hospital, nearly 600 employed physicians, and 7,100 contracting physicians.

• Allina, which consists of almost 2,700 hospital beds, 500 employed physicians, and nearly 8,000 contracting doctors. Allina also owns Medica, as well as SelectCare, the second-largest PPO in the market.

• Fairview, which has over 2,000 hospital beds, approximately 350 doctors who are either salaried or have exclusive contractual arrangements with the system, and 8,000 contracting physicians. Fairview, which is affiliated with the Lutheran Church, runs Preferred One, a 200,000-member PPO.

- HealthEast, which has 600 hospital beds, 78 employed physicians, and almost 550 contracted physicians. The system has a near-monopoly position in St. Paul.
- HealthSystem Minnesota, which has 355 hospital beds and 500 employed physicians.
- The Mayo Clinic, which controls over 2,200 hospital beds and has 1,000 employed physicians.

According to the health plans, the consolidation among providers has resulted in a near-monopoly position for some providers in certain markets, particularly in rural areas. As a result, prices and health plan premiums are higher in some rural areas than in the metropolitan area.

The managed care plans in the Twin Cities have significant overlap in their provider networks, excluding physicians who are employees of health plan–owned groups. For instance, HealthPartners has about 40 percent of its members in its own clinics, which operate very much like a group model HMO. The rest of the plan's members receive care from any of the seven thousand physicians who contract with the plan. Virtually all of these doctors are also in the provider networks of the other large HMOs.

Despite this concentration, the health insurance market is very price competitive, especially in the public employer market, where many cities and counties put their business out to bid on a regular basis and award a single contract to the health plan with the lowest price. However, private sector employers have also been very aggressive in attempting to control health care costs. A coalition of thirty of the largest employers in Twin Cities, coupled with another fourteen self-funded employers in Sioux Falls, Iowa, have adopted a coordinated approach to purchasing health care involving direct provider contracting. This involves bypassing the HMOs and allowing consumers to choose among groups of care providers based on cost and quality. The resulting Buyer's Health Care Action Group (BHCAG) product, Choice Plus, was founded on four principles:

- Minimize or eliminate unnecessary care through continuous quality improvement.
- Streamline administrative costs.
- Increase consumers' ability to take responsibility for their own well-being and for using their health plan appropriately.
- Develop a partnership between providers and employers.

Choice Plus members enroll in one of twenty-eight "care systems," each of which includes primary care clinics, primary care physicians, specialists, hospitals, and other health care providers. Primary care providers may belong to only one care system, a feature intended to create greater accountability at the primary care level. If the member receives care from within the care system, cost-sharing is minimal for most services. If the member visits a provider outside the care system, cost-sharing is significantly higher.

In the Twin Cities, total BHCAG enrollment is approximately 150,000, making it the seventh-largest health plan in the state. Observers of the Twin Cities health care market differ in their assessment of how the BHCAG model has worked. According to some health plan employees, the model has not worked as well as hoped because of the monopoly position of many provider systems and the systems have raised their cost bids annually because they know consumers cannot realistically change to another provider. "BHCAG gets a lot of publicity nationally," said one health plan executive. "But it only covers about 5 percent of the market in the Twin Cities, so it's really not very important."

HEALTH PLAN INVOLVEMENT IN COMMUNITY HEALTH

The public health structure in Minnesota has several levels, including the state Department of Health, forty-nine regional community health boards, eighty-seven county health departments, and a large number of city health departments. Among the responsibilities of the state Department of Health is to establish statewide health goals every four years. Each area of the state has a community health board that identifies and prioritizes public health goals for its area. These boards receive advice on local goals and priorities from a community health advisory board, which has representatives of the entire community.

Local Discussion and Interaction

The health plans, public agencies, and other organizations have a variety of forums for discussion of public health issues. Two of the most important are the Center for Population Health and the Minnesota Health Improvement Partnership.

The Center for Population Health came about after a series of meetings among state and local public health organizations in 1993 and 1994 focused on how various public and private organizations could collaborate to achieve community health goals. The group issued a report in April 1995 that recommended, among other things, the continuation of a forum to serve as a convening point for joint efforts among public health agencies, managed care plans, and community health organizations. The Center for Population Health was established to serve this purpose in the Twin Cities area.

The Center's mission is to "maintain and improve the health of the population through public-private initiatives." It is governed by a council of representatives from partner organizations, which include the state and county health departments, health plans, health and hospital systems, academia, and community-based health organizations. The Center does not replace the functions of other groups but facilitates coordination and communication of population health initiatives between the public and private sectors and among various private organizations.

The Center has worked on a number of initiatives, including the development of a metro-wide population-based immunization registry and a community-wide plan to prevent the use of tobacco. "So far the Center's initiatives have been things that are easy to implement, require little money, and are not threatening," commented one participant. "But it's been a good way to build relationships. Plus even issues that are not so hard, like immunizations, have so many problems: the overlapping provider networks of the plans, which plan should work with which providers, who should pay—the public or private sector, the state or the county?"

The second organization, the Minnesota Health Improvement Partnership (MHIP), is an advisory group to the Minnesota Department of Health (MDOH), with representation from a broad base of constituencies including local public health, health plans, providers, and consumers. The group advises MDOH on selected issues, including the update of the Minnesota Public Health Goals and issues that affect the development of collaborative partnerships to achieve public health goals in the state.

Legal Requirements for Plan Participation in Public Health

Although the managed care plans in the Twin Cities have long been involved in health improvement efforts, many observers, particularly in the public sector and advocacy community, point to two key events as the catalysts for the plans to move much more aggressively into community health improvement work. The first was the enactment in 1994 of a state law requiring health plans to submit public health "collaboration plans" to MDOH. The second was the passage of 1997 legislation empowering counties to include local public health goals in contracts with health plans for the Medicaid program.

All managed care organizations are required to submit a "Local Public Accountability and Collaboration Plan" every two years to the state commissioner of health. The plans must describe "the actions the managed care organization has taken and those it intends to take to contribute to achieving public health goals for each service area in which an enrollee of the managed care plans resides," and must be developed in collaboration with local public health, regional boards, and other community organizations. Local public health agencies also have an opportunity, along with other community groups, to submit written comments on whether the plan meets the needs of the community.

Besides submission of collaboration plans, health plans have had to respond to counties that have become more involved in health purchasing, particularly for public program recipients. This came about, in part, because of the counties' desire to ensure that medical care is coordinated with other necessary social services and to improve health through better coordination of health care and public health responsibilities. But, according to a local public health official, "Counties also saw their revenue streams for funding essential public health services drying up when the Medicaid money started going into managed care plans. . . . Counties are important and powerful in Minnesota and they each want to have their own goals."

As a result of county efforts, a law was enacted in 1997 that allows county boards to request that state Medicaid contracts with health plans include requirements related to the achievement of local public health goals. As a condition of contracting with the State of Minnesota employee group, health plans are required to contract with the state Medicaid program. As a result, most HMOs in the state, including HealthPartners, serve Medicaid members.

In its most recent contracts with managed care plans, the state Department of Human Services included specific public health goals. HealthPartners, for example, had Twin Cities area goals to encourage its clinics to identify and refer victims of domestic violence, to work with other organizations to develop and implement a regional immunization registry, and to promote tobacco use prevention and control policies and practices.

Some health plans take a dim view of the regulatory requirements. "There was a lot of good, voluntary collaboration going on before the state requirements," according to one health plan representative. "But the whole tone changed once things were regulated. There is more antagonism. Plus it is hard enough to do meaningful collaboration in the metro area. . . . It is impossible to work with eighty-seven counties. . . . The requirement has not really changed what we are doing." But another health plan employee said, "The process has educated the counties more about our business environment and the fiscal realities we are under. They are beginning to see that there is no new money. They are also realizing that we have very limited ability to change how the providers operate."

Public health officials are generally more positive. "We have spent the last two years building trust and knowledge and coming to agreement about the appropriate roles and responsibilities of all the parties," said a state official. "I can't point to any hugely different outcomes as a result of this collaboration. But at least we all have a better mutual understanding of the concerns and the possibilities. We don't have enough time or money to be unclear or duplicative." A local public health official agreed: "These regulatory provisions have had some benefits and some limitations. They have gotten the health plans and others to the table, and they begin to define health plan accountability. Plus they help level the playing field for all health plans. . . . But they do not ensure adequate resources will be available from the health plans to do the work, and now limited resources are directed at required and not voluntary collaboration efforts." Another official commented, "The collaboration plans so far are a bunch of crap. But the value is that it requires people to meet and share data. And it's not just the health plans with local public health, but it's the local public health people talking to one another. Until there were the collaboration plans, the local departments never talked to one another."

But legal requirements are not the only reason for health plans to support public health work, according to staff at the Council of Health Plans. "Involvement in public health makes business sense for the plans," said one staff member. "It builds trust and goodwill in the community, which can fuel membership growth. . . . The plans are serving an increasingly diverse and complex membership. . . . It's less expensive for plans to purchase outreach and related services from public health than to build their own services . . . and including the public health system in case management of complex patients will save costs and improve outcomes. . . . Plus if health plan goals are more closely aligned with public health goals it may lessen the perceived need for government regulation."

HealthPartners and Community Health Improvement Programs

HealthPartners was formed in 1992 from the merger of two HMOs, Group Health Inc., a staff model plan, and MedCenters Health Plan, a group model HMO. HealthPartners uses a variety of care delivery systems, including HealthPartners Medical Group and Clinics, Regions Hospital (the largest provider of charity care in St. Paul), and more than thirty contracted care delivery systems or medical groups. Like all HMOs in Minnesota, by law, HealthPartners is a nonprofit company. It is also a consumer-governed organization, with a board of directors elected by the members of the plan.

HealthPartners is involved in a wide variety of efforts to "make a positive difference" in its community. These efforts include some of the community benefits traditional for hospitals, such as providing uncompensated care and services to other vulnerable populations at Regions Hospital (a former county hospital), and offering or supporting unique and important community services such as trauma and burn care, as well as giving financial and in-kind support (including employee volunteer time) to a large number of community-based organizations. HealthPartners has also undertaken a range of community health improvement initiatives, both individually and in collaboration with other organizations.

PARTNERS FOR BETTER HEALTH. Partners for Better Health is one of HealthPartners' major health improvement initiatives. It has eight major health improvement goals for the population served by Health-Partners:

- *Breast cancer:* Improve the early detection of breast cancer, reducing by 50 percent the cases that reach an advanced state before being detected. Increase to 85 percent the biannual mammography rate for women aged fifty to seventy-four.
- *Childhood injuries:* Decrease by 25 percent those childhood injuries severe enough to require medical care and to reduce by 10 percent the injuries so severe that they need hospitalization.

- *Dental cavities:* Reduce by 50 percent new dental cavities in all age groups.

- *Diabetes:* Improve the early detection of diabetes by screening 90 percent of high-risk members; reduce by 25 percent the progression from a high-risk state to active disease; and reduce by 30 percent the onset and progression of eye, kidney, and nerve damage resulting from diabetes.

- *Family violence prevention:* Help identify members who may be victims of abuse and continually link them with appropriate services and prevention resources at HealthPartners and within the community.

- *Heart disease:* Reduce the number of heart disease events among members by 25 percent. This includes myocardial infarction, angioplasty, coronary artery bypass, and congestive heart failure.

- *Immunization rates:* Increase from 75 percent to 95 percent the number of children who are fully immunized by age two.

- *Infant and maternal health:* Reduce by 30 percent infant and maternal complications among members. This includes preterm deliveries, infants affected by smoking or substance abuse, and repeat teenage pregnancies.

"We set highly ambitious targets," said one HealthPartners executive. "We wanted goals that would be challenging, not ones we knew we could do. We already had the best medical results in the state in these goal areas. But we knew that real breakthroughs in these areas would not come from minor changes to the status quo. So we got the best caregivers together, from within and outside of Minnesota, and asked them to think aggressively to come up with truly meaningful goals." Another added, "Partners for Better Health is directly related to our mission. Our responsibility as a health organization is to pay a 'health dividend.' What we learn and what we earn gets reinvested in health. . . . And we've seen our competition begin to offer similar prevention programs, which fits with the second half of our mission, to improve the health of our community."

Partners for Better Health is based on a health improvement model, which breaks the population into people who are at no or low risk, at risk, at high risk, have early symptoms, or have active disease. HealthPartners has tried to develop a range of clinical and nonclinical approaches that target individuals at each point in the risk spectrum.

Much of the health improvement work of HealthPartners is focused on areas related to achieving the Partners for Better Health goals. It has created dozens of specific programs and communication approaches targeted at its eight improvement goals: member newsletters; video programs that provide information about the benefits and risk of various treatment options, including those for breast cancer; a provider-based computer database to collect information on risk factors associated with the development of cavities; allowing physicians to write prescriptions for at-risk members to meet with a dietitian; smoking cessation programs; sponsorship of walking programs in local communities; and a range of disease management programs, including ones targeted at preterm birth prevention and congestive heart failure. For some time, HealthPartners also sponsored "The Better Health Restaurant Challenge," an annual competition in which local restaurants compete to create low-fat menu items, but it recently ended this sponsorship.

The goals and progress of the Partners for Better Health program are reviewed on an annual basis by an interdisciplinary group of physicians, health educators, health plan members, employers, and members of the community.

PARTNERS FOR BETTER HEALTH EMPLOYER INITIATIVE. In 1995, HealthPartners launched the Partners for Better Health Employer Initiative (PBHEI). The goal of the program is "to improve organizational and individual health" of employees and dependents by working in collaboration with employers, clinicians, and individuals. PBHEI brings health improvement programs to individuals at home, the worksite, and the physician's office. The approach includes a phone-based health risk survey, administered to individuals on a voluntary basis, and provides individual results to the participant, aggregate results for all survey respondents to the employer, and feedback to the employee's physician. Individuals are advised by HealthPartners about steps they can take through the HealthPartners system to reduce their risks. If an individual has indicated a willingness to be contacted directly, clinical staff from the individual's physician or HealthPartners health education staff follow up to discuss identified health risks. After an assessment of the individual's readiness to change, the counselor or physician and the individual develop a health promotion plan. The program has demonstrated considerable success in a number of areas, including weight reduction and increase in physical activity.

PBHEI also creates a management report for the employer that defines the health risks of the employee population and recommends strategies to address the risks. The report also includes an analysis of the employer's claims experience and a "preventable cost" analysis. Based on this information, HealthPartners and the employer determine what on-site health promotion programs should be implemented.

More than eight hundred employers have enrolled in PBHEI. HealthPartners bears the cost of the health risk assessment and shares the costs of any programs implemented with the employer. ("The program is a real market differentiator and helps us sell accounts," said a HealthPartners staff member.) Based on results from the first three years of PBHEI, from more than five hundred employers and 130,000 members, the top preventable conditions for HealthPartners members were cardiovascular disease, mental health problems, women's health issues, back problems, and lack of self-care.

HealthPartners is also working to create the "Partners for Better Health Registry." This registry will be an integrated health database combining data from the health risk assessment with data from medical claims, laboratory and pharmacy data, and other clinical information.

INSTITUTE FOR CLINICAL SERVICES INTEGRATION. HealthPartners regards its leadership in establishing the Institute for Clinical Services Integration (ICSI) as another of its major community health improvement activities. ICSI is an organization founded in 1993 by HealthPartners, the Mayo Clinic, and HealthSystem Minnesota. The organization was initially conceived in 1992 at the time of the merger of Group Health and MedCenters. This proved to be a prescient idea "because the first request for proposals from BHCAG required successful bidders to have a guidelines organization that was physician controlled," one observer pointed out. "So we were fortunate that we had already had the idea of creating a separate structure."

The mission of ICSI is to "champion the cause of health care quality and to accelerate improvement in the value of the health care we deliver." ICSI provides health care improvement services to seventeen participating medical groups affiliated with HealthPartners. Most of the groups are multi-specialty practices and range in size from fourteen practitioners to more than a thousand physicians. The combined medical groups represent nearly twenty-five hundred doctors. All but two of the large medical groups in the Twin Cities metropolitan area are members of ICSI. HealthPartners and BHCAG accept membership in ICSI as meeting their requirements for continual improvement processes, and they accept ICSI guidelines.

ICSI undertakes activities to standardize health care processes, improve health care outcomes, and reduce health care costs. It is an independent, nonprofit organization, governed by a board that includes representatives from the founding organizations, as well as two other medical groups and two other purchasers. "The independence of ICSI is critical to its success," said an ICSI employee. "We wanted to get beyond the trust problems of physicians with managed care plans. Physicians come to the table with managed care plans assuming they will lose money or patients. As a result, they don't come in good faith or with energy."

However, financial support comes from HealthPartners. "I think we will eventually have other cosponsors," according to an ICSI spokesperson. "But HealthPartners has not been willing to give up its exclusive arrangement with ICSI until recently. It uses this association in its sales meetings with employers, and providers regard the Health-Partners sponsorship of ICSI as evidence of the plan's commitment to quality. But I think the HealthPartners leadership believes that ICSI is a vital community resource and is willing to broaden its base. Plus, they will get a good public relations hit when they eventually give ICSI to the community."

The major focus of ICSI initially was to develop best practice guidelines, which now total more than forty in a number of disease areas, and technology assessments, which evaluate the effectiveness and safety of emerging and controversial medical technologies. A number of the ICSI guidelines relate directly to the Partners for Better Health goals: heart disease (including stable coronary heart disease and tobacco cessation), preterm birth prevention, initial treatment of breast cancer, management of Type II diabetes mellitus, pediatric immunization, and domestic abuse.

Physicians and other professionals from participating medical groups (and more recently, patients) participate in work groups to develop guidelines, which are reviewed by participating physician groups before being adopted. The workgroup that developed each guideline meets annually to review the guideline and revise it as appropriate.

Medical groups must apply to become ICSI members. "We look at their ability and willingness to do quality improvement work," said an ICSI staff member. "The main motivation of the groups is professional, but there is also prestige among their peers if the group belongs." As a condition of belonging to ICSI, participating medical groups must agree to use ICSI guidelines, as well as commit to specific improvement efforts on select topics.

In the last two years, ICSI has worked more on guideline implementation, using a number of "collaborative forums" where clinicians and staff can share information and strategies on implementing guidelines. "We want them to share not only their successes but their failures as well," said ICSI spokesperson. As of April 1999, ICSI had five action groups under way (diabetes, preventive services, ADHD, asthma, and secondary prevention of cardiovascular disease). Individual physician groups were working on an average of three to five specific improvement areas, the most common of which were diabetes, preventive services, stable coronary disease, and asthma.

ICSI views one of its central roles as being a "champion for quality," by informing the community about evidence-based medicine and the benefits to the public of providers' health care improvement efforts. "We see one of our major roles as improving community health through education and advocacy," said an ICSI executive. In furtherance of this role, ICSI sponsors a national colloquium on clinical quality improvement, conducts seminars and other educational forums, publishes newsletters and articles in professional journals, and conducts public awareness and legislative campaigns on topics that support continual improvement. ICSI has made its guidelines available on the Internet at http://www.icsi.org; fifty-six separate entries were available as of April 2003.

DOMESTIC VIOLENCE. Domestic violence has been a major focus of HealthPartners' community health work. The plan has worked on a number of initiatives to improve identification and referral of victims of domestic violence, including the ICSI domestic violence clinical care protocol and production of a videotape training program to help doctors, nurses, and other staff identify and help victims of domestic violence.

"This is a difficult issue because we are selling what nobody wants to buy," said a HealthPartners staff member who works on the program, who continued,

> I worked for nine years with victims and perpetrators, so I thought this would be easy. I was wrong. . . . It took two years for the whole system to understand this issue and to chip away at the resistance.

None of the providers thought they saw these women. . . . The only people who were aware of the magnitude of this problem were the receptionists at the clinics. We had to get the providers information specific to their practice. So we did things like putting tearaway cards in safe locations in the clinics, including the bathrooms, that said, "if you're a victim of abuse, here's what to do." In the first few months, more than four thousand cards were taken. We sent the clinics data on the number of women seen by the local shelter in their area and told them that they could assume that at least some of these women were their patients . . . and we pulled charts of women who had a diagnosis of depression or injury. We found that only 2 of the 270 cases mentioned the possibility of domestic violence in the record. . . . It was not identified as a problem even in one case where the woman told the doctor she had been beaten up by her boyfriend.

HealthPartners has also been an active participant on the statewide Health Care Coalition on Violence, which has asked hospitals to voluntarily use "Ecodes" (External Causes) on billings to permit better statistics to be collected on causes of injury for patients seen in the emergency room or as inpatients. This information will be used to develop a better understanding of patterns of violence in the Twin Cities and how to address them.

SMART. In the past three years, HealthPartners has undertaken a major initiative to support early childhood brain development, called Stimulate Minds At the Right Time, or SMART. Based on research showing how vitally important brain stimulation and nurturing are during the first three years of life, HealthPartners has engaged in a number of efforts to educate parents and providers about the need to stimulate infants and toddlers in appropriate nurturing ways. "We have a permanent underclass in the United States," said one HealthPartners executive. "The majority of kids who drop out of school have IQs of under 85. If we can increase IQs twenty-five to thirty points, it can be the difference between Yale and jail, between welfare and a job. . . . The state and Medicaid should be demanding this type of program from all its contracting health plans."

One of the earliest components of this initiative was sponsoring a community dialogue about the importance of supporting early childhood brain development. Since then HealthPartners developed and distributed "Food for Thought," a video that explains the link between stimulation, reading, brain development, and intelligence, and a children's book to all new parents who are HealthPartners members, as well as to the general public through a wide range of organizations, including all licensed in-home day care centers in the Twin Cities, as well as public libraries, teen parents, and adults through school and community early education programs and reading readiness programs. The video is also available at no cost from participating video rental stores. HealthPartners is working to expand the program, collaborating with the Minnesota Department of Health to distribute SMART material as part of the statewide birth packet given to all new parents.

PREVENTING TOBACCO USE. HealthPartners has devoted considerable resources to preventing tobacco use. A major counter-tobacco advertising campaign aimed at teens was initiated by the plan in 1996. The campaign, called Garbage Face, used radio and television ads to try to convince teenagers that they would suffer all types of social opprobrium, including not being able to get dates, if they smoked. The plan also distributed over one million copies of "Sure fire, fifty-day way to stop smoking" calendars as inserts in local newspapers. In addition, HealthPartners has partnered with schools, clinics, community groups, and public health agencies to offer smoking cessation activities in community settings, including schools, and worked on statewide collaborations to support passage of laws that restrict youth access to tobacco.

A Few Examples of Collaborations

The Minnesota Council of Health Plans, working in partnership with the Department of Health, recently developed and distributed an immunization packet to all pediatric providers to help them set up patient records that will be compatible with a centralized patient immunization registry. The Council also developed a Health Record Folder that is being distributed to all new parents to educate them about the need and timing of necessary immunizations and help them keep immunization records for their children.

In an example of collaboration between two plans, HealthPartners and Blue Cross undertook an AHCPR-funded project to improve preventive screening, called IMPROVE (for "IMproving PRevention through Organization, Vision and Empowerment"). The project recruited forty-four clinics, which were randomly assigned to either an intervention group or a control group. The intervention group received training in a variety of continuous quality improvement techniques aimed at improving the delivery of eight selected preventive services (for example, breast exams, mammograms, pap smears, flu shots for elders). According to one study of the project, "Although there is much debate about the role of competition in health care, collaboration has in this case led to benefits for clinics, health plans, and the community. Collaboration on IMPROVE has been a bridge over troubled waters, reminding us that the enemy is neither ourselves nor others. The common enemy is disease" (Magnan and others, 1998, p. 578).

Another successful collaboration between the health plans and the public sector was the development of the "Minnesota Pregnancy Assessment Form." This project was initiated by the Minnesota Council of Health Plans so that the health plans and the Minnesota Department of Human Services could accept the same screening tool from all obstetrical providers for women covered by publicly financed health care programs, including Medicaid. As part of the initiative, a resource and service guide was developed for obstetrical providers to help them connect pregnant women with needed medical or social services. "We had to broaden beyond the screening tool because doctors did not want to ask questions like, 'Are you getting adequate nutrition?' if they could not intervene," said one health plan representative.

One of the public-private community health improvement projects in the Twin Cities that took a broad perspective on community health improvement is the Philips Partnership, a collaborative venture spearheaded by the Allina Health System, in collaboration with Honeywell. The groundwork for the Philips Partnership was laid in 1996, when Minneapolis was dubbed "Murder-apolis" by the *New York Times* after the city had a record high ninety-three murders in 1995 (Johnson, 1996). Many of the murders occurred in the Philips neighborhood, home to Honeywell's world headquarters and two Allina facilities, Abbott Northwestern Hospital and Philips Eye Institute. "Patients and employees were worried about coming to the hospitals," said an Allina executive. "So we had a vested business interest in the safety of the neighborhood. We needed to make the hospital a good place to come to work and a safe place to seek health care. But that's a critical component of successful collaborations—you have got to align the community and business interests of the organization."

The upsurge in crime in the neighborhood was linked to epidemic use of crack cocaine. Working as part of Minnesota for Hope, Education and Law and Safety (HEALS), a statewide public-private partnership to reduce crime, the group developed a better understanding of the causes of rising crime, including the rise in crack cocaine use and gang activity. The group bulldozed crack houses, improved coordination among law enforcement officials, and even changed school days to a later start time to minimize unsupervised afternoon hours when most robberies happened.

The Philips Partnership grew out of HEALS in the spring of 1997. The Partnership, a collaboration of Allina, Children's Hospital, Fannie Mae, Honeywell, the Minneapolis Foundation, Norwest Bank, US Bank, the City of Minneapolis, and Hennepin County, aims to improve the long-term livability of the Philips neighborhood. "Our goal is to help the community to heal so that vitality and overall 'health' can be restored to the neighborhood," said Mike Christenson, Allina's head of Community Investments and the Allina Foundation. So far, the Partnership has focused on four areas: safety, jobs, housing, and infrastructure.

A job training initiative has been undertaken to improve the work readiness skills of area residents and help with job placement at Abbott Northwestern Hospital. The Partnership has brought more than $25 million to the neighborhood to improve rental housing and create new home ownership opportunities. So far, construction of more than eighty new townhomes and houses is under way, as well as the rehabilitation of a number of severely degraded apartment buildings and the building of new parks and recreation facilities. Allina is also making grants available to employees who want to buy homes in the neighborhood. The Partnership is also working to improve the accessibility of the neighborhood by developing new ramps that will provide direct access from major freeways.

"Crime is down, property values are rising, and for the first time in decades new homes are being built in the neighborhood," said an Allina official. He admits that it could become harder to convince Allina to make such investments if health care resources grow more constrained. "The payoff for the work is long term and many people wonder why we are fixing up houses when we need more nurses on the floors. With the recent Medicare payment cuts, this tension will increase even more. But we need to take a much broader vision of health—it's not just what happens in a doctor's office or inside a hospital."

Barriers and Challenges

Opinion in the Twin Cities differs about how successful the involvement of managed care plans in community health improvement has
been. Even people who point to successes also acknowledge significant challenges remain. In these conversations, some common themes
emerge.

The efforts of the health plans are disparate and uncoordinated: Many
public health officials and providers complain of lack of coordination
among the health plans. According to one observer:

> The community health issues are all being divided up. Each plan has
> staked out its own territory, and usually in areas that will accrue com-
> petitive advantage for them with employers. . . . HealthPartners is gen-
> uinely interested in improving health but it has really focused on
> *individual* health and health promotion, not community health . . .
> things like diabetes and heart health that are just good medical care.
> Maybe not typical medical care, but still a medical model. . . . Allina's
> approach is to give out money to projects that support its strategic pri-
> orities. A lot of their community health efforts are fluff to build up
> their marketing. . . . BCBS's big issue has been smoking. But their com-
> munity health people are buried in the organization and don't have
> much presence.

The health plans believe that they have collaborated well on many
initiatives. "The health plan market is very competitive," said one
health plan employee. "But the competition is at different and higher
levels in the organization. There is no competition at the program
level. We all cooperate because we all want to improve the health of
the community." But the view is somewhat different outside the health
plans. "This is a very competitive town," said a public health official.
"We talk a lot about collaboration and how we are so different in
Minnesota, but the fact is that each plan usually picks its own initiatives and does its own thing. All the health plans do things to help the
community and most of these efforts do have spillover effects that end
up benefiting everyone, but there is little true collaboration . . . and
when it occurs, like in the area of immunizations, it's only because collaboration is the only way to get improvement . . . and because it's an
area that purchasers are paying attention to." Another observer agreed,
"It is hard for the managed care companies to collaborate. They all

have different interests, different market positions, and unequal financial resources. . . . There are lots of good areas for clinical collaboration but the health plans don't really want to do it because each of them wants to be able to say that its program is the best."

Several observers noted inconsistencies in the behavior of health plans as competitive businesses and as champions of community health improvement. "The overriding economic incentive for the health plans is still to want to keep high-risk people out of their plans in order to keep premiums lower," said one employer. "So HealthPartners talks about its diabetes care management programs but it denies nongroup insurance coverage to people who have diabetes. And it charges a $10 per vial copayment for insulin. . . . Until we fix the ways in which health plans are paid, by paying risk-adjusted premiums, we cannot fix any of these public health problems."

Tensions between the public and private sectors: Some health plans expressed a number of frustrations in dealing with the public sector in their community health efforts. "There are lots of turf issues with the public health folks," complained one health plan employee. "They tell us 'we do public health, so you can do this, but not that.' It's all about control and money." "It should be the responsibility of government to lead these efforts," said one health plan executive. "But the state health department is bureaucratic and political and is not driving the effort. No private managed care plan can make up for ineffective government in public health."

Many in the public health agencies seemed sympathetic to these complaints. Said one public health official,

> We are lucky in the Twin Cities because people in the health plans and government have long personal relationships and there is a lot of movement between the public and private sectors. We have a small and intimate health care community and a long history of working together. But even so, doing public health in Minnesota is like herding cats. I think the managed care plans are feeling overwhelmed. There is so much to do and so many people they have to deal with, in both the public sector and the community. . . . Minnesota has so many different levels of government and they are not at all integrated, even at the same level of government. For example, if you have a meeting with the Hennepin County health department, you have to invite at least five different people.

Another public health official agreed: "There is tremendous variability in public health across the state and no common expectations. The managed care plans need a road map to help them figure out where and how they can best plug in and really make a difference."

What is the value added by managed care plans? The question of what unique competencies managed care plans bring to community health seems to be pondered frequently. "There is a real question of where health plans can bring value to this work," said one provider. "I think managed care has a limited ability to contribute to many of these public health issues. Where they can add value is in datasets, helping to understand prevalence and connecting data across plans . . . and improving the internal operations of providers and helping to develop and implement best practices and clinical guidelines . . . and improving care for people in public programs like Medicare and Medicaid . . . but they don't really know anything about communities." Another person from a community-based organization echoed this assessment, saying, "Health plans do not know much about sitting down with communities and helping them create their own priorities and identify their own approaches for solving community problems. They often disempower people or they don't want to get involved in what communities really want and need because it isn't what the health plan thought the community would need. . . . They don't get why a community park might make a much bigger contribution to health in a low-income, high-crime community than any other intervention."

The key determinants of health: People in the Twin Cities often acknowledge that many of the determinants of health are outside the control, and perhaps influence, of managed care plans. "The types of work being done by the health plans are frustrating the more you know about the factors that influence health," said one provider. "The reasons for poor health have little to do with medical care. They have to do with poverty, poor education, segregation, unemployment, alienation, lack of transportation. It just feels like these problems are far beyond the ability of the health care system, let alone just managed care plans, to solve."

This fact is acknowledged by at least some health plan staff. "It's clear that member-based programs are not enough to achieve public health outcomes," said one health plan representative. "We need new approaches that integrate public health investments, market health and prevention to entire communities, and draw upon the health industry's ability to innovate and deliver."

But many remain skeptical that private managed care plans will ever be willing or able to develop these new approaches. "There is enough money in the system to meet the needs of everyone," said one consumer activist. "One less MRI would pay for lots of early childhood education, which would do a lot for health. But it would mean reallocating money. This is highly charged politically and we have no structure for getting those kinds of questions answered. So the only collaboration that has happened in the market is about innocent stuff that no one to the left of Genghis Khan would object to, on issues that don't cost much and do not rearrange the power and money."

Willingness to continue community health investments: Whether health plans will continue to support community health work is an open question for many people.

"The local mood is that 'we cannot afford to do community health,' and the managed care plans and many providers are at the point of disengaging," said a hospital official. "The hospital association has disbanded its committee on community health. The HMOs are all losing money and community health is the first thing to go when organizations are doing poorly. So the health plans are downsizing their efforts, staff is disappearing, and budgets are being cut. The community health advocates have been complete failures at convincing people of the overall value of these efforts. So I fear that community health improvement is just another fad that will die and recede."

Many employers seem skeptical about the involvement of health plans in community health activities. "There's a split among businesses about these issues," reported one employer representative. "Some of them think business needs to be accountable to the community. But this is not a core business for the employers and many are very frustrated with the health plans. They do not want the plans focused on public health. They want them to focus on taking care of sick people and show good performance doing that.... They don't want business to have a public health agenda—that's government's role. The obligation of business is to keep its health insurance premiums down to be accountable to stockholders."

This tension is becoming evident to public health officials also. "We are seeing more push-back from the managed care organizations, even if they buy into community health in the long term, because they say employers won't pay," observed one government official. "The Minnesota Public Health Association proposed doing an annual report on HMO investments in population health and community health. At first the plans were interested and thought they would get some good press but then they decided it was too risky because it might antagonize business and cause them trouble on the pricing side. Employers would ask, why am I spending any money on this stuff? HealthPartners has done well to stay focused on the Partners for Better Health program, but they see that program as a marketing advantage."

The Future

HealthPartners remains committed to its health improvement agenda. "It's clear to all of us that there needs to be a shift between health and health care," said a plan executive. "The need is bigger than ever. Managed care has squeezed out all that it can from medical management. How will we reduce the need and demand for health services in the future and address the demands of employers for affordable health care coverage? The answer has got to be improving the health of the entire community."

But not everyone is certain about the future role of health plans in community health improvement. According to one public health official:

> So far, we have picked small, low-risk ventures to work on with the managed care plans. We are still dating and we have not decided whether to have sex yet. One of the questions for public health agencies is, Will the health plans be here in five years? What will they look like? At the moment, there is a lot of uncertainty about the future of managed care plans. The providers will be here, the state will be here, the counties will be here, and the local public health departments will be here. The purchasers will be here. But will the health plans?

~~ Epilogue: The New Mission of HealthPartners—A Perspective on Progress

George Isham, M.D., and Maureen Peterson
HealthPartners

HealthPartners revised its mission in 2000, expanding it to read as follows: *"The mission of HealthPartners is to improve the health of our members, our patients, and the community."*

The reason for adding "our patients" to the mission statement is to emphasize the importance of caring for the chronically ill as well as preventing illness in those who are well.

As of 2002, HealthPartners' membership was 665,000 members, and the plan contracted with more than eight thousand physicians. George Halvorson resigned in May 2002, and the Board of Directors appointed Mary Brainerd as the new president and CEO. Since 1994, she had been second in command there, most recently as executive vice president and chief operating officer.

ORGANIZATIONAL STRUCTURES

Several organizational structures that support HealthPartners community health improvement work have changed since 1999.

Health Promotion/Disease Prevention Council

The Community Health Council, created to guide HealthPartners involvement in community health initiatives, has evolved into the Health Promotion/Disease Prevention Council (HP/DP). The mission of the HP/DP is to provide coordination, integration, tracking, and prioritization of systemwide health promotion and disease prevention activities that reach members, patients, and the community. The committee focuses its work on primary prevention activities and tracks HealthPartners' involvement in multiple community and statewide health promotion initiatives. The membership of the Council has been expanded significantly to include such areas as Corporate Communications, the chief health officer and two associate medical directors, the vice president of Customer and Member Services, and the vice president of Health Services Analysis. The Council has proved to be an effective tool for outlining issues, prioritizing, and integrating efforts in the areas of health disparities, member, clinic, and worksite HP/DP activities, and Partners for Better Health goals achievement activities. The Council sponsors discussions with key local and state public health leaders on opportunities for collaboration.

Partners for Better Health

Partners for Better Health continues as one of HealthPartners' major health improvement initiatives. In 2000, a new set of goals, Partners for Better Health 2005, was created. PBH 2005 builds on the knowledge gained since the program was launched in 1994, focusing on diseases, lifestyle and behavior issues, populations, process-oriented improvements, and customer-oriented improvements. PBH 2005 goals recognize the important role social determinants and public programs have on health and also address issues such as socioeconomic status, race, and ethnicity. These areas of focus represent a way of emphasizing population-based and lifestyle-oriented goals. Once again Health-Partners has set measurable goals for improving health in specific areas including heart health, diabetes, depression, healthy eating, physical activity, and tobacco control. Exhibit 9.1 lists the PBH 2005 goals—the objectives are to be achieved by 2005—in full.

Research Foundation

The HealthPartners Research Foundation continues to fulfill the important role of seeding new ideas and collaborating with public

Exhibit 9.1.   Partners for Better Health 2005 Goals.

A. HEART HEALTH

Goal Statement #1: PREVENT THE CLINICAL EXPRESSION OF ATHEROSCLEROTIC DISEASE IN THE AT-RISK POPULATION.
Objectives

1.1 Individually contact 100% of our adult membership to assess risk for cardiovascular disease, with a completion rate of 50%.

1.2 Among individuals at risk for atherosclerotic disease, increase by 50% the number of people who have all their modifiable risk factors in control.

1.3 To decrease by 50% the risk of atherosclerotic disease by favorable impact on modifiable risk factors.

Goal Statement #2: REDUCE REOCCURRING EVENTS AND COMPLICATIONS IN PATIENTS WITH KNOWN CARDIO-VASCULAR DISEASE.
Objectives

2.1 Increase by 50% the number of patients with atherosclerotic cardio-vascular disease who have all their modifiable risk factors in control.

2.2 Reduce by 50% the rate of CHF-related hospitalizations and all Emergency Department visits for patients with CHF.

Goal Statement #3: OPTIMIZE LIFETIME FUNCTIONAL CAPAC-ITY FOR INDIVIDUALS WITH CARDIOVASCULAR DISEASE.
Objective

3.1 By 2005, 75% of individuals with cardiovascular disease will self-report being satisfied with their functional capacity.

B. DIABETES

Goal Statement #1: DECREASE THE RATE OF DEVELOPMENT OF TYPE 2 DIABETES IN OUR MEMBERS, PATIENTS, AND COMMUNITY BY REDUCING OR PREVENTING MODIFIABLE RISK FACTORS.
Objectives

1.1 Individually contact 100% of our adult membership to assess risk for diabetes, with a rate of risk assessment completion of 50%.

1.2 Increase the percentage of members, patients, and community who are engaged in physical activity and healthy eating by 20% for each behavior.

(Continued)

Exhibit 9.1.   Partners for Better Health 2005 Goals. (*Continued*)

1.3 Reduce the incidence of diabetes in high-risk members by 25%.

1.4 Decrease the mean weight by five pounds among members who are at high risk for the development of Type 2 diabetes and whose BMI is > 25 kg/m.

Goal Statement #2: INCREASE THE QUALITY AND YEARS OF HEALTHY LIFE FOR OUR MEMBERS, PATIENTS, AND COMMUNITY AFFECTED BY DIABETES.

Objectives

2.1 Increase by 50% the percentage of members and patients with diabetes receiving comprehensive clinical care needed to manage the disease and its complications.

2.2 Ensure a holistic approach to care for individuals with diabetes as evidenced by an improvement of 50% over baseline of members indicating their spiritual, emotional, and clinical needs have been supported.

2.3 Engage 90% of members and patients with diabetes in self-care activities.

2.4 Decrease the risk of heart disease events in our patients and members with diabetes by 25%.

2.5 Decrease the risk of end stage renal disease, lower extremity amputations, and blindness in our members and patients with diabetes each by 30%.

2.6 Measure and record the number of heart disease events, end stage renal disease, blindness, and lower extremity amputations.

2.7 Develop, strengthen, or improve the health care systems that support diabetes care for all HealthPartners members.

C. DEPRESSION

Goal Statement #1: IMPROVE THE UNDERSTANDING, RECOGNITION, DIAGNOSIS, AND TREATMENT OF DEPRESSION ACROSS THE RISK CONTINUUM.

Objectives

1.1 Increase by 50% the proportion of the general population who identify that depression is a treatable disease.

1.2 Increase by 50% the number of members at risk for depression who are identified and who receive appropriate intervention.

1.3 Become the benchmark health plan for HEDIS regarding the percentage of members with depression who are accurately diagnosed and who receive appropriate treatment and management.

1.4 Decrease by 50% the number of suicide attempts and suicides among HealthPartners members.

Goal Statement #2: INCREASE COLLABORATION AMONG COMMUNITY SYSTEMS, FAMILIES, AND HEALTH CARE TO MEET THE NEEDS OF PEOPLE ACROSS THE DEPRESSION RISK CONTINUUM.

Objectives

2.1 Increase effective educational, health improvement, and depression support initiatives that are created and delivered via collaborative partnerships between HealthPartners, worksites, schools, and other community organizations.

2.2 Increase coordination, communication, and continuity of care relative to depression between primary care, specialty care, and behavioral health.

D. HEALTHY EATING

Goal Statement: IMPROVE THE FOOD CHOICES OF OUR MEM-BERS AND PATIENTS TO PROMOTE HEALTH AND QUALITY OF LIFE.

Objectives

1. Double the number of members who consume recommended amounts of specific food groups by focusing on the following populations:

    Members with diabetes, heart disease and depression

    Members with a BMI of greater than 25 kg/m

    Senior members ages 65–75

    Adolescents

    Apparently healthy adults

2. Among young children and women of child-bearing age, decrease by 25% the incidence of iron deficiency anemia.

3. Reach 90% of women of childbearing age with messaging regarding the benefits of adequate folate/folic acid consumption.

(Continued)

Exhibit 9.1.   Partners for Better Health 2005 Goals. (*Continued*)

4. Reach all pregnant women, their partners, and providers, with messaging regarding the benefits of breastfeeding for one year.

5. Reduce the proportion of individuals who self-report a BMI of > 29.9 kg/m to no more than 25%.

6. Among all adult members who have completed a Health Risk Assessment and exceed a BMI of 25 kg/m, reduce average weight by five pounds.

E. PHYSICAL ACTIVITY

Goal Statement: INCREASE THE PROPORTION OF INDIVIDUALS AMONG OUR MEMBERS AND OUR COMMUNITY WHO CHOOSE TO LIVE A PHYSICALLY ACTIVE LIFE.

Objectives

1. Among our adult members, increase the average number of physically active days by 2 days per week by focusing on the following groups:

   apparently healthy adults

   members with chronic diseases of diabetes, heart disease, and depression

   members with a body mass index greater than 25 kg/m

   senior members ages 65–75

2. Among our adolescent members, increase the average number of days of physically active days by 2 days per week.

3. Among our senior members ages 75 years and older, reduce the prevalence of completely sedentary behavior by 50%.

4. Increase to 90%, the proportion of individuals who can identify twice as many pros as opposed to cons to being physically active among

   apparently healthy adults

   members with chronic diseases of diabetes, heart disease, and depression

   members with a body mass index greater than 25 kg/m

   parents with children of ages 0–18

   adolescent members

   senior members ages 65 years and older

   health care providers

F. TOBACCO CONTROL

Goal Statement: REDUCE THE PREVALENCE OF TOBACCO USE AND REDUCE CHILDHOOD AND ADOLESCENT EXPOSURE TO TOBACCO AMONG HEALTHPARTNERS MEMBERS AND PATIENTS.

Objectives

1. Reduce prevalence of tobacco use among adults, age 18 years of age and older, from 25% to 15%.

2. Reduce the prevalence of tobacco use among adolescents, 13 through 17 years of age, to 15% and secondhand smoke exposure to 12%.

3. Reduce secondhand smoke exposure among children, birth through 12 years, from 24% to 12%.

---

health organizations to improve health. External government sources of funding provide the largest share of the over $9 million in grants and contracts received in 2001. Major collaborations with eleven other research organizations within managed care are producing advances in cancer research through a $20 million cooperative agreement with the National Cancer Institute. Several projects were awarded funding to address the issues of errors and quality in medicine. Support from the federal Agency for Healthcare Research and Quality and the Robert Wood Johnson Foundation are generating novel efforts to detect and improve the safety of care delivery through the Pursuing Perfection initiative (described later in this chapter). Utilizing research in practice and informing research from practice is an increasing theme for the HealthPartners Research Foundation's work.

ICSI

The Institute for Clinical Services Integration (ICSI), now renamed the Institute for Clinical Systems Improvement, broadened its reach considerably in 2001. Under a new agreement, Minnesota become the first state in the nation where medical care is built around the systematic use of science-based best practice protocols developed by physicians and supported by all major health plans. In March 2001, Blue Cross and Blue Shield of Minnesota, Medica, Preferred One, and UCare Minnesota joined the original sponsors (HealthPartners, Mayo Clinic, and Park Nicollet Health Services) as ICSI sponsors and will use the care protocols developed by the Institute. This means that collaboration not competition is the goal of Minnesota's leading medical groups and health plans when it comes to quality of care. ICSI currently has twenty-eight member organizations located in Minnesota, Wisconsin, and North Dakota. Currently 50 percent of physicians in Minnesota practice in member organizations, and that total is expected to increase to 60 percent by the end of 2002.

BHCAG

Total BHCAG enrollment has dropped from approximately 150,000 to under 100,000. (For more information on BHCAG, see Lyles and others, 2002, and Christianson and Feldman, 2002.)

SUMMARY

The key issue has moved from whether health plans should be engaged in improving the health of their members to how proper incentives can be created for improving health and health care.

HealthPartners is involved in two major projects to further explore this issue: "Making the Business Case for Health Care Quality," and "Pursuing Perfection: Raising the Bar for Health Care Performance."

Making the Business Case for Health Care Quality

The Commonwealth Fund and the Institute for Healthcare Improvement have launched a project titled "Making the Business Case for Health Care Quality." This project aims to build a baseline of evidence in the form of several case studies to illustrate how the flow of resources in the U.S. health care system presents both barriers and incentives to quality improvement while simultaneously illustrating the systemwide benefits of innovative, improved patient care. The cases will be widely disseminated and used to form recommendations to better align payment systems with health care quality improvement. HealthPartners is one of two health plans selected for the case study on chronic care, specifically, diabetes management. HealthPartners was selected because it has successfully implemented a diabetes management program to improve the quality and reduce the cost of caring for diabetic health plan members.

Pursuing Perfection

HealthPartners Medical Clinics (HPMC) has shown its leadership position nationally as a clinical site to develop the next generation of high-performing care systems. It was one of twelve health care organizations chosen as part of "Pursuing Perfection: Raising the Bar for Health Care Performance," a $20.9 million nationwide initiative aimed at improving the quality of health care sponsored jointly by the Robert Wood Johnson Foundation and the Institute for Healthcare Improvement. HealthPartners was chosen for the first phase of this project from a field of over 250 health care organizations. In April 2002, HealthPartners was one of seven organizations nationwide to receive an implementation grant of $1.9 million to develop systems that improve care.

During the first phase, each of these organizations developed "promises" to their patients and a business plan to markedly improve care systems with "perfection" as their ultimate goal.

"Pursuing Perfection" is a program that challenges health care organizations to create best practices for patient-centered, timely, efficient, equitable, effective, and safe care. HealthPartners chose several areas of health care, including care for diabetes and access to information and care, where it will drastically change the system of delivery.

These initiatives will both explore reimbursement for improvement issues. HealthPartners will focus on improving the entire model of health care delivery, including the flow of patient care and relationships between personnel and patients.

Once the new model has been planned and implemented, Health-Partners will share its learnings with other health systems across the country. It will make use of both ICSI and community partnerships to translate the means to attain the six aims throughout the community.

PUBLIC HEALTH LINKAGES

The Minnesota Council of Health Plans has strengthened its community health committee with membership from all the health plans, and the group facilitates interplan activities and communications on public health issues. The committee worked with the Minnesota Department of Health on developing new guidelines for the Public Health Collaboration Plans, that is, each organization's plans for how its staff will work with local and state public agencies to improve population health. The committee also works with public health leaders directly to help set priorities, share information, and support public policy. The health plans recognize that they have a role in not only improving member health but in improving population health in the communities they serve. Major areas for collaboration with public and private sectors have included two significant initiatives. "Cover All Kids" is a collaborative to increase health insurance coverage and access to preventive care for children; it has been a successful program for the past two years. A second major focus has been on behavioral health care improvement, by working together to create a better continuum of community and inpatient care for adolescents and adults experiencing serious mental illness. The health plans came together in 2002 to establish the Community Mental Health Trust Fund to seed community alternatives to care and to improve crisis response.

Lastly, HealthPartners has developed a real-time bioterrorism surveillance system in partnership with MDOH. This involves the collection of CPT 4 diagnosis codes for patients who are seen in HPMG clinics. The codes are transmitted nightly and analyzed by a Department of Health epidemiology technician to detect possible bioterrorism-related illness symptoms. This is an important partnership between the public and private health systems to improve the local response to bioterrorism events should they occur.

References

Christianson, J. B., and Feldman, R. "Evolution in the Buyer's Health Care Action Group Purchasing Initiative." *Health Affairs,* 2002, *21*(1), 76–88.

HealthPartners. "Partners for Better Health 2005 Goals." Corporate publication.

Johnson, D. "Nice City's Nasty Distinction: Murders Soar in Minneapolis." *New York Times,* June 30, 1996, Sec. 1, p. 1.

Lyles, A., and others. "Cost and Quality Trends in Direct Contracting Arrangements." *Health Affairs,* 2002, *21*(1), 89–102.

Magnan, S., and others. "IMPROVE: Bridge over Troubled Waters." *Joint Commission Journal on Quality Improvement,* 1998, *24*(10), 566–578.

Minnesota Department of Health. *Public Health Interventions.* Minneapolis: Minnesota Department of Health, Oct. 1997.

CHAPTER TEN

The UAW Bargains for Health Benefits

I n 1996, the United Auto Workers (UAW), the union representing skilled trade and production workers in the automobile industry, and the Big Three auto manufacturers, Chrysler Corporation, Ford Motor Company, and General Motors (GM), were preparing to negotiate their triennial national bargaining agreements. (Note: for the sake of simplicity, throughout this chapter, the term *UAW workers* refers to UAW members who work for the Big Three unless the context clearly indicates otherwise, even though almost half of UAW members actually work for other companies.) The current UAW contracts with the companies were due to expire at midnight on September 14. Despite widespread predictions that the UAW would pick Chrysler as the target company with which to begin negotiations, as it had in 1993, the union chose Ford. Although the UAW would still negotiate separately with each company, this meant that the agreement

---

This case was originally written by the authors in 1997. Funding was provided by Astra USA. The authors thank William Hoffman and Chuck Gayney of the UAW for their interest and assistance in preparing the case.

with Ford would set the national pattern for the contracts with GM and Chrysler.

The UAW decision to target Ford, a company that was doing particularly well financially and with which the UAW had a generally good relationship, was, according to some observers, of particular concern to GM, which was steadily losing share in the U.S. auto market, had the highest labor costs of any of the Big Three, and the most adversarial relationship with the UAW.

The 1996 contracts would be the first to be bargained under the leadership of Stephen Yokich. Elected union president in June 1995 after fifteen years as a UAW vice president, Yokich had directed many of the union's major departments. He and his team needed to negotiate several key issues, including job security and employment guarantees, restrictions on outsourcing of parts production to nonunion external suppliers, wages, and pensions. The UAW's main goal for the contract, as laid out by its collective bargaining convention, was job security, an issue of widespread concern to union members given the climate of downsizing and outsourcing. The outsourcing issue has been contentious, particularly at GM, where UAW members struck local plants a number of times in recent months before winning outsourcing battles. "These negotiations are about jobs," said UAW VP Richard Shoemaker, "about saving what good-paying jobs there are left and trying to find ways to create new ones." His fellow UAW VP Jack Laskowski added, "Our members could do an even better job if the outsourced parts they assemble on vehicles were produced in-house, so they could be monitored more closely to ensure top-notch quality." However, health benefits for UAW workers and retirees were also high on the list of issues that would be discussed at the negotiating table.

In the 1990 and 1993 contract negotiations, health care had been one of the most significant and contentious issues. In fact, in 1990, health care had been *the* issue. Despite the intense desire of the auto companies to impose cost-sharing requirements or mandate managed care enrollment for UAW members, or both, the UAW made it clear that its members were prepared to strike to resist any such changes. Again in 1993, the Big Three pressed hard for concessions in health care, particularly GM, reeling from a three-year $17 billion loss in its North American operations. However, the companies again backed away from their demands when it became clear that failure to do so would have resulted in a strike.

BACKGROUND

Automaking is one of the largest industries in the United States, accounting directly and indirectly for one out of seven U.S. jobs. In 1995, the Big Three U.S. automakers—General Motors with 34 percent, Ford Motor Company with 21 percent, and Chrysler Corporation with 9 percent—accounted for more than 60 percent of total new cars sold in the United States. The robust performance and condition of the Big Three in 1996 was a far cry from the desperate financial condition of the companies in the previous decade, when the U.S. auto industry lost dominance and market share to foreign competitors. In recent years, the total market share of the Big Three has been quite stable, with gains by Ford and Chrysler largely offset by declines at GM.

The Automakers

General Motors is the world's largest industrial enterprise and the biggest manufacturer of cars and trucks. The company directly employs almost 2 million people and, by its purchasing and sales activities, determines the employment of another 7 million. GM's total output is nearly 4 percent of the U.S. gross domestic product (GDP). In 1995, the company estimated that it spent $3.5 billion on its health programs ($1.8 billion for active employees and $1.7 billion for retirees), and in addition accrued $1.3 billion for its liability for future health benefits. GM's health program is so large that there are only three major zip codes where GM does not have a person covered.

GM is the most vertically integrated and the least profitable of the Big Three. During the 1980s—while Ford and Chrysler were busy scaling back and outsourcing—GM continued to build new factories and roll out ever more labor-intensive car models. During this time, the company lost 15 percentage points of market share. As a result, the company is under tremendous pressure to reduce its workforce and cut costs. Some industry analysts estimate that GM would need to regain all 15 points of market share to justify the size of its current hourly workforce.

GM is widely perceived to have the most adversarial relationship with UAW workers of the Big Three. "They have a culture of arrogance," said one UAW official. "They missed the window of opportunity during the last few years of profitability to rebuild labor relations. Ford and Chrysler made major changes, like decentralizing authority on the shop floor and having union people running quality circles. . . . GM prefers to rely on slogans. There is no trust—a GM plant manager in New Jersey who was complaining about the quality of vehicles built there would not allow in the UAW quality experts to help. They neglect investments in plants that are losing money, even where the investments might improve productivity or quality." UAW concerns about the company's treatment of workers, including unsafe working conditions and inadequate staffing to keep up with production, have triggered a number of local labor actions, including more than fourteen major work stoppages in last decade. By contrast, there has been only one major work stoppage at Chrysler in the last fifteen years and none at Ford for at least twenty years. In 1996, the UAW struck at two GM plants in Ohio over a variety of problems, including workloads, outside contracting, and health and safety matters. The strike lasted seventeen days and idled twenty-four of the company's twenty-nine plants in North America.

This lack of trust sometimes carries over into the company's health programs. "GM misses opportunities to do new programs because there is no trust on the shop floor. Shop floor relations are so bad that workers won't even fill out the questionnaires for the LifeSteps program," according to one UAW staff member. (LifeSteps is a GM-sponsored individualized risk assessment and appraisal program, under which workers with certain risk factors can be eligible for payment of otherwise noncovered health services.) At least one GM official acknowledged this problem: "I believe the UAW and GM share the same values. . . . We both recognize that the economics are that if more money is spent on health programs, there is less at the bargaining table for wages . . . we have to be equal partners in improvement . . . but we realize that the UAW needs to be convinced that new programs are not just a cleverly disguised way to reduce costs and benefits."

Ford is the number two automaker but the world's largest truck manufacturer. The company retrenched in the 1970s and 1980s, cut its workforce by 33 percent, and closed fifteen plants. It also diversified its operations, with purchases of businesses such as agricultural equipment manufacturers and financial institutions. Buoyed by the 1988 introduction of the highly successful Taurus and Sable models, Ford's market share has been growing steadily over the last decade.

In the view of several union officials, Ford was regarded as generally reasonable. Particularly on health issues, Ford officials downplayed any differences with the UAW:

We think Ford and the UAW have the same goals. It is like a good marriage: we have sharp differences but we stay together. In fact, I think we are closer on health care than we have ever been. We need to spar occasionally so we don't look too cozy. Union leadership has been crucial. They understand the world and that it is in the interests of everyone to align incentives in health care. Health care is not an area where we need to fight—there are many other areas that are inevitably contentious, but this is not one of them.

The smallest of the Big Three automakers is Chrysler. The company's steadily declining market share in the 1960s and 1970s led to losses of more than $1 billion in 1979 and 1980. Facing bankruptcy, Chrysler negotiated $1.5 billion in federal loan guarantees. Under Lee Iacocca, the highly visible CEO who assumed control in 1978, Chrysler reorganized, closed plants, cut its workforce, and lowered production costs. By 1983, the company had repaid all its federal loans ahead of schedule. But the company slid into red ink again in 1991 as a result of the recession and weak consumer demand. Chrysler sold off nonautomotive assets, replaced Iacocca, and continued to shed noncore businesses. By 1994, the financial condition of the company had rebounded, spurred in large part by the popularity of the minivan, which it pioneered.

Chrysler was regarded by several observers as having the best relationship with the UAW. "They have always had the humility to know that they can't work alone," said one union official. "They are also more dependent than GM or Ford on domestic workers, so they have to get along better."

The United Auto Workers

The UAW (officially the "International Union, United Automobile, Aerospace and Agricultural Implement Workers of America") is one of the largest and most diverse unions in North America, with members in virtually every sector of the economy, from aerospace to colleges and universities. The union has approximately 775,000 active members and nearly 500,000 retired members in 1,130 local unions. It negotiates more than two thousand contracts with about fifteen hundred employers in the United States, Puerto Rico, and Ontario, Canada.

Of active UAW members, approximately half work for the Big Three. The UAW represents 215,000 skilled trades and production workers at GM, some 66,000 at Chrysler, and around 111,000 at Ford; in addition, it represents several thousand salaried workers at the Big Three, including 6,000 at Chrysler.

The union's active membership has been shrinking, and is predicted to fall even more in the coming years. For instance, of GM's 240,000 hourly workers, fully half will retire in the next ten years. A major factor in membership decline has been the trend, beginning in the 1950s and accelerating in the 1980s, for the companies to outsource parts manufacturing to nonunion suppliers. By 1995, less than 20 percent of workers at independent auto parts makers were represented by the UAW, down from 65 percent twenty years before.

The UAW has a long history of social activism, especially in the health care arena. In the 1940s, the UAW pioneered the idea that employers should pay for workers' health care. The union was one of the earliest advocates for national health insurance, and continues to support a single-payer system. In the 1960s, the UAW was a key member of the coalition that successfully fought for the creation of Medicare and Medicaid, and has recently worked actively to oppose cuts in those programs. The union was also a pioneer in the HMO movement, supporting the original HMO Act in 1973 and sponsoring one of the first HMOs in Michigan, the Health Alliance Plan.

The UAW Health Benefit Program

The UAW–Big Three workers have one of the most extensive health insurance programs of any U.S. industry. It is also one of the most complicated: the health program portion of the 1993 UAW-GM agreement ran to 237 pages. Members are eligible for medical, dental, and vision benefits. Most UAW members can choose from a range of options, including traditional indemnity, PPO, HMO, and prepaid dental plans. While most members have a choice of two to eight local medical plan options (from a total of more than a hundred managed care plans offered nationwide), the specific choices available to a UAW member depend on the availability of approved options in the member's geographic area and the member's Medicare status.

Regardless of the options selected, UAW members make no contribution to premiums; the entire cost of the UAW health program is borne by the automakers. The Health Care Agreement does contain a provision that the companies may require a UAW member to pay a portion of the premium for any HMO, dental, or vision plan whose premium exceeds the cost of the indemnity plan. However, according to the union, this provision has "little practical effect, as the UAW won't approve an HMO on that basis." The agreement includes a detailed methodology for comparing indemnity and HMO premiums, designed to adjust for any differences in the mix of single, two-person, and family contracts between the indemnity and HMO plans. HMOs and PPOs can also be eliminated as options if they are more costly than the indemnity plan, which has happened to about a dozen plans in the last few years.

TRADITIONAL INDEMNITY OPTION. This plan, which is offered to all UAW members, is a freedom-of-choice product that provides coverage for hospital, medical, and surgical services, as well as prescription drugs and hearing aids. Benefits are comprehensive, with the exception of exclusion of coverage for preventive care or routine physician office visits for children or adults. (Certain screening tests are covered, however, including Pap smears and mammograms.) Hospital or physician services have no deductibles or copayments; copayments for prescription drugs range from $2 for mail-order prescriptions to $5 for retail prescriptions.

The indemnity option is self-funded by all three automakers, and in most locations, the plan is administered by Blue Cross Blue Shield of Michigan (BCBSM) and participating plans in other states. The UAW-automaker agreements specify that BCBS will be the carrier for the plan. The indemnity plan has some predetermination and review requirements, including prior authorization of nonemergency inpatient admissions, second opinions for selected procedures, concurrent review, and a Case Management Program. According to the Health Program Agreement, benefits for certain covered services that require predetermination but are obtained without preapproval will still be paid at 80 percent of reasonable and customary charges, after the first $100 of expense. If annual coinsurance payments in such situations reach certain levels ($750 per individual and $1,500 per family), benefits are paid in full.

MENTAL HEALTH AND SUBSTANCE ABUSE. These benefits are carved out of the indemnity and PPO plans and delivered through a restricted provider network, administered by different vendors for each of the Big Three.

OTHER CARVE-OUTS. Other benefits are also carved out from the indemnity plan and provided by vendors with specialized expertise. These benefits vary by automaker, as do the vendors that are used, but

---

Exhibit 10.1.   Carve-Out Programs, Chrysler/UAW, 1996

Drugs: Prescription drugs are provided by a national managed care pharmacy program, PCS Health Systems, Inc. All mail order prescription drugs are covered by Health Care Services, Inc.

Foot Care: Foot and ankle care is provided by the National Foot Care Program, Inc.

Lab: Lab services are provided by Universal Standard Managed Care, Inc.

DME/P&O: Durable medical equipment and prosthetic and orthotic appliances are provided by The Support Program.

MH/SA: Mental health and substance abuse care is provided by Help-Line.

Vision: Vision care is provided by CO/OP optical or Davis Vision of BCBS (local plan)

Note: Medicare enrollees are not eligible for foot care, lab, and mental health and substance abuse programs.

---

may include lab services, durable medical equipment, and foot care. (As an example, see Exhibit 10.1 for a list of the carve-outs and vendors for UAW-Chrysler members in selected states.)

PPOs. The PPO plans offered to UAW members provide the same benefits as the indemnity plan, with the addition of coverage for preventive and routine office care. In-network benefits are covered in full (except for office visits, which are covered at 70 percent); out-of-network services are covered at 80 percent; once a PPO member has incurred $500 (individual) or $1,000 (family) in out-of-pocket payments to non-network providers, services received out-of-network are covered at 100 percent. Routine and preventive services are covered only if received from network providers. The copayment for prescription drugs is $3 per prescription.

HMOs. Under the UAW agreements, the types and scope of coverage offered by HMOs may differ from those required in the indemnity and PPO plans, and may vary among HMOs. However, HMOs generally offer benefits that are more comprehensive than the indemnity plan, including coverage for preventive services and routine office visits. HMOs may have no copayments for office visits, and copayments for prescription drugs range from nonexistent to $2.

Each of the Big Three selects and negotiates with its own managed care plans, and each has a different method and process for picking plans. The UAW must approve any managed care plan offered to UAW members, including HMOs, PPOs, prepaid dental plans, vision care networks, foot care networks, or mental health and substance abuse carve-outs. The union has developed detailed standards for evaluating plans, which vary by type of plan. For most types of plans, the standards cover areas such as minimum levels of benefits, access, provider contracts, financial stability, consumer representation on the plan's governing body, utilization management programs, and quality. Both the automakers and the UAW have begun to rely more on NCQA accreditation, and the UAW's 1993 contract with GM requires "all HMOs and PPOs made available to UAW members to apply for accreditation by an accrediting agency mutually agreed upon by the Corporation and the Union, such as NCQA, no later than January 1, 1996; and it is expected that all such HMOs and PPOs will have received accreditation by January 1, 1997."

ENROLLMENT IN MANAGED CARE PLANS. Although UAW members have no incentive to join a managed care plan in terms of premium contribution or cost-sharing, the benefits in the PPO and HMO plans are more comprehensive. For example, GM estimates that on average the benefits in its HMO plans are 23 percent richer than those of the indemnity plan. Enrollment of UAW members in managed care plans has been growing at all the Big Three companies, although the percentage of active workers in managed care varies somewhat by company. In total about 60 percent of active UAW members at the automakers belong to managed care plans, split evenly between HMOs and PPOs. (See Table 10.1.) Penetration is highest at Chrysler, with 69 percent of active workers enrolled in HMO or PPO plans, followed by GM at 58 percent and Ford at 56 percent. HMO enrollment is highest at Ford, with 38 percent. The proportion of retirees selecting managed care plans is low at all three companies, ranging from 16 percent at Ford to 20 percent at GM to 22 percent at Chrysler.

In general, both the UAW and the automakers have been supportive of managed care, and believe the UAW managed care options have improved quality for UAW members. There is also a widely held belief that a focus on quality will result in lower costs. An often-cited example is the selective network for foot care, instituted in the mid-1980s, which is credited with eliminating unnecessary procedures,

Chrysler, Hourly and Salary

Contract Type:	Trad. (#)	Trad. (percent)	PPO (#)	PPO (percent)	HMO (#)	HMO (percent)
Active	21,256	32	32,555	49	13,282	20
Retiree	51,940	78	8,639	13	5,806	9
Total	73,196	55	41,194	31	19,088	14

Ford, Hourly

Contract Type:	Trad. (#)	Trad. (percent)	PPO (#)	PPO (percent)	HMO (#)	HMO (percent)
Active	43,900	44	18,100	18	37,400	38
Retiree	83,500	84	5,100	5	11,400	11
Total	127,400	64	23,200	12	48,800	24

GM, Hourly

Contract Type:	Trad. (#)	Trad. (percent)	PPO (#)	PPO (percent)	HMO (#)	HMO (percent)
Active	95,554	42	67,547	30	64,792	28
Retiree	206,219	80	16,211	6	34,729	14
Total	301,773	62	83,758	17	99,521	21

Table 10.1.   Health Coverage in Force, UAW Big Three: Number of Contracts per Category (July 12, 1996).

reducing costs, and enhancing the quality of care provided to UAW members. Auto assembly workers have a high need for foot care services because they are standing all day on concrete floors; foot problems are as common as back problems among auto workers. However, after the automakers analyzed podiatric claims data and shared it with the UAW, a consensus developed that the cost and use of podiatric care was a major problem in many locations, especially Michigan. The UAW podiatric benefit was generous, payment was on a fee-for-service basis, and there were many podiatrists in Michigan. As a result, podiatric use rates were out of line compared to other parts of the country (including a high incidence of what several UAW officials referred to as "serial podiatric surgery"), adversely affecting work attendance and productivity. After the managed foot care selective network plan was instituted, and podiatrists were required to obtain precertification for foot surgery (including submitting X-rays), utilization rates fell by 35–60 percent.

There is also agreement that the mental health and substance abuse carve-out has reduced substance abuse recidivism rates and reduced costs. However, some observers criticize the fragmented nature of the health programs. One notes, "All of these different plans and vendors are confusing to UAW members and act as an impediment to good service by the carriers. There is a lot of time spent making the interfaces work—it's very expensive and time consuming."

However, opinions differ somewhat about how much HMOs have reduced costs. Most observers believe that the HMOs and PPOs have experienced positive selection, enrolling UAW members who are, on average, younger and in better health. In addition, as the indemnity plans have instituted utilization management programs, the utilization rates in the UAW indemnity plan and many of the managed care plans are converging.

The Concerns of the Automakers

Despite sales growth and record corporate profits, health care costs remained high on the Big Three agenda, a focus rekindled by Congress's recent failure to act on health care reform at the national level. Although the companies had seen two years of fairly stable health insurance premiums, the level of overall health care costs were a significant concern. "While everyone else is declaring victory over health costs, that is not at all how we view it," said one GM official. "Health care costs are a fundamental competitive issue for us."

According to company figures, health spending was a major factor in the cost of each new vehicle, although totals varied widely among the Big Three: GM estimated health care costs at $1,200 per vehicle, $700 more than it spent on steel. Chrysler estimated its health care spending at $700 per car, and Ford spent $510 per car. The lower costs for Chrysler and Ford were the result of having younger workforces and fewer retirees. In particular, the automakers contend that their health care costs put them at a real disadvantage with foreign competitors, which they contend pay far lower percentage of their workers' health care costs—or none at all in countries with national programs. They estimated that the comparable cost per vehicle made in Japan was $200, and as low as $100 for cars made in the U.S. factories of foreign automakers, who have young, relatively healthy workers and hardly any retirees. The automakers contended that these cost differences would be exacerbated by an aging workforce. The average

age of UAW workers at the Big Three was forty-nine, much higher than that of the national workforce.

Although encouraged by the recent financial performance of the industry, Big Three management knew that financial results were cyclical and they believed that additional cost cutting was imperative for continued long-term success in the highly competitive industry. Analysts were predicting that auto sales would decline in 1997, reflecting both the declining affordability of vehicles and a slow-growth economy, which had resulted in sluggish growth in disposable personal income. High levels of consumer installment debt and volatile consumer confidence levels were also expected to adversely affect automobile sales in the coming months.

The automakers wanted to introduce cost-sharing into the UAW health program. In 1993, in what many saw as a move to position itself for the 1993 UAW negotiation, Ford became the first of Big Three to require active salaried employees to pay contributions toward their health insurance premiums. In 1996, the active salaried employee contributions ranged from $17 to $45 per month. In addition, newly hired salaried employees no longer had the option of enrolling in the traditional indemnity plan but instead had to select a managed care plan.

The companies believed that financial incentives were an important tool in facilitating worker acceptance of managed care. Despite the existing benefit incentives for workers to join managed care plans, the automakers contended that benefit design differences were less effective than requiring employees to pay a portion of the premium. They also believed that financial incentives could be used in combination with more sophisticated assessments of plan performance to encourage employees to join more cost-efficient HMOs. GM, for example, was developing contribution strategies that gave incentives for salaried workers to select those HMOs that GM determined were "higher quality" managed care plans. "We want to move our employees up the continuum of managed care plans," said a GM health benefits manager. "We think that the savings are in getting our people with the greatest medical needs—like retirees—into the highest-quality systems of care . . . and then to step up to the plate and be willing to pay risk-adjusted premium rates for higher-cost people."

The divergence between the health programs for unionized and salaried workers were creating a serious employee relations problem for the automakers. In fact, a class action suit, *Sprague* v. *GM,* was filed by seventy thousand GM salaried retirees alleging a breach of contract as a result of GM's unilateral changes in their health coverage. "Frankly, our salaried workers are really angry that the UAW does not have the same health benefits—they have a better package." (In response to this observation, one union official remarked wryly, "If they are upset, they should unionize.") However, this issue has not inhibited company action. Said a GM manager, "We would like our salaried and UAW plans to be consistent but if we can go faster in salaried, we will."

The automakers wanted to negotiate similar cost-sharing requirement in the 1996 agreements with the UAW, in addition to imposing other requirements to further promote the growth of managed care. The companies knew that the UAW, in holding out for 100 percent company-paid health insurance coverage, was bucking a far-reaching national trend.

In 1990, approximately 30 percent of large employers paid all health insurance premiums for single coverage and 15 percent paid fully for family policies. Those proportions were now down to only 10 percent for single and under 6 percent for family. Employer contributions varied by industry and region; contribution rates were more generous in financial services, while manufacturing and retail companies were less so. Reductions in employer contributions were largely an attempt to combat double-digit escalation of costs.

While premium costs had leveled or actually gone down in recent years, most employers believed that future reductions were uncertain, especially as an aging workforce and growing number of actual retirees would demand more medical care.

Despite these national trends, the automakers were also well aware of the union's long-standing opposition to these types of changes. They had also closely watched the recent experience at Boeing, where similar demands by the company had pushed the International Association of Machinists to embark on a lengthy and ultimately successful strike.

Managing Care in the Indemnity Plan

Beyond increased cost-sharing, there appeared to be opportunities to improve care in the traditional indemnity plan. "The indemnity plan has been the equivalent of handing providers the corporate checkbook and saying, 'please spend wisely,'" said one Big Three representative. "We want to improve delivery in the indemnity plan also. We may need to take baby steps because there's a lot of history and it takes a long time to get things done. But we are moving away from just writing checks to writing them with an attitude." One automaker had recently done a study of the use of beta blockers after acute myocardial infarction (AMI) in the indemnity and HMO plans, and found only 14 percent compliance in the indemnity plan, compared to 30–80 percent compliance in the HMOs.

As part of the 1993 agreements, the UAW and automakers had agreed to evaluate, and if mutually agreed, implement a disease management program being developed by BCBS of Michigan called Coordinated Care Management (CCM) for members of the indemnity plan. The CCM was just one of more than twenty items specified in a separate section of the contracts on similar terms, with the goal of identifying "activities that may have high potential for costs savings while achieving the maximum coverage and service for the employees covered for health care benefits for the money spent for such protection." Other activities included considering the development of pilot "Centers of Excellence" programs; investigating and implementing network pilots for diagnostic imaging, durable medical equipment, and prosthetic and orthotic appliances; and working to review and revise the utilization review programs already in place in the indemnity plan.

Although the UAW originally envisioned that the CCM would be a broad initiative, it was eventually implemented as a small pilot program for UAW members with severe cardiovascular disease who lived in seven counties in Michigan. "We had to battle like crazy to get the automakers to agree to the CCM," said one UAW official. "But it makes more sense than cost-sharing. Cost-sharing may have a superficial appeal, but at the end of the day, the vast proportion of health care cost is incurred by a relatively small portion of the population. Cost-sharing does nothing to change that." The decision to focus the CCM pilot on cardiovascular disease was based on the fact that 35 percent of the automakers' total health care expenditures for non-Medicare-covered individuals were for cardiovascular-related services.

The CCM program attempted to enhance patient care and decrease costs by identifying individuals with severe cardiovascular disease (defined by certain diagnosis, cost, and utilization criteria); development of an individualized treatment plan by a care manager, in consultation with the individual's primary treating physician (which could include payment for otherwise uncovered services such as nutrition counseling, smoking cessation, stress management, and weight reduction); facilitation of coordination of care; and follow-up by a care manager to assess progress and the need for additional services. The goal of the program was to achieve cost savings and better care through medical management (improved coordination, earlier identification and treatment of co-morbidities, reduced need for and use of inpatient services), and risk reduction.

The program was BCBSM's first foray into disease management. "We want to focus on longitudinal management of a cohort of patients . . . but we need to learn how to intervene with patients who have existing disease states in a continuous rather than episodic fashion," said a BCBSM executive. The structure of the indemnity plan benefit package was identified by some observers as a barrier to longitudinal care. "The UAW benefits have no coverage for office visits, which leads to all kinds of perverse treatment patterns, including inappropriate use of the ER and inpatient setting, and no incentives to do secondary prevention," said one physician. The UAW took issue with the physician's assertion about inappropriate ER use, however, noting that its standard contracts contained "prudent layperson language," under which a member had to pay for any unnecessary ER use.

Although both the UAW and the automakers were optimistic about the potential of the CCM program, it was too early to know what kind of effects the cardiovascular pilot might have on costs and quality.

Preparing for the 1996 Bargaining Table

As in previous years, the UAW adamantly opposed any reductions in benefits, including increased cost-sharing by its members, in the form of instituting worker contributions to premium costs or any increases to the modest copayment in existing plans. "Opposing cost-sharing is as high a priority as we have, ahead of wage increases," said one union official. "It is an article of faith for our members. The membership has to ratify any agreement and would view cost-sharing as a violation of the faith. It would never be implemented without a strike." The UAW felt particularly strongly that any cost-sharing was not acceptable in 1996 because health care costs for the Big Three had been increasing for several years at rates below the national average.

The strong sales performance and profits of each of the Big Three were also uppermost in the minds of the UAW negotiators and rank-and-file members as they developed their bargaining positions.

"The continuing efforts of our members, particularly in improving manufacturing quality and efficiency, have contributed substantially to the Autos' success," said a senior UAW official. "These agreements are being negotiated in the context of wealth. All three companies can afford to treat their workers well." Added another senior UAW official, "What we are trying to do in these talks is to ensure that workers get a fair share of their employer's business and financial success."

According to the UAW Research Department, the combined after-tax profits of the Big Three in 1994 and 1995 were the best back-to-back annual results on record. The union estimated that the companies made an average profit of $980 per vehicle sold during the second quarter of 1996, up from $840 per vehicle a year earlier. The UAW believed these profit increases could—if the companies chose—be translated into both higher wages and improved benefits for workers and lower prices for consumers. The union noted that auto executives' pay and benefits had grown dramatically during the period of improved profitability. As one union official noted in our interview with him, the Big Three "have had little reluctance" to increase CEO compensation. He pointed out that the average annual CEO compensation at the Big Three reached $5.7 million in 1995, compared to the average $45,131 earned by the typical auto assembler in wages, lump-sum bonuses, and profit sharing. This resulted in a ratio of CEO compensation to assembler compensation of 128:1, compared to 93:1 in 1981–1985. The UAW communications on health issues also often noted that CEOs of managed care companies were among the best paid in business.

The union also contested the automakers' contention that health care costs were a major source of competitive disadvantage for the companies. In particular, the UAW took issue with the health care cost figures often used by the Big Three, claiming that the total average labor cost per hour figures used by the companies included wages and benefits paid to active workers plus the costs of all benefits paid to laid-off and retired workers and surviving spouses. The union also contended that hourly labor costs for autoworkers were higher in both Germany and Japan. For example, the UAW estimated that in 1994 German autoworkers' wages and benefits cost 44 percent more than UAW wages and benefits, and Japanese autoworkers' wages and benefits cost 15 percent more. The union also cited data from the U.S. Commerce Department showing that total labor costs as a percentage of the cost of new domestic cars decreased from 26.5 percent in 1980 to 15.5 percent in 1994.

The union based its opposition to cost-sharing on a number of long-held beliefs in addition to its current arguments regarding the financial position of the automakers. First, it argued that copayments and deductibles did not reduce costs overall, they merely shifted costs. In fact, the union believed that, to the extent that higher copayments and deductibles discouraged people from seeking care until their conditions became serious, increased cost-sharing would actually cause higher health care costs, as well as higher costs for lost work time and disability payments. "Copayments and deductibles are a pennywise, dollar-foolish approach to controlling health care costs," according to the UAW.

The union also criticized the automakers for their hypocrisy in vehemently and publicly opposing cost-shifting by the federal Medicare and Medicaid to employers and other private payers, while at the same time attempting themselves "to shift costs to the backs of the workers." Noting the significant amounts of fraud and abuse among health care providers, the UAW argued that "the focus should be on the providers who are perpetrating the abuses. Only when the abuse is out of the system should we consider cost-sharing."

While affirming union support for managed care, the UAW leadership also opposed any changes that would require members to select managed care plans. "We believe managed care plans save money, and would like to encourage people to enroll in them," said one senior UAW officer, who added,

> But most of our members deal with the medical care system only when they get sick, and we can't rely on benefit information and education strategies, combined with choice only of managed care plans, to be right for everyone. A lot of the influence on employee choice of plan comes from the benefit reps on the shop floor. For instance, when the Greater Detroit Area Health Council put out informational materials on the importance of going to a high-volume hospital for a coronary artery bypass graft (CABG), it was not terribly influential in terms of workers' choices. Choice is guided by what they hear on the shop floor. We would not want to hide useful information but we have to make sure it is useful and understandable. And we need the safety valve of an indemnity option for people who want it.

The union leadership was, in the view of some outside observers, in a difficult position. According to one, "The basic position of the union is that 'the world will end if the automakers try to come after our health care.' But I think the leadership is more sophisticated than that . . . but they can't sell changes to the membership. They are elected by the rank and file and they would never stay in office if they backed off this position." Another outsider said,

> The UAW believes that managed care is a better way to deliver health care. But they have to deal with member concerns about access and choice . . . although the access issue is overstated: the use of out-of-network services in most PPO plans is only 6–7 percent. . . . The UAW leadership also finds it hard to maintain the balance between appropriate use and their members' sense of entitlement to anything they want. This is an issue for everyone, but is heightened in the UAW population. The attitude is, "if my wife wants a hysterectomy, she will get it, and she will stay in the hospital as long as she wants." So their membership is more resistant to managed care mechanisms.

POSSIBLE ALTERNATIVES TO COST-SHARING AND MANAGED CARE PLANS. The UAW had long supported a range of alternatives to higher cost-sharing and benefit reductions, including wellness programs, employee assistance programs to help workers overcome alcohol and drug dependencies, and workplace health and safety programs. Some observers criticized the UAW for not doing enough to focus on behaviors that contribute to health care costs. An example cited by one health plan executive was smoking: "Cigarette smoking is a big health problem for auto workers. . . . But what is the UAW doing to help? It does not want to deal with smoking for fear of alienating members, so it defers culpability by beating up on the health plans and asking why our outcomes are not better for respiratory and cardiovascular disease." A UAW official acknowledged that this was a difficult issue for the union: "If you have members working all day in an environmentally challenged plant—noisy, smelly, and hot—asking people to stop smoking is kind of cynical. Plant workers are more likely to smoke but the incidence has come down a lot. Besides smoking is a plant-by-plant bargaining issue, not a national one."

But the union also has a long history of advocating for more systemic changes to the health care system as a way to help control health care costs. As one union spokesperson pointed out,

The UAW's experience has been that benefits do not drive the cost of health care. If they did, you would see uniformly high costs in communities with large concentrations of UAW members. That's not the case. Instead, health care costs vary significantly from state to state, and from community to community within a particular state. . . . We believe that health care costs tend to be significantly lower in states with strong regulatory controls curtailing unneeded medical technologies, and in areas with an appropriate ratio of specialists to general practitioners, and where there is healthy competition between fee-for-service and managed care plans.

Consistent with this position, the UAW and the Big Three started working together in 1994 on a new health care approach, called community health care initiatives (CHCIs), to improve the quality, accessibility, and cost-efficiency of health care delivery systems in communities with large concentrations of UAW workers. CHCIs were designed to involve all sectors of a community—employers (union and nonunion alike), unions, health care providers, local government, consumers—in a collaborative effort to improve the quality, cost, and accessibility of the community's health care delivery system. (See Exhibit 10.2 for a copy of the vision and mission statement for the CHCI program.) "We believe strongly in the need to focus on changing the organization and delivery of care," said one UAW official. "But employers have a false idea that competition will lead to efficiencies in the delivery system; there's no evidence of that. HMOs sell cost containment, but then they skim good risks, cost-shift, squeeze the providers, and increase administrative costs. HMOs and competition are not changing the system. . . . The appropriate way to focus on delivery system issues is not competition but cooperation and collaboration among all stakeholders." At the time of the negotiations in 1996, pilot community health initiatives were already under way in three communities: Flint, Michigan; Anderson, Indiana (both with GM); and Kokomo, Indiana (with Chrysler and GM/Delco).

THE FLINT CHCI. The first Community Health Care Initiative was a joint program of the UAW and GM, begun in 1995 in Flint, Michigan, a city of 140,000. The program, which was jointly run by a UAW representative and a GM manager, originated in part from an analysis of GM claims data that compared the amount of money the company spent in ten U.S. cities to provide UAW workers and their families with

---

Exhibit 10.2.   Community Initiatives Vision and Mission Statement.

We are firmly committed to encourage the development of community health care delivery systems that provide high quality health services, promote disease and accident prevention, expand health education, improve community health status and enhance the quality of life, while reducing costs by efficient and appropriate cost-effective delivery of services.

The Community Initiatives process will stimulate community activity, including coalitions and other consensus building forums, to encourage collaboration and cooperation of consumers, purchasers, caregivers, and providers to improve the health care system by promoting:

- the delivery of high quality health care;
- a culture of "best practice";
- state-of-the-art data collection and information systems; and
- a balancing of the health care resources of the community with the community's health care needs.

Community activity supported by information acquired through the assessment of community needs and resources and a survey of national and local "best practices" will generate the development and implementation of action plans to ensure that health care resources in the community are used efficiently and effectively to meet its needs. This commitment to community activity and collaboration will be ongoing and emphasize continuous improvement of the delivery system. An immediate goal will be achieving a voluntary community commitment to a moratorium on expansion that does not have a consensus of need.

---

the same health care benefits. The analysis revealed wide cost variations; for example, GM's per capita costs in Flint were 66 percent higher than in Rochester, New York. GM estimated that it could reduce its annual health care costs by $800 million if it could lower its costs in all cities to the Rochester level.

The data were useful in persuading GM to consider a more collaborative approach. "In the 1980s and early 1990s, we tried and used up all the easy approaches to cost containment. As we studied our own data on health care spending, we saw how our size can make us vulnerable to potential abuses by medical providers serving members who have no limits on health care spending," said a GM manager. Another noted that GM immediately understood the value of a collaborative approach because "they are used to working with coalitions on a local level—it's how they have to deal with their suppliers, on a case-by-case basis."

In addition to its high costs, Flint was a good target for a pilot program because it was essentially a GM town. The area has forty-three thousand GM workers, about 22 percent of the county labor force. Local providers, employers, and public officials had formed the Greater Flint Health Coalition in 1992 to work on a range of community health issues, including lobbying for no-smoking legislation in the county, reducing C-section rates, and improving health care access. Although GM and the UAW had initially been involved in this effort, their participation waned as these efforts stalled. The Coalition became inactive in 1993.

With the impetus of the UAW and GM, the Coalition was restructured and revitalized in the spring of 1996. The union and GM, through their Corporate-Union Committee on Health Care Benefits, had commissioned Lewin, a consulting company, to undertake an assessment of the health care system and health care outcomes in the Flint area as a starting point and, hopefully, galvanizing force for the community initiative. Lewin's assessment, in the form of a 432-page document titled "Community Assessment Factbook: Genesee County, Michigan," was presented to the Committee and then to the Flint community in May 1996. The analysis, which compared capacity, use rates, costs, and other health indicators in Flint to a variety of national and local benchmarks, concluded that "quality of care is mixed," "there tend to be more invasive procedures than the national average," and "costs are higher due to high rates of service utilization." The following points were among the report's specific findings:

- The Flint community was at risk for health status problems due to local socioeconomic characteristics, including lower incomes, less education, higher unemployment, and higher rates of crime and violence than Michigan or U.S. averages.

- Genesee county residents engaged in a variety of unhealthy behaviors (smoking, poor diet choices, substance abuse, and lack of exercise), although at rates consistent with local and national norms.

- Health status was relatively poor on the majority of the indicators analyzed (including a very high rate of teenage pregnancy).

- Residents were dying at a higher rate than benchmark populations: the overall mortality rate in the county was 11 percent higher than the state average and 14 percent higher than the U.S. average; the mortality rates for many conditions, including heart disease, diabetes, and chronic obstructive pulmonary disease, were even higher.

- Hospital capacity was likely to exceed projected needs, especially if utilization rates declined to benchmark levels.

- Total physician supply was average compared to U.S. levels; the primary care physician supply was 30 percent higher than the national level and the specialist supply was 24 percent lower than the national average. Physician capacity significantly exceeded levels that would be required by HMO staffing patterns.

- Utilization rates significantly exceeded benchmark norms for most diagnostic categories and many procedures (including coronary artery bypass grafts, C-sections, hysterectomies, and cholecystectomies).

- Average costs (per unit of service) were generally comparable to benchmarks.

- Quality was mixed, with unfavorable performance on many indicators (for example, emergency room use, pediatric asthma admission rates, diabetic inpatient rates, lung cancer mortality rate, infant mortality rate, low-birth-weight infant rate, AMI inpatient admission rate).

Table 10.2 provides selected excerpts from the Lewin Community Assessment Factbook.

As part of its Community Health Care Initiative, the UAW and GM were working as members of a restructured and revitalized Greater Flint Health Coalition to address many of the health problems in Flint. The Coalition included participants from the three local hospitals, physicians, local government, labor, employers, and teachers, in addition to GM and the UAW. Through a formal governance and operating structure the Coalition had identified several priority projects, including reducing C-section rates, developing consensus guidelines for cardiac catheterization, and improving diagnosis and treatment of *H-pylori*-caused stomach ulcers.

The Coalition also hoped to work on rationalizing capacity and infrastructure in Flint. Even before the CHCI, the three hospitals in Flint had begun to experiment with some joint programs. Hurley Medical Center, a public hospital that cared for most Medicaid

Cause of Death	County Compared to State	County Compared to United States
Major cardiovascular disease	Less favorable	Less favorable
• Diseases of the heart	Less favorable	Less favorable
• Cerebrovascular disease	Less favorable	Less favorable
Malignant neoplasm	Less favorable	Less favorable
• Colon	Less favorable	Not known
• Lung and bronchus	Less favorable	More favorable
• Breast	Comparable	Comparable
• Prostate gland	More favorable	Not known
Chronic obstructive pulmonary disease and allied conditions	Less favorable	Less favorable
Pneumonia and influenza	More favorable	More favorable
Diabetes mellitus	Less favorable	Less favorable
Chronic liver disease and cirrhosis	More favorable	More favorable
HIV-III/LAV infection	Comparable	More favorable
All accidents	Less favorable	Comparable
• Motor vehicle accidents	Comparable	Comparable
Homicide and legal intervention	Less favorable	Less favorable
Suicide	More favorable	More favorable
All causes of death	Less favorable	Less favorable

Table 10.2.   Genesee County Age-Adjusted Death Rates per 100,000 Persons by Cause of Death, 1992.

Source: 1992 data, Office of the State Registrar and Division of Health Statistics, Michigan Department of Public Health, and 1992 data, U.S. National Center for Health Statistics.

Note: Death rates age-adjusted for 1992 population.

recipients and uninsured individuals, had agreed with Genesee Medical System to jointly operate a cancer center. Hurley and McLaren Medical Center had agreed to exchange services, with Hurley shutting its open heart surgery program and McLaren closing its inpatient pediatric unit.

Both the UAW and GM were initially criticized by some members of the Flint community for "coming late to the table." "They were not interested several years ago when local providers and public officials formed the Coalition," said one critic. GM conceded that this feeling was valid: "We have realized that dictating to the community will not work. Being the eight-hundred-pound gorilla hasn't gotten us much up until now. We all need to sit at a community table and work out the issues. We know that we need to take costs out of the system. If we don't they will just come back at us later."

In late 1995, the UAW and Chrysler had begun a similar CHCI in Kokomo, Indiana, a city where seventy-four hundred Chrysler employees worked at a company engine and transmission plant. An initial assessment of Kokomo, also conducted by Lewin, found Chrysler's health care costs were much higher than in Syracuse, where Chrysler also had a transmission plant: $1,611 per worker in Kokomo compared to $901 in Syracuse, that is, 79 percent more in Kokomo than in Syracuse. The Lewin analysis found major differences in a variety of indicators, including hospitalization rates 46 percent higher in Kokomo than Syracuse, and back strain incidence 60 percent higher—and almost twice the rate in Michigan. GM, which had fifty-five hundred workers at a Delco plant in Kokomo, later joined the initiative. GM's costs in Kokomo were even higher, $2,445 per capita, the highest of any city in which GM operated, although Indianapolis at $2,430 and Detroit at $2,120 were not far behind. Kokomo also had a significant excess number of hospital beds, an oversupply of specialists, and extremely high utilization and unit costs compared to other benchmarks.

A similar GM-sponsored initiative in Anderson, Indiana, had begun in 1995, again with the first step being a community health assessment as a means to produce an objective fact base that could be the basis for community discussion and action. This analysis also found tremendous variations in cost and practice.

The UAW and the automakers were cautiously optimistic about the potential for the CHCIs to produce significant improvements in health care quality and costs for the companies and the communities. "This is a paradigm shift to a civic model, in the middle between the market and the regulatory," said a union official, commenting on the Flint initiative. "It recognizes that health care is a community resource and it can't be approached like two auto companies competing to produce cars. . . . The CHCI program represents the coalescing of the UAW's long-standing philosophical approach toward systemic change and cooperation with the views of the sharp-pencil folks at General Motors."

⸺ The Results of the 1996 Negotiations

Health care did not become a major issue in the 1996 negotiations. For the most part, the UAW successfully resisted any attempt by the Big Three to make reductions in the health care programs. There were no changes in cost-sharing nor any requirement that UAW members pay any portion of health insurance premiums. (According to some accounts, the issue of cost-sharing simply did not arise.) Coverage was enhanced in several areas, including small increases in vision, dental, durable medical equipment, and drug benefits. In exchange, the UAW agreed to a requirement that all new hires at the Big Three must enroll in an HMO when they become eligible for coverage (seven months after hiring) and maintain that membership for their first two years of coverage, after which they will be able to select any health care option. (One observer said this requirement came about "because Ford had not settled yet and the company needed some victory on the health front." The mandatory HMO enrollment requirement was similar to one imposed by Ford on salaried workers beginning in 1995.) In addition, the two sides agreed to require all HMOs offered to UAW members to have some type of NCQA accreditation by July 1, 1998. The union also agreed to a new national vision network, while gaining minor expansions in dental and prescription drug benefits.

Quality Initiatives

Instead of benefits and cost-sharing, quality was the key issue in the 1996 agreement. According to a UAW official:

> Generally, during negotiations we try to build on things we already have. Our tactic was to try to remove health care from the contentious issues by focusing on quality. We carved health care out from the fisticuffs and stressed that if we focused on quality, costs would follow. This approach positioned the companies so that they would either have had to attack quality or come along. . . . The Autos were not prepared to take on a big fight on the quality issue . . . it's a very emotional, human interest type of approach and they did not have a good response. . . . Fortunately, the focus on quality also happens to be a good public health approach and good social policy.

The major substantive health provisions of the new UAW contract were an expansion of two quality initiatives already operating on a pilot basis, CCM and CHCI, along with a new clinical protocol tool, the Care Management System (CMS).

Coordinated Care Management

As a result of the negotiations, the UAW and the Big Three agreed to support expansion and development of the Blue Cross Blue Shield CCM program for indemnity plan members beyond its previous focus on severe cardiac cases in parts of Michigan. Provisions included

- Expansion to cover all cases of pediatric and adult asthma and diabetes in Michigan
- Expansion of disease management initiatives based on risk assessment to all cardiovascular cases regardless of severity or dollar expenditures
- Expansion of the CCM to select participating plans outside Michigan to attempt to cover 90 percent of eligible UAW members

As described earlier in the chapter, the CCM is a disease management program developed by BCBSM that attempts to delay or prevent further disease progression in individuals with chronic conditions, improve health status and quality of care, and reduce costs. BCBS tries to identify patients with a given chronic condition as early as possible through multiple sources (such as physician referrals,

claims data, and precertification programs). Patients are then stratified according to health status severity, using criteria such as total
health care expenditures, use of services, and multiple admissions.
(These criteria vary from condition to condition.) Those categorized
as severe or high-risk require more intensive case management, while
those classified as moderate or mild can be managed with less intense
interventions. For individuals who choose to participate in the program, a care nurse develops an individualized care plan in consultation with the patient's primary treating physician; the primary
physician must also agree to participate in the CCM program.

Individuals with severe disease are actively managed and monitored
by a care manager and the treating doctor, and are eligible for a wide
range of interventions, including many ordinarily noncovered services.
Progress is monitored by regular telephone contact between the patient
and the care manager. Those with moderate to mild conditions generally receive a variety of self-care and education material (diet, exercise),
as well as occasional calls from the nurse case manager to check health
status and provide further education about the patient's disease and
appropriate care. For patients in both groups, the interventions become
less intensive and phase out over a three-year period.

The UAW and Big Three, in consultation with BCBSM, decided to
expand the CCM to asthma and diabetes because the two conditions
are widely prevalent in the UAW population, and are both expensive
if patients are not well managed but generally easily managed through
existing outpatient interventions and programs with demonstrated
outcomes. The goal is to implement the CCM for all three diseases in
Michigan in early 1997, and to expand the program as soon as possible to include UAW workers with traditional indemnity coverage who
reside in selected states with BCBS participating plans (that is, in states
other than Michigan where BCBS administers the UAW's indemnity
health program). Participating plans will be included if they have large
numbers of UAW members potentially eligible for the CCM, have current disease management capabilities, and have the provider network
and operational capability to administer the program.

"There is a lot of cultural anthropology at work here," said
one physician about the CCM. "We all need to adopt new ways of
thinking. For the carriers and the providers, it is taking a longitudinal
approach, focused more on episodes of care and secondary prevention. For the UAW, it is to get the rank and file to understand that
more is not always better. The workers are often in a mindset that they
are always getting screwed. They know they are limited on the wage

side but there are no limits on health care. I think the workers would often rather have the doctor charge the expletive out of the Autos, even if the care is not needed, especially because the union workers don't have to pay anything."

Some observers are skeptical about the CCM program because, they contend, they see no real evidence that disease management systems have had a significant impact on costs. Others support the program in concept but worry about the ability of BCBS to fully implement CCM, based on the company's historical performance. "BCBS has an inability to develop innovative programs or to deliver on existing ones," said one auto official. "We want our carriers to be ahead of us, but we always have to push them, not the reverse. BCBS is not on the cutting edge of quality; they are more focused on costs. That's understandable historically—the Autos asked for cost cutting, so that's what we got." Although the UAW also has its criticism of the Blues, it has always had a strong symbiotic relationship with them. One observer of the UAW and the Blues characterized the relationship between the two somewhat differently: "Blue Cross Blue Shield is like a sharecropper to the UAW—the UAW gives work to them and keeps control." Forty percent of BCBSM's 2 million members are enrolled through the automaker accounts, and UAW has bargained into the agreements that BCBSM is to be the carrier for the indemnity health program. The UAW has four seats on BCBSM's thirty-five-member board; each of the Big Three also has one seat.

This close relationship is sometimes frustrating to the automakers. "We would like to remove the carriers and build our own network capacity," said one auto official. "Blue Cross has no managed care expertise or infrastructure . . . and the Autos have strong information management and technology management capacity. But the UAW is skeptical about our proficiency to build our own plans. And the UAW wants to keep BCBS, in part because they don't think BCBS has ability or incentives to deny care or manage care the way the managed care plans can." Another company said, "We would consider bypassing Blue Cross and all the managed care companies too, and doing direct contracting; we already do that with some of the carve-outs. Although direct contracting would probably be a cost-efficient option in only a few locations, we are reevaluating the wisdom of our health benefits strategy in every way. . . . Claims payment is becoming a commodity. If Blue Cross wants a role, it needs to focus on what adds value—its care management—that's where the comparative advantage will be for carriers."

The UAW seems to take a more measured perspective on Blue Cross. One union official commented,

> The Blues' strengths are their provider arrangements, discounts, and market presence; it would be very hard for the companies to match them if they wanted to get rid of Blue Cross. The UAW has had service issues sometimes. . . . The Blues don't always do what they say they will. They have also not taken a leadership role in most cases—they are usually reactive rather than proactive, and the union has been pushing them to take the lead more, which they have been trying to do. But the Autos are not their only customer and the Autos have to deal with that. . . . The company is in a hard situation often, caught between all the players.

The union also opposes the direct contracting approach, "We do believe the carriers add value and expertise," said a UAW official, "and we certainly would not want the companies doing the direct contracting. So that means there would have to be a joint UAW–Big Three effort and no one around here would want to serve on that committee!"

Care Management System

The second major quality initiative in the 1996 bargaining agreements was support of a new tool for promoting the use of best practice clinical guidelines, called the Care Management System (CMS). CMS is an automated system of clinical guidelines, called Specifications of Acceptable Care (SACs), developed by a private consulting firm, Preferred Health Systems (PHS) and financed by BCBSM. PHS contends that the SACS have been developed in a different way from other clinical guidelines, using expert physician panels, drawn from over 120 "world class physicians" under exclusive contracts to PHS. The SACs are revised at least quarterly, based on the most recent clinical literature in the appropriate area. So far, SACs have been developed in seven areas: cardiovascular (covering fifteen conditions), cancer (covering eleven conditions), diabetes (covering twenty-two conditions), asthma (covering eleven conditions), behavioral health, women and newborn health, and musculoskeletal health. PHS estimates that these SACs cover approximately 60 percent of pathological conditions, and more SACs are being developed. (As a result of a recently concluded agreement, Magellan has taken over all development and maintenance of the SACs from PHS, which went out of business. The Blues will have ultimate responsibility for the system.)

The CMS is structured to be used in a decision-making environment. The SACs are accessible on PHS's Web site, and will be available electronically to physicians in their offices or from other remote locations if they belong to health plans or other clients that have purchased the rights to use the system. All physicians participating in the indemnity plan would have access to CMS through BCBSM. The Web site also includes links that allow the user to access references and abstracts of the clinical literature used to develop the SACs. (Eventually PHS hopes to provide access to the actual literature. A long-term goal is to enable physicians to meet continuing medical education requirements by studying interactive tutorials and taking tests through the Web site.)

The primary goal of CMS is to have clinicians use the guidelines to screen, diagnose, stage, treat, and follow up on patients. "Physicians, and particularly primary care physicians who operate as gatekeepers for managed care plans, are seeing a spectrum of human disease that is completely overwhelming to them," said a PHS executive. "Most doctors want to do the right thing and they are looking for tools to help them." BCBS and PHS also hope to link CMS to other programs, including BCBSM's utilization and disease management programs (for example, automatic precertification of cases in which care meets the SACs; use by care nurses in developing individualized care plans for patients enrolled in the CCM). BCBSM also hopes to collect data from physicians who use CMS on a real-time basis by having them enter clinical data for patients they have treated while (or after) accessing the CMS guidelines. These data would be used to do retrospective studies, such as assessing physician compliance with the SACs, and to track outcomes (for example, to assess whether asthma patients of physicians who used the SACs had lower rates of emergency department use than did patients of other physicians).

The CMS is being piloted in Michigan during 1997 in a limited number of locations, including as part of the Flint CHCI. According to a BCBSM official, "Flint is . . . our first real case of demonstrating the program and trying to get physicians to buy into the guidelines." As an initial step in Flint, BCBS performed a small analysis of treatment received by GM employees with cardiovascular disease, compared to the SACs, using detailed chart review. The analysis found enormous variation in treatment, including many invasive diagnostic tests leading to invasive therapies. "For example, there were a lot of forty-five-year-olds with angina who got cardiac caths and CABGs as first-line treatment instead of medical treatment," said a BCBS executive. "For many of these patients, the care did not meet indications for testing and procedures. The complications are worse after these procedures, they have to be redone ten years later, and then the person never goes back to work again. It's often better to treat patients medically and wait to do the first bypass later—outcomes are better and it allows the patient to go back to work. But you have to look at the actual content of care to find these opportunities. Most current utilization management would not identify these issues. For example, in the Flint study, all of the CABGs had lengths of stay within standard boundaries."

Chrysler data have also been used to assess care received by employees against the SACs for diabetes and asthma. In both cases, the analysis found tremendous variations from the guidelines and the potential for improved quality and significant cost savings. PHS and BCBSM intend to pilot the CMS in other locations during the next year, and are developing plans to expand the program nationally later in 1997 or early 1998 to other BCBS participating plans that have large concentrations of UAW workers.

All involved in the CMS project agree that the system must have certain attributes to make physicians willing to apply it, including ease of use and clinical value. In the words of one physician: "Engineering the information and presentation is a real art. . . . The information must be right there because doctors will not be willing to go through lots of layers to find what they need." Another clinician agreed, "The system has to be easy, but it also has to add value by telling you more than you already know. If you check it two times and learn nothing new, you won't use it the third time."

But some observers doubt whether CMS will be valuable or used by most physicians. The issue of physician acceptance of the guidelines was a commonly sounded concern. Another was the cost and redundancy of effort: "Doctors can't figure out all these guidelines," argued one clinician. "There are seventy-five groups developing *the* best practice and they all say they do it differently and better. Physicians don't want to treat patients differently based on what insurance plan they are in. . . . Enough already of all these private efforts . . . there needs to be some centralized common set of guidelines that can be used for all patients, maybe developed by NCQA and administered and monitored by local plans." Several observers questioned the usefulness of any system that relies on claims data for clinical information: "It's hard for me to see how CMS can work outside of an organized system of care that has electronic medical records," commented a managed care executive. Another physician noted that even the clinical data input by physicians may be inaccurate: "Sloan Kettering Medical Center in New York City has a system similar to CMS but they had to stop letting doctors enter data and instead had to hire other people to do it because much of the information the doctors entered was wrong."

Perhaps the biggest problem with CMS is developing incentives for physicians and other clinicians to use the system. The suggestion of one Big Three official that "the incentive to use CMS ought to be as simple as to live up to the oath they took in medical school" was not seen by most observers as being sufficient. The UAW, at least, believes there needs to be a stronger carrot, or rather a bigger stick, and is considering requiring that physicians agree to use the CMS as a condition of serving UAW patients: "We hope in the future to make CMS part of the physician contract. Physicians will have to agree to participate in the program or they will not get a contract. BCBSM tells us they don't expect much resistance," said a UAW official.

Even if physicians embrace the CMS, its potential to affect costs and quality is unclear. "We have to manage expectations," warned a BCBS executive. "CMS will not result in dramatic changes overnight. If that is the expectation, we will be disappointed." At least one UAW official cautioned that best practices alone will not be enough: "I think the CMS has tremendous potential . . . but of course, once we have best practices, all of the social issues emerge again, like capacity, reduced incomes for providers, and access."

Community Health Care Initiatives

During the negotiations, the union and company conducted extensive discussions regarding the continued development of the Community Health Care Initiatives process. The contract "reaffirms that the CHCI process has the potential to promote high quality, cost-effective health care delivery systems for the entire community and thereby enhance the effectiveness and value of the health care benefits provided to UAW-represented employees under the Health Care Program." In the contract, the parties agreed to continue the pilots in Flint, Kokomo, and Anderson, and to expand the program to other areas.

Although it still too early to tell how the initiatives are working, the politics and reaction of the constituencies in the different communities appear to vary. According to one UAW member,

> Bringing hospitals together is murder. They know there is overbedding and they need to come to terms with it, but they are not ready to

do it. . . . Flint has no excess hospital beds, so it has been easier to bring the hospitals to the table. . . . Anderson is overbedded, and there are too many specialists, so the provider community has been very political and factionalized. . . . In Kokomo, Chrysler announced that it was building a new plant in town six months before the CHCI initiative began, so the view is that since the company is making an investment to keep the local economy strong, it is not unreasonable that they would want quality health care in return.

However, according to one Big Three manager, it was only the threat by Chrysler to build its own medical clinics in Kokomo that brought some of the providers to the table. And the UAW acknowledges that the potential effect of the initiatives on provider employment is a difficult issue for labor. "Employment by providers is central in all communities . . . but that's why there needs to be a slow and careful process to delivery system change. . . . You can't just use a machete," remarked one UAW member involved in the initiatives. The automakers give the union a great deal of credit for being willing to take on the providers. "Health system change, particularly closing hospitals, will cause people to lose their jobs," said one Big Three official. "The vision has to be that there are lots of jobs that have not been created yet and needs that can be addressed. The UAW has the vision to see that things in health care have to be changed and that there are opportunities to refocus and build in different ways. . . . The reality is that there are no safe jobs anywhere anymore."

While there appears to be strong support at the UAW and the automakers for the CHCI program, opinions differ about how effective this approach will ultimately be at improving quality and controlling costs. The experience of Rochester, New York, which has had a successful community health planning process for thirty years, is often cited as the prototype for the CHCI program. But many believe the Rochester experience will be hard to duplicate. "Rochester is no model; neither is Minnesota," according to one Big Three official. "There's high HMO penetration and community rating in Rochester . . . and both areas are too rich, too homogeneous, and they are not urban-challenged. . . . I give them no respect in terms of replicability. If we can succeed in Chicago, Cleveland, or Pittsburgh, then we will have something." "These are worthy experiments," suggested another manager. "But although I think we will make inroads in the community, those efforts are unlikely to make a real difference. The only places where the approach will have any difference are ones where the Autos are dominant, and there aren't that many communities where that is the case." Officials at Ford noted that they have moved slowly into the CHCI program in part because "we operate in many more bigger cities where we are a big fish in a big pond. We are not able to dictate to the community in the same way that GM and Chrysler have been able to in Flint, Anderson, and Kokomo. So we have to find other types of leverage."

There is also debate about whether the CHCI approach will be a more effective approach than relying on managed care. "While the CHCI is a reasonable strategy, the outcome is up for grabs," said one physician. "I don't think the initiatives will have the effect that they want. . . . Providers need to be part of organized delivery systems that have risk and accountability for costs and outcomes. This is too global and too diffuse. . . . A better approach would be for the UAW to educate its members about the good things in managed care." But an automaker official thought the two approaches were compatible: "The initiatives are not meant to stop market forces and managed care but to help direct and rationalize them. Managed care does reduce capacity, but at the moment it is not the right providers that die, it is the weak ones. . . . Changes do not have to be brutal and horrible, they can be controlled and measured. . . . The CHCIs might be the anesthesia that is needed for the pain of making system change."

In fact, the UAW sees the CHCIs as a way to achieve many of the same results as managed care. Explained one UAW official, "We see the CHCIs as a way to get managed care into high-density areas without having to bargain it. . . . Politically we can't agree to require workers to join HMOs, but we can try to remake the community into a system that acts as an HMO in terms of best practices, capacity, collaboration." But others doubted the UAW's stance. One automaker official said,

> While I think this is a worthy effort, I think it has resulted largely from the UAW's unwillingness to really support managed care with its membership . . . and I don't see the UAW doing much to push HMOs in the near future. They have no need to make the tough call because everyone is doing well, at least in Detroit. No one is really suffering. The Autos are well, unemployment is low, inflation is low, and most of the providers are doing well . . . but that will change eventually and the UAW will be faced with the same issues again.

‐‿‿‐ Epilogue: Practical Results

Kiran Verma
Harvard School of Public Health

General Motors workers are living longer, healthier lives, according to a recent GM-UAW report on community Health. The study found the mortality rate of GM workers has dropped 35 percent and health screenings have increased since the formation of the Greater Flint Coalition in 1992.

"The coalition plays a major role in improving the value of Flint health care services for UAW and GM employees," said James Cubbin, health care Czar for GM. "This collaboration has provided many solutions to tackle difficult healthcare issues. Yet more can and will be done to improve the quality of health care in Flint" [Kirkendoll, 2000].

As discussed earlier in the chapter, the Greater Flint Coalition was the first Community Health Care Initiative, a joint program of the UAW and GM to address many of the health problems in this Michigan city of 140,000. Flint was chosen as a site for a pilot program to develop a collaborative approach to achieving cost savings through improved quality. This innovative approach to controlling health care costs reflected in part the major shift in focus from cost-sharing to quality. One of the major health provisions of the 1996 UAW contract was to expand the two quality initiatives already operating on a pilot basis, CCM program and the CHCI program, along with a new clinical protocol tool, the CMS.

The 1999 contract agreement between the UAW and the Big Three auto manufacturers further reaffirmed the belief that CHCI programs have the potential to promote high-quality, cost-effective health care systems for the whole community. Accordingly, the union and the automakers agreed to expand the program to additional communities and further develop activities to "achieve demonstrable improvements in health status, quality, and cost effectiveness of the health care delivery system over time." New CHCI locations were to be determined by the Corporate-Union Committee on Health Care Benefits. In addition, it was to oversee the CHCI initiatives and develop mechanisms to evaluate the programs. Based on the agreement, the automakers (in collaboration with the UAW) started a number of initiatives in several communities, as shown in Table 10.3.

In addition to the CHCI-related agreements, in the 1999 agreement the UAW was successful in resisting the corporations' attempts to increase copayments for prescription drugs. Apart from some changes in benefits such as dental allowances, childhood immunizations, and ambulance services, the basic features of the health benefit for unionized employees remained essentially the same as had been agreed in 1996—that is, with no cost-sharing in the form of copayments or coinsurance for the participants, and only a two-year mandatory enrollment in an HMO for new employees. The following paragraphs update the story of the Flint CHCI, which was introduced in the preceding section of the chapter, and give brief descriptions of some of the other initiatives.

Community Health Care Initiative Site	Automaker	Date Implemented
Flint	General Motors	1995
Anderson	General Motors	1995
Kokomo	DaimlerChrysler	1996
Warren Youngstown	General Motors	1998
Delaware	DaimlerChrysler	1998
Kansas City	Ford	1998
Kenosha	DaimlerChrysler	2000
Louisville	Ford	2001

Table 10.3.   Spread of CHCI Agreements.

CHCI IN FLINT

The Flint Coalition, a group of providers and businesspeople, was formed by community leaders in 1992. GM and UAW joined the coalition in 1994 with a mission to improve quality of care and access to care.

Robert N. Alpert, executive director of the UAW's Center for Community Heath Care Initiatives, said, "We made a commitment to actively seek, with the companies, the highest quality health care through best practices and cost-effectiveness. These community initiatives are not a selective contracting process, they are not a competitive approach, they are a collaborative, a cooperative process." He noted, however, that the programs were not a magic wand: "It's hard work to bring people together. But cooperation is key to bringing down health care costs. Quality and cost-effectiveness need to be addressed in the communities. Unless we can eliminate duplications and redundancies at the local level, health care costs will never be brought into balance."

Anthony Stasmus, a GM employee who serves as a director of the greater Flint Coalition, noted, "As the largest local employer, GM can put some pressure on people to begin and continue discussions. However, being the eight-hundred-pound gorilla is not enough by itself. Consumers, payers, and providers need to together set goals, develop ways to improve quality, and reduce costs." Given that in 1995 GM spent $3.6 billion on health care for more than 1.6 million people, including workers, their families, and retirees, controlling costs was a big issue.

Some impressive improvements have been attributed to the work of the Coalition. A 1999 study jointly conducted by the GM and UAW to evaluate the Coalition's work noted the following positive outcomes (Kirkendoll, 2000):

- Death rates of hospitalized GM workers dropped by 35 percent after the initiative began.
- The number of cardiac catheterizations was reduced and the positive outcomes from this procedure had improved by 10 percent.
- Breast cancer screening covered 70 percent of women.
- Cervical cancer screenings had increased to 65 percent of women.

The impressive decrease in hospital deaths was being attributed to two changes made during the last five years. The first was a reduction in duplicate hospital-based services. Genesys Health Systems consolidated its inpatient services to the new health park campus, eliminating five hundred beds; Hurley Medical Center moved its coronary artery bypass surgeries to McLaren Regional Medical Center; and Hurley and Mott Children's Heath Center joined pediatric units. This allowed each of the resulting combined specialty services to become more focused and efficient. Consolidating specialty programs resulted in increased volume leading to more experience, enhanced skills, and greater expertise for physicians and other health care providers in the specialty.

The second contributing factor was the implementation of an evidence-based medical care practice, leading to vast improvements in the diagnosis, treatment, and outcomes for cardiac catheterization patients. A cardiac catheterization protocol was developed by the health coalition's cardiac task force. The protocol included standards for appropriate cardiac catheterization that, when followed by physicians, reduced unnecessary procedures and improved the quality of care received by those whose condition warranted the more extensive CABG surgery.

Along with recognizing successes, the report also noted that work still needed to be done. Diabetes testing was inadequate, and the number of hysterectomies was too high, as were the medical error rates.

Although the report discussed health care achievements and future challenges in some depth, missing was an evaluation of any associated cost savings. Some savings have come from lowering the number of cardiac catheterizations—a $4,000 test—given to local patients. But a Flint area cardiologist wondered where the savings had gone. He noted, "If money is saved and workers don't see it, then it is not a job accomplished" (Kirkendoll, 2000).

The Coalition has consistently resisted pressure to focus only on the bottom line and is looking at the next set of issues such as racial gaps in health care, infant mortality, and the uninsured.

OTHER COMMUNITY HEALTH CARE INITIATIVES

Since 1995, the CHCI movement has grown from the first two, in Flint, Michigan, and Anderson, Indiana, to a total of eight communities, including Kokomo, Indiana (1996), Warren Youngstown, Ohio

(1998), Wilmington, Delaware (1998), Kansas City (1998), Kenosha, Wisconsin (2000), and Louisville, Kentucky (2001) (personal communication, Robert N. Alpert, UAW, January 10, 2002). All are seeking to improve medical practice in their communities through the application of best practices and evidence-based care, in collaboration with their local medical communities. The projects begin with community health assessments facilitated by outside consultants, and lead to lengthy community dialogs about health status, access, wellness, fitness, and quality of care. Several of the communities have reached consensus on specific disease initiatives, such as improving care for asthma and reducing the rate of inappropriate hysterectomy (Anderson), promoting healthy lifestyles and improving drug prescribing practices (Kokomo), and developing guidelines for managing congestive heart failure (Kansas City) (Greater Kansas City Area Community Healthcare Initiative, n.d.).

As one community health initiatives participant explained, "Our aim is to bring people together in one room and try to reach a consensus on clinical guidelines, to work through issues of commonality and come up with what is doable for doctors and patients" (Bloice, 2001). She went on to say that community health initiatives were part of a larger "social reform movement" that presented an effective approach for addressing such issues as health disparities and the uninsured, using better data to measure and improve the health of the community.

References

Bloice, C. "UAW, Big Three Take Initiative for Community Health." *KC Press*, Mar.-Apr. 2001.

Kirkendoll, S. M. "GM-UAW Coalition Charts Better Health for Workers." *Flint Journal*, Apr. 25, 2000.

Greater Kansas City Area Community Healthcare Initiative. "Other Community Healthcare Initiatives," n.d. Available online: http://kchealth.org/other.html (access date Mar. 31, 2003).

Lewin Group. "Community Assessment Factbook: Genesee County, Michigan." Unpublished report presented to the Corporate-Union Committee on Health Care Benefits, May 16, 1996.

CHAPTER ELEVEN

The Next Wave of General Practitioner Fundholding

Welcome or Farewell?

Why eliminate fundholding and demotivate the only group of doctors who are motivated in the NHS?

> —*Physician from Castlefields Health Centre*

The question for the future of General Practitioner Fundholding is: How much can we expect from primary care? The top 15 percent of GPs are excellent and enthusiastic. But what about the others? . . . We don't have the consistency in GPs to rely on them to be the purchasers.

> —*Official for North West Regional Office*

We are getting better service and care since GP fundholding went into effect and we want to keep it. But if it's abandoned, we know that Castlefields Health Centre will make the most of whatever is put in its place. We can only keep our fingers crossed that it will all work out OK.

> —*Patient of Castlefields Health Centre*

This case was originally written by the authors in 1996. Funding was provided by Astra Zeneca. The authors thank Dr. David Colin-Thome and his colleagues at Castlefields Health Centre for their tremendous assistance.

reat Britain will hold a general election in the fall of 1996 or early in 1997. The future role and structure of managed care and competitive forces in the British health care system will be a major issue in the election and a significant policy issue facing the next government. In particular, there is considerable controversy over the future of General Practitioner Fundholding (GPF or "GP fundholding"), one of the initiatives enacted by the Conservative government as part of its sweeping 1991 health reforms. The goals of GPF, as set out in the 1989 National Health Service (NHS) working paper on the issue, are "to offer GPs an opportunity to improve the quality of services they offer to patients, to stimulate hospitals to be more responsive to the needs of GPs and their patients and to develop their own practices for the benefit of their patients. It will also enable the practices that take part to play a more important role in the way in which NHS money is used to provide services for their patients" (Department of Health, 1989).

Under the fundholding initiative, certain general practitioner practices are allowed to become "GP fundholders," with control of their own budgets for a specified range of primary care, specialty, hospital, and other services. Application for fundholder status is voluntary and has occurred in several "waves"; as of July 1996, approximately half of GPs and patients in England are covered by GPF.

The fundholding initiative was one of a number of reforms designed to provide more services at less cost and improve quality of care by inducing competition among providers. The major components of the 1991 reforms were to separate purchasers of care from providers of care by having District Health Authorities (DHAs) and GP fundholders negotiate contracts with hospitals and other providers, and to allow hospitals and other community health organizations to become autonomous trusts that compete for contracts from local health authorities and GP fundholders.

The 1991 reforms were opposed by many factions, including the Labour Party and much of the medical profession and media. Opponents alleged, among other criticisms, that the government was privatizing and corporatizing the NHS; that decentralization of purchasing would raise administrative costs and make it difficult to achieve rational health objectives; and that the changes were one more step to increase the "managerialism" of the NHS at the expense of providers and clinical care. GPF was criticized based on various concerns, including that GPs would become managers rather than doctors; that the initiative would create a two-tier system of care in which the patients of non-fundholding GPs would have less access to care; and that GP fundholding would fragment the ability to do rational health planning on a regional and national basis.

But many advocates of reform, including many family physicians, believed that fundholding provided an opportunity to raise standards of clinical practice and improve quality of care. Supporters also hoped that reforms would reduce the serious disparities and resource imbalances among regions, and, in particular, shift resources out of London, with its vast number of teaching hospitals, to other parts of the country with significant health care needs.

The results of the 1991 reforms have sparked considerable controversy. Anecdotes about positive and negative effects abound, but formal evaluation of most of the changes has been scarce and the data that are available are limited and often of poor quality. In fact, one of the criticisms of the reforms is that they were made before data collection and information systems were in place to support and evaluate them. In addition, change has been constant since 1991, making evaluation difficult. In general, the results of the reforms seem to be somewhat mixed; neither the dire predictions of opponents nor the high hopes of advocates have been realized. Instead, it appears that changes have been made slowly by providers and purchasers, and that competition has been limited and rather tightly controlled within a highly regulatory structure. It is also clear that the changes are still in the early stages of development and that it is too soon to tell what the long-term impact of the reforms will be.

Although fundholding was viewed as one of the minor reforms in the 1991 law and was expected to have only modest results, it has proven to be a significant change and, in the minds of many, a successful innovation. Its proponents believe GPF has had many desirable effects, including making a start at ending the dominance of hospitals and specialists and shifting resources to primary care and other community services, as well as creating more coordinated continuums of care across sectors; encouraging more cost-conscious practice by clinicians; empowering GPs to demand more responsiveness and accountability from specialists and hospitals, which has shortened waiting times and improved access and service for patients; and encouraging innovation, such as consultant services at GP sites, case management programs, and the development of other new services.

However, fundholding also continues to have many critics. Among the most often stated concerns:

- Fundholding has fragmented district budgets and weakened the ability of health authorities to purchase for the needs of all residents in their area, and to implement public health programs for entire populations.

- Fundholding has resulted in discrimination against the patients of non-fundholders, including concerns that overfunding of fundholders has reduced the resources available for other patients and that shorter waits for the patients of fundholders have been achieved at the cost of longer waits for patients of non-fundholding GPs.

- The increased administrative costs of fundholding have reduced resources available for clinical care.

- Many GP fundholders have profited personally from fundholding surpluses by investing in their practices and by referring to providers in which they have a financial interest.

Ironically, one of the major criticisms of fundholding, and the health reforms generally, is the absence of any systematic evaluation of their effects. Despite the few independent assessments of fundholding, a soon-to-be released national audit report evidently will conclude that fundholding has resulted in minimal cost savings because most of the savings from fundholding have been reinvested in the practices of GP fundholders.

Although the Labour Party now appears to concede that many of the 1991 reforms have had some positive effects, Labour has been steadfast in its opposition to fundholding. If the Labour Party wins the next general election, as is widely predicted, it will need to decide whether to continue, abandon, or modify GPF.

BACKGROUND

The British National Health Service has long been envied by many observers for a number of characteristics and achievements, including universal coverage, regardless of age, income, or health status; equitable financing; strict national budgets; a well-developed health infrastructure, and a particularly strong primary care system; and administrative costs among the lowest of any national health system in the developed world. Since the NHS was established in 1948, it has always provided nearly free health care to all citizens. The system is funded almost entirely through general taxation, with some limited revenue from payroll levies and small user charges. Coverage is comprehensive, with minimal copayments for a limited range of services, including drugs and dental and eye exams. Copayments are waived for the poor, elderly, and mothers and children.

The NHS operates on a top-down budgeting system in which government controls the overall level of spending. The budget is determined at the national level, and is allocated to regions based on needs, according to a formula that takes into account historic activity as well as regional variations in demographics and socioeconomic factors. Efforts to make the formula "needs-based" have resulted in a shift of resources from certain parts of the country to others, including shifting resources out of London. As of April 1, 1996, the formula eliminated the so-called deprivation allowance, which gave additional resources to regions that had relatively high rates of unemployment and poverty. This change significantly reduced resources available in the North West region of England.

Each of the NHS regions distributes resources to the local level based on a similar needs-based methodology. (Until 1994, there were eighteen NHS regions. The number of regions was reduced to eight in 1994, and as of April 1996, the separate Regional Health Authorities were reorganized as regional outposts of the NHS Executive.)

The global budget approach has been a successful cost-containment method. Britain spends approximately 7 percent of GDP on health care, an amount that has been falling in real dollar terms for the past ten to fifteen years and is considerably lower than spending in comparable countries. The costs of nonemergency care are controlled, in part, by waits, which can be up to a year for certain types of elective procedures. Although a major goal of the 1991 health reforms (which are discussed in more detail later in this chapter) was to improve service and reduce waiting times, waiting lists continue to be a major feature on the British system and one that has created a demand for private insurance. There is a great deal of discussion and debate in Britain about whether the NHS is underfunded.

Physicians

Britain has a well-developed primary care system. GPs provide 90 percent of all episodes of care and act as gatekeepers for secondary care. The system is unique in having a registered population—every covered individual is on the list of a primary care physician. This registration system is a critical component of the move to a population- and community-based primary care system, with defined accountability at the local and practitioner level for the health needs of an entire population. The geographic distribution of GPs varies widely, with twice as many GPs in the south of England as in the north, where there are major concentrations of population. "GPs like to practice in Cornwall," remarked one physician in the north.

Many GPs are in solo or two-person practice. "GPs in Britain are fiercely independent and the system is quite fragmented," according to one observer. "GPs want to control their own practices. Many of them are in solo practice because they could not get along with their partners."

General practitioners are self-employed independent contractors who are paid by the NHS through a negotiated national contract. Traditional GP payment has fixed and variable components: a capitation payment based on the number of patients on the physician's list and varying by the age and sex of each patient; an additional payment, calculated through a complex socioeconomic formula; and special fees for providing certain other services (such as clinical assessments of new patients, health promotion clinics, training medical students). Under the requirements of the most recent national GP contract, which went into effect in 1990, the performance of each individual GP in providing certain primary and preventive services (for example, pap smears, immunizations) is monitored, and performance must be within certain bands to receive full payment. Physicians working in areas classified as "deprived" receive additional payments (although as one clinician at Castlefields noted, "the performance targets for preventive and primary care services are not lower in the areas where access to primary and preventive services is more limited, so the government gives with one hand and takes with the other.") GPs also receive funding from the NHS for staffing and other expenses of the practice, including office space and computer systems.

People have freedom of choice of primary care provider and are permitted to switch GPs at will, with minimal administrative burden, However, this choice is rarely exercised and patient turnover among GPs is very low. GPs can close their practices when they reach capacity, and some geographic areas have few open GP practices where patients could choose to enroll.

Specialists, or "consultants" as they are known, are salaried employees of the NHS. Salaries are based on specialty and seniority, and range from approximately $75,000–$115,000. Specialists are expected to work twenty-two hours per week, and are permitted to work privately the rest of the time. According to several observers, most specialists earn two to three times their NHS salaries seeing private patients. Patients may not self-refer to specialists but must be referred by their GP. Consultant capacity is tight in Britain. The number of general practice and consultant positions is centrally controlled by limiting the number of medical students and foreign trainees and by matching the number of resident positions to the number of GP and consultant posts available. According to several observers, a significant problem facing Britain is the large number of medical students who leave the health system after finishing medical school, either to move to other countries or to give up practice entirely.

Hospitals

Virtually all hospitals are now organized as autonomous hospital trusts, which compete for contracts from GP fundholders and District Health Authorities. The vast majority of hospital revenue is derived from contracts with DHAs. Hospitals are typically paid in these ways:

- *Block contracts:* The hospital is paid a fixed amount to provide any covered services required by any patients of the purchaser. These contracts generally allow some additional payment for volume that exceeds projected levels, although payment is less than the hospital's full cost. Most hospital revenue is from these block grants, which is how most DHAs and GPFs pay for most hospital care.

- *Cost and volume contracts:* Payment is fixed for volume within certain limits. If volume increases beyond the limit (for example, by 2.5 percent of the expected level), additional payment is made at marginal cost.

- *Cost per case contracts:* Payment is made on an individual case-type (that is, diagnosis-related group or DRG) basis, and is the method GP fundholders use to shift specific case types out of one hospital and into another. Only a small proportion of hospital revenues (10 percent or less) is earned from cost per case contracts.

Hospital occupancy causes considerable debate in Britain. Over the past decade, lengths of stay have fallen and care has been shifting to outpatient settings. In response, the NHS has closed hospitals in some areas, raising concerns about inadequate inpatient capacity in certain regions, especially for accident and emergency admissions. In a number of highly publicized cases, people have died as a result of being turned away from hospitals that did not have ICU beds available.

Drugs

Physicians are required to prescribe from a limited list of drugs established by the NHS. The patient copayment for prescription drugs is about $8; however, more than half the population is exempt from copayments, and copayments are made for only 12 percent of prescriptions. The prescribing habits of non-fundholding physicians are monitored by District Health Authorities through the use of individual indicative budgets, which are based on current prescription costs and the average for similar practices. If the GP exceeds the assigned indicative budget, the DHA gives advice. If necessary, the GP may be subject to peer review and financial penalties. British physicians tend to be conservative prescribers compared to their counterparts in many other countries, and drugs account for approximately 10 percent of total NHS expenditures, one of the lowest expenditures per capita in the European Union. According to one study, GP fundholders spent 7 percent less on drugs than did non-fundholders in 1993, and they also made greater use of generic prescriptions. Thus fundholding appears to reinforce the already conservative prescribing habits of British GPs.

Private Health Insurance

Approximately 16 percent of the British population has private insurance coverage in addition to their coverage by the NHS. Half of private insurance is provided through employers as a fringe benefit. The other half is purchased directly by individuals, many of whom purchase coverage for their children but not themselves because of the cost. Since the NHS provides easy access to primary and emergency services, demand for private insurance stems from a desire for quicker access to nonemergency services that have long waits (such as elective surgery) and for unrestricted access to and choice of specialists.

Privately insured individuals usually receive care in small limited-service private hospitals (that is, hospitals with no ICUs or ERs) that offer greater amenities than most NHS hospitals. Although the proportion of the population with private coverage is quite low, it has been growing somewhat, and is taken by some observers to be an indication of the failure of the nation to address the problems of waiting lists and inadequate funding of the NHS.

THE 1991 REFORMS

"What makes the British case special . . . is the ambitious scope of the reforms and the relentless determination with which Mrs. Thatcher's government implemented them. . . . Disdaining consensus, experiment, and incrementalism and overriding strident opposition from the medical profession and others, it introduced and implemented systemwide changes: a big bang approach to health care reform," says Rudolf Klein of the University of Bath, England (Klein, 1995, pp. 299–300).

In 1991, Britain enacted the National Health Service and Community Care Act, legislation that made some of the most far-reaching changes to health financing and delivery the country had seen in decades. Health policymakers and politicians have a variety of differing opinions about the reasons for the act; there seems, however, to be general agreement that it was in large part a response to mounting political tensions about perceived underfunding of the NHS and growing inequalities in health and income. Despite widespread continuing public support for the NHS, and particularly for universal, comprehensive coverage, discontent was growing over the waiting lists and other by-products that successful cost containment had created for the government.

Given the unwillingness of the government to increase the NHS budget in an era of financial pressures or to deal with the socioeconomic issues facing the country, Prime Minister Margaret Thatcher chose to deal with these political pressures by targeting inefficiency in the NHS. Her solution, which was consonant with the free market, procompetition approaches favored by her Conservative Party and several other countries, including the United States, was to introduce more competition and greater market forces into the NHS. The goals of the reform were to get "more value for the money" by making the health system more efficient, making providers more cost conscious and more responsive to consumers, and increasing quality of care. Mrs. Thatcher's approach was also influenced, at least indirectly, by Alain Enthoven, the U.S. economist from Stanford University, who authored an analysis of the NHS in 1985 in which he argued that the system was replete with perverse incentives that hampered efficiency and cost containment, including salaried physicians and hospitals operating within fixed budgets. Although Enthoven recommended some reforms similar to those enacted by Thatcher's Conservative government, he advocated a more incremental, pilot approach rather than the "big bang" approach that was adopted.

The Act made three major changes: it split purchasing from providing, permitted the establishment of trusts, and created the GP fundholding system. As a group, these reforms are often characterized as creating "internal markets" because providers and purchasers compete within a system that continues to be constrained by overall district and national budgets. In addition, it included the "Patient's Charter," a law that establishes performance standards for the NHS and providers in certain areas, including waiting times for emergency, outpatient, and inpatient care. For example, the target waiting time for an outpatient specialist appointment is no more than thirteen weeks after written referral by the patient's GP. National and regional data on performance against the Patient's Charter standards are published regularly by the NHS.

Split Between Purchasing and Providing

The financing and purchasing of health care were separated from its provision. Prior to this change, District Health Authorities, funded by and accountable to the central NHS, were responsible for providing health services needed by their populations, and they directly managed all hospitals and community health services. After 1991, local health authorities, funded on a per capita formula weighted for population characteristics, are responsible for purchasing care from providers instead of for managing the providers. A central goal of the purchaser-provider split is to have resources follow patients instead of being attached to providers. District Health Authorities are required to develop needs assessments of their populations and an annual purchasing plan that spells out the services they intend to buy. (This purchasing role, whether performed by health authorities or GPs, has come to be referred to as *commissioning*, a word that is intended to connote the active role that purchasers are expected to play in shaping the configuration of services and delivery system for their populations.)

The reforms have also made many changes to the structure and organization of the NHS at the local and regional level over the last five years. As of 1996, District Health Authorities, which had been responsible for secondary care, and Family Health Service Authorities, which had been responsible for primary care management, will combine into a single DHA with responsibility for efficient provision of total patient care. As of April 1996, the name, status, and function of the Regional Health Authorities changed. The newly titled "Regional Offices" of the NHS no longer have budget or management authority, which has devolved to the DHAs. Instead, the role of the Regional Office is to provide strategy, support, and monitoring, including monitoring the progress being made by DHAs in meeting health needs, and to provide support to encourage providers and purchasers to work together. In the words of one public official, these changes "have created an identity crisis for the Regional Offices," although observers generally believe this change will further centralize the NHS.

Establishment of Trusts

Hospitals and other health care organizations, which had been run by local health authorities, were allowed to become self-governing trusts, with greater management and financial autonomy as well as the need to sell their services to purchasers, including local authorities, GPs, and private insurers. In creating a trust, the assets of the organization are transferred to a new organization, governed by a separate Board, with debt due to the federal Treasury. Trusts are still public organizations but are accountable directly to the NHS Executive, which monitors financial and business planning and performance but does not manage the organizations. Hospital trusts have more authority over personnel and capital, including freedom to seek private financing. Trusts must still operate within certain guidelines, including meeting a target return on assets of at least 6 percent and not borrowing beyond an external financing limit. Most capital spending must be reviewed and approved by local authorities.

Among the explicit goals of creating trusts were to dismantle the close relationships that had developed between the providers and the District Health Authorities so there would be less conflict in roles, and to free trusts from the bureaucracy of the NHS so they can innovate more easily and be more responsive to local needs. Conversion to trust status is voluntary, and has occurred in several stages, or "waves." In the first wave in 1991, hospitals representing 12 percent of inpatient beds converted; by 1993, two-thirds of beds were converted; and by 1995 essentially all hospitals had become trusts. In addition to acute care hospitals, many other providers that deliver community services have converted to trust status.

Creation of GP Fundholding

GPs meeting certain criteria were allowed to assume budget responsibility on behalf of their patients for certain services and to purchase those services from any provider. Originally only practices with at least nine thousand patients were eligible to become fundholders, but the size has been reduced steadily and is now five thousand patients. The first wave of fundholders was approximately three hundred practices, representing 8 percent of the population. As of April 1996, approximately 51 percent of GPs, representing 53 percent of the population, were fundholders. The percentage of GPs who are fundholders varies significantly by region; fundholding is more prevalent in suburban and rural areas and underrepresented in inner cities.

The range of services included in fundholder budgets varies, depending on the type of fundholding arrangement. In the original version of the program, referred to as "standard" fundholding, GPs assumed budget responsibility for services that accounted for approximately 20 percent of hospital and community health spending, including a defined set of surgical inpatient and day surgery cases covering most elective procedures, outpatient services, prescription drugs, diagnostic tests, specified services for individuals with mental health and learning disabilities, and the costs of certain GP practice staff. The range of services in standard fundholding was expanded in 1992 to include community services (such as district nurses, speech therapy, podiatry, psychology, and community mental health nursing). Standard fundholders are not at risk for obstetrical cases, accident and emergency care, acute medical admissions, or inpatient mental health services.

In the first two years of fundholding, budgets were based exclusively on each practice's historical uses and costs. According to one CHC clinician, "The 1991 data were so bad that those of us in the first wave of fundholding really lost out. The later waves received budgets that were based on much more accurate data, and their payments were higher as a result." The formulas used to determine fundholding budgets vary; subsequent years' budgets are subject to benchmarking to reduce variability. In addition to the capitation payments, fundholding practices also receive financial assistance with start-up costs, including the costs of purchasing computer hardware and software.

GPs in fundholding practices are not at personal financial risk for fundholding services. The fundholding practices are responsible for budgets for covered services, which are negotiated with and paid by the DHAs, which hold the funds. Fundholding practices are protected by individual stop-loss coverage, with the DHA assuming responsibility for costs above $7,500. Any losses are covered by the DHA; surpluses are retained by the GP practice but cannot be used to increase the income of the fundholding physicians—the funds may be invested in new services or used to improve the fundholding practice. The DHA must review and approve the use of fundholding surpluses. Fundholders are accountable to the NHS Executive, through the DHAs, for the effective and efficient management of funds. Among the obligations of fundholders is to produce an annual report on their performance.

Since 1991, several other types of fundholding have been developed. "Community fundholding" is available to GPs with at least three thousand patients and is the same as standard fundholding with the exception of the exclusion of hospital services. Another option, "total fundholding," which was added in 1993, allows practices or groups of practices with at least sixty thousand patients to assume budget responsibility for most services, with the exception of certain high-cost cases (such as organ transplants). Total fundholding was first implemented on a pilot basis in 1993 in four sites, three of which are consortia of at least eight practices with a total of seventy thousand to eighty-five thousand patients each. (Two of the three original total fundholding sites cover entire towns.) The other pilot site was the Castlefields Health Centre in Runcorn, which had a population of only twelve thousand patients. Although well below the required patient list size to be financially viable for total fundholding, the CHC practice proposed that it be funded on a rolling five-year budget, which means that it must meet its total fundholding budget over the five years of the project but is not held to budgets in each separate year.

Its total fundholding budget also includes a "social deprivation" adjustment that was developed to recognize the higher levels of health need and chronic disease in the CHC population. The following section discusses CHC's operations in more detail.

The program was greatly expanded as of April 1996, when an additional fifty practices became total fundholders. (The recommendation of the NHS Executive was that subsequent total fundholding sites have a minimum of thirty thousand patients, although other models with fewer patients have been permitted.) Total fundholding is one component of a move by the NHS toward "Locality Purchasing," in which DHAs work in partnership with local GPs to purchase health care on behalf of a given population. Unlike other aspects of the NHS reforms, the total fundholding initiative is undergoing a formal independent evaluation commissioned by the government, although there is some concern that the program will be expanded further before the results have been studied. "The Tories are pushing total fundholding like crazy, although they have no explicit vision or strategy," observed one health policymaker.

THE VIEW FROM THE NORTH WEST

There is much discussion and concern about the future of fundholding throughout Britain, and especially in the North West region of England, an area that has been at the forefront of many of the health care financing and delivery reforms enacted in 1991. This region has some of the earliest and most enthusiastic and creative GP fundholders, including the Castlefields Health Centre mentioned in the preceding section. CHC is a six-physician primary care group practice in Runcorn, a town in the northwest part of England, midway between Manchester and Liverpool. It has approximately twelve thousand patients, many of whom are residents of the Castlefields industrial estate in which the Centre is located. The size of CHC is typical for Runcorn, although many GPs in the North West are in solo or two-person practices. The CHC practice is unusual in its inclusion of a number of nurse practitioners and other midlevel clinicians as part of the practice's Primary Care Team. CHC operates a satellite practice at another housing estate that is staffed by NPs. "I think we can eventually move to a practice model that has a ratio of two NPs to one physician," said one CHC physician. "NPs are excellent clinicians, and better than physicians at many aspects of care, including prescribing and maintaining relationships with patients."

Since its founding twenty years ago, CHC has had an explicit mission of serving and being an advocate for the community. The Centre's mission statement, as described in its most recent annual report, says: "We aim to provide the best possible care for our patients at all times by responding to their needs, providing accessible reactive and anticipatory care of the highest quality. We aim to provide a resource for the local community." Eighty-five percent of estate residents are CHC patients. (As one clinician remarked, "The residents are poor and have no cars, so they are stuck with us.") The CHC's Patient's Forum, an advisory group open to all patients and residents of the Castlefields estate, is regarded as a leader nationally for how to involve consumers in health care.

CHC has been a fundholding practice since 1991, and became the fourth total fundholding site in 1994, although implementation of total fundholding will not occur at CHC until the 1996–97 fiscal year. The practice's 1996 GPF budget is approximately $2.7 million; its non-GPF budget is approximately $6 million. Although CHC's current GPs are supportive of GPF, the issue was contentious when it was first discussed, and one GP left CHC because of his belief that fundholding was unethical and would result in a two-tier system of care.

Although CHC has long had a reputation as an innovative practice, the Centre has implemented a number of creative changes in contracting, care management and coordination, staffing, and quality measurement and improvement since it became a fundholder. CHC has invested considerable time and resources in data collection, medical audit, and the development of clinical protocols. "We are trying to clarify the 80 percent of medicine that is not understood," said a CHC physician. The practice operates on a paperless basis, with all information computerized. In its annual report, the practice describes one of its missions as, "Audit everything that moves. If it doesn't move, audit it to find out why it doesn't!" The clear focus is on using clinical data to look carefully at practice patterns and change behavior to improve outcomes for CHC patients. "I scare the pants off the consultants and hospitals because I have the numbers. They can't argue with the data," crowed a CHC physician.

Fundholding and health authority commissioning have also unleashed a great deal of interest at local hospitals in reengineering, benchmarking, and evidence-based medicine. According to one hospital administrator, "There is no doubt that GP fundholding has made hospitals think about why and how things are done."

Hospitals are devoting particular attention to the development of clinical protocols and care pathways, write-ups that detail the type and process of care that should be given to patients with particular illnesses or conditions. "Care pathways are a means to break down professional tribalism," said one hospital administrator. "They get everyone to focus on the same targets and outcomes and provide a predefined means to get there. We are developing them for all of our high-cost, high-volume, and high-variation services. At the moment, half of care is being provided according to pathways, and we expect to reach 80 percent by the end of the year," she added. In fact, many providers seem to have an almost evangelistic enthusiasm for care pathways. At a recent presentation on care pathways at a local hospital, one speaker discussed how care pathways can become the "clinical arm of purchasing" and help purchasers move away from a "macho dictator" mode of purchasing to a more outcomes-oriented model. She listed the following attributes of care pathways:

- They provide clear descriptions of care.
- They are a currency for contracting that makes sense (as opposed to the current use of "finished consultant episodes").
- They promote care that is supported by guidelines (as opposed to referring to "protocols"—a very sensitive term for clinicians).
- They are a description of best practices that can be used to assess provider performance.
- They can be adapted to local standards of practice.
- They are auditable.
- They lend themselves to research and development because different approaches can be tried within a pathway.
- They are dynamic and can facilitate change in clinical practice.
- They provide more information to patients and establish clearer expectations about care.
- They support multidisciplinary care.
- They help clarify roles and responsibilities, both for caregivers and patients.
- They are useful for simple and complex cases.

• They are useful for budgeting and costing because they help identify the resources needed to provide care and make it easier to have resources follow the patient.

• They require less documentation (for example, only one set of clinical notes).

• They increase accountability by making roles and responsibilities clearer.

• They open the door to case management.

• They increase consistency of care, so that fewer patients fall through the cracks.

Others are, however, somewhat more cautious about care pathways. One hospital administrator said, "The perception here was that care pathway development was not a worthwhile exercise. The hospital can only develop them for secondary care but not primary or follow-up care. It is a frustrating exercise without those elements. The consultants here want to avoid a lot of process and paper generation and are still cynical about the value added by pathways." Even an enthusiastic advocate of pathways agreed that getting clinician buy-in is a difficult process: "The number one issue with pathways is culture change," said this administrator. "It needs a huge investment in training and education." There were also disagreements over the appropriate role for GPs. Noted one hospital manager, "Working with GPs is like herding cats. But they have to be involved in developing the pathways or they won't use them." Other observers wondered how much of a role GPs, who generally see patients with chronic lifelong conditions (such as diabetes, asthma, COPD, and hypertension), can reasonably play in developing guidelines for the care of more acutely ill patients in the hospital setting.

Like most fundholders, CHC has, so far, maintained most of its historic relationships with hospitals and consultants. ("Most GP fundholders have been too nice to hospitals," observed one physician at CHC.) However, the practice has shifted some of its business. For example, community nursing services were shifted from the local trust to another trust based eighty miles away. The practice moved its ENT business to a different group of consultants because it was concerned about inappropriate utilization; one of the results was an 80 percent reduction in the number of grommets for pediatric ear infections, with no difference in outcomes. According to one CHC staff member,

"We have only moved a limited number of contracts. But just the possibility that we might move our contracts has been very effective at getting the attention of the hospitals and consultants."

Although local hospitals agree that GP fundholders have generally maintained historic care patterns, the shifts have had an effect. "There has not been wholesale shifting of care; it's been more like chipping away, a process of attrition," commented one hospital manager. "But it's hard to plan when you don't know what your volume will be. Losing a bit from a number of GP fundholders adds up to a lot." Consultants have felt the effects of contract shifts as well. According to one consultant, "GP fundholding has disrupted referral patterns. I often cannot refer patients where I want because there is no contract between the consultant I want to use and the GP fundholders. Even the contracts we have with the fundholders create problems. . . . Consultants have no idea what our costs are, and the hospital never involves us in negotiating the contracts. So the hospital signs all these contracts for more volume but we never get more resources."

Many hospital managers and consultants questioned whether competition among hospitals that are operating at capacity is an effective strategy for improving efficiency and quality of care. "There is no leeway on the staff side. The number of managers has increased but the skill mix of the clinical staff has been downgraded to save money. All the nurses are tired and demoralized. There is just no margin; everyone is working at capacity," said one consultant. An administrator at another hospital agreed, "It is hard to become efficient when occupancy is 100 percent because we are always working at the margins and cannot manage well."

But the CHC doctors were skeptical about the hospitals' complaints. "I have been in the National Health Service for thirty years and there is low morale reported every year. It's hard to separate the myth from the fact," said one physician. Another noted, "Hospital occupancy is high in the winter but not at other times. Hospitals are not run efficiently. Many people are overtrained for the jobs they are doing, and resources could be used better. For example, surgery suites could be used around the clock. But a movement to a more radical model will never happen in the current political environment. Hospitals will lose money if they start being analytical about quality because they will reduce volume."

Fundholding is widely believed to have shifted the balance of power between GPs and other providers. "The GP is now our customer," said one hospital manager. "We market actively to the GPs in all kinds of ways. If we don't do outreach, we will lose the patients." One hospital consultant quipped, "The GPs used to send Christmas cards to the consultants; now the consultants send them to the GPs," adding that it was a popular joke these days. A CHC physician described the change somewhat differently: "The relationship between GPs and consultants used to be one of child and parent. Consultants did not have to listen and there was no opportunity for dialogue. Now we are beginning to talk adult to adult."

Although the staff of CHC have been strong advocates of GPF, they have been frustrated by certain aspects of fundholding. In particular, they believe that resources have not directly followed changes in care and that GPs have not been allowed to have actual control over a significant enough portion of health spending. One of CHC's staff explained some of the practice frustrations: "We can move fundholding services and budgets but not the budgets for non-fundholding services. For instance, of our £80,000 [$120,000] urology budget, we can only shift the £30,000 [$45,000] that is non-urgent. . . . That's a problem for quality, continuity, and coordination of care. . . . We are about to do utilization management in the hospitals and we know we will free up a six-figure sum. But the problem is that there is no way under our current structure of GP fundholding for CHC to get the money back for other uses."

CHC's frustrations over the scope of standard fundholding led the group to lobby actively for the total fundholding pilot project, which it believes will improve its ability to develop new approaches for improving the health of CHC patients. However, the budgets in the total fundholding program are only indicative budgets, which means that CHC does not completely control the money. "The health authorities will not give total fundholders the real budgeted resources because other non-fundholding GPs would have to reduce their use for the authority to stay within its overall budget," explained one CHC staff member. "Total fundholding is a problem for health authorities because it reduces the DHA's budget for other services. And if the total fundholder underspends, it makes the DHA look bad, as if it is not an effective purchaser," he added.

Despite its concerns, CHC believes that GPF has been an important force for change, and it fears that a Labour government would abandon fundholding, to the detriment of patients and health care. "Fundholding has been a powerful way to challenge providers, particularly hospitals and consultants, on clinical and quality issues," said one CHC clinician. "But a Labour government will reduce the ability to move forward with fundholding. Labour seems determined to disempower the achievers to the level of the nonachievers," he lamented, adding, "Too bad none of the election will be about the real issues, like poverty, unemployment, AIDS, and chronic mental illness."

But not everyone in the North West believes that fundholding should be continued or expanded. Despite widespread praise of CHC and its achievements as a fundholding practice, many were quick to note that CHC was not a typical practice. "The doctors at CHC are unusual," said one district health official. "They have a much more open and holistic view of health and are supportive of establishing linkages to other services. They are much more challenging of the system and question everything, including whether they are needed. . . . Most other fundholders think of fundholding not as a way to improve quality but as a means to get freedom from the health authority." A hospital manager echoed this view:

> The GPs at Castlefields are very good, and are focused on quality, but that's not true in most other places. Most GPs are not ready to be purchasers. There are lots of indicia of poor GP practice and preparedness, including the prevalence of solo practice, many lock-up surgeries, little or no practice coverage in many practices, and lots of physicians with a poor command of English. Plus, GP fundholding is so bureaucratic with so much data and such high transactions costs. Most fundholders have not really focused on clinical issues, and most are not ready to make purchasing decisions. The trick with GP fundholders is to have good relationships. But collaborative relationships are not the same as improving patient care. We need to develop more pump-priming programs that can train and educate GPs on how to be effective managers and purchasers.

A regional health authority official agreed: "No one has looked at efficiency in primary care. GPs need to challenge their own practices before they begin on hospitals and consultants. The focus should be on making them better GPs first, not better purchasers. They need to use more nurse practitioners, change their prescribing habits, and learn to say no to patients."

Although some observers believe that the Labour Party might be supportive of geographically based local purchasing initiatives, including total fundholding, this approach is not seen as a viable over-all strategy by some local NHS officials. "Fundholding is very limited in its ability to save money or restructure services in cost-effective ways," said one. "After all, most of the costs and potential savings are still in the district health authority budgets. . . . Of our £190 million [$285 million] budget, only £14 million [$21 million] goes to GP fundholding and only £3 million [$4.5 million] for total fund-holding. . . . Total fundholding could be one approach, but frankly, most GPs don't want to become total fundholders—they didn't go into medicine to be managers or businessmen."

A colleague added:

> There will be no strategic direction if we move to total fundholding for all services. We need to shift contracts based on price, quality, and other considerations, not just price like most GPs are doing . . . and work with providers at the local level to bring up standards. One of the challenges is how to be strategic and not fragmented. These decisions need to be made in a larger context. Who controls the money and what are the goals; those are the critical questions. We want a cooperative not a competitive model, but we don't want to go too far so the providers are all working together and create a monopoly to drive up prices.

Despite the uncertain future of fundholding, CHC is committed to moving forward to develop a total fundholding project that will with-stand any changing political winds. And, as appears to be typical of the community organizing spirit of the practice, one CHC physician advo-cated a proactive strategy for shaping the future of GP fundholding:

> The task in the coming months is to make GP fundholding so wide-spread that it will be difficult to dismantle when Labour wins. We need to get as many GPs into fundholding as we can. . . . Labour's opposi-tion is ironic because fundholding is really consistent with Labour views. A primary care model, like fundholding, is radical because it gives power to the people and to the community. . . . We can't let the genie be put back in the bottle. If we do, the levers we have created to improve quality of care and improve the delivery system will be gone, and there will only be sporadic attempts in the foreseeable future to improve practice.

References

Castlefields Health Centre. "Annual Report." Runcorn, England: Castle-fields Health Centre, 1995.

Department of Health. *Practice Budgets for General Practitioners.* London: National Health Service, 1989.

Klein, R. "Big Bang Health Care Reform—Does It Work? The Case of Britain's National Health Service Reforms." *Milbank Quarterly,* 1995, *73*(3), 299–337.

CHAPTER TWELVE

PCGs and PCTs

Can You Make an Elephant Dance Like a Bee?

The NHS is responding to the pressures and dilemmas which face every health system in the developed world. We can no longer afford to be large lumbering organisations, slow to dance to the tune of the people we serve. As a metaphor for modern health care systems, elephants just don't work. Honey bees as a metaphor work better. Honey bees working effectively in colonies of one million can dance. They live in colonies where everyone has a part to play and their nests have vertical and horizontal combs. They are organised and constantly communicating with each other in a creative hum. . . . The NHS needs to be like the honey bee. We need to be explicit about our purpose and the results we are trying to achieve and we need to have strategies for delivering them. We need to encourage innovation, diversity, and responsiveness, experimentation, evaluation and more effective communication. . . . The NHS won't be a multi-product, multi-market system in constant flux and shaped by consumer preference like the managed care companies in California. We will never be that light on our feet. On the other hand we will not see the inequities that such a system produces.

—Alan Langlands and Jennifer Dixon, 1999

This case was originally written by the authors in 2000. Funding was provided by Astra Zeneca. The authors thank Dr. David Colin-Thome for his tremendous assistance with the case.

T he British National Health Service is in the midst of its biggest restructuring and reform since it was founded in 1948. In March 2000, the Labour government, headed by Prime Minister Tony Blair, promised to increase spending on the NHS in real terms by a third over the next five years from £50 billion to £69 billion by 2004, representing an increase from 5.9 percent of GDP to 7.6 percent. (Total 2000 spending on health care is 6.8 percent of GDP, including 0.9 percent private spending.) Annual spending increases will rise to 6 percent in real terms, double the historic trend. This investment in the NHS is equivalent to an increase over the next four years from £1,800 per household to £2,800. "This is quite simply the most important step in providing excellent public health care since the National Health Service was set up more than fifty years ago," stated Secretary of Health Alan Milburn.

As this case is being written, the government is about to announce its plan for spending the extra funding promised to the NHS over the next five years. This plan will be the culmination of a months-long consultation process, in which the government has solicited views from people who work in the NHS as well as from the general public (via public forums, a Web site, and the distribution of 12 million survey leaflets to the general public, asking "What are the top three things that would make the NHS better for you and your family?") Six modernization action teams have been established that include health professionals, patients and user groups, academics, policymakers, and health care managers, each led by a government minister. These teams will come up with suggestions for improving performance.

While the promise of a better-financed NHS has been almost universally well received, the government has made clear that the quid pro quo is an expectation of better performance. "The values of the NHS are every bit as relevant today as they were fifty years ago," Prime Minister Blair said to the House of Commons on March 22, 2000, when he announced the new funding. "But they have to be applied in a different way for a new age. The NHS is one of the great institutions that binds our country together. It is one of the great civilising achievements of the 20th century. It is our task as the Party which created the NHS to renew it for the 21st century and defeat the pessimists and the privatisers who would see it dismantled." And some in the NHS did not applaud the new resources. For example, one GP said, "I belong to a small group of people who think the health service is adequately funded. There are a lot of clinical interventions, even in a cheap health service, that are so unnecessary and so wasteful that we could free up lots of resources by challenging clinical activity. Then we could use the money that's just been given to the health service for other things, like housing and education, that would improve health more than more medical care."

This new plan comes on top of an aggressive program of reform already under way since the Labour Party took office in 1996. In the past three years, the government has enacted a dizzying array of new health initiatives. Primary care is one area where a number of important changes are happening. Among the new initiatives has been the establishment of Primary Care Groups (PCGs) and Primary Care Trusts (PCTs), which have replaced the fundholding initiative adopted by the previous Conservative Party government.

Since April 1, 1999, all GP practices (and their patients) have been part of a PCG. The groups work together with patient and local health authority representatives to take delegated responsibility for the health care needs of their community. According to the government's 1997 health care White Paper, *The New NHS: Modern Dependable,* "[PCGs] are intended to bring GPs, nurses and other local stakeholders together and give them a lead role in the planning, provision and development of local health services. In doing so, Primary Care Groups ensure that they pursue the development of the highest quality of provision for *all* patients within their area, whilst also acting to ensure the best value for money from the resources available to them."

According to Alan Langlands, chief executive of the NHS, "PCGs move towards a national system of managed care, but care managed by primary care physicians and their teams of nursing and paramedical staff, not by a third party."

Hopes are high among many NHS providers and managers that the reforms under way, particularly the new resources and the creation of PCGs, can create a truly primary-care-driven NHS. But many NHS employees also fear that success is critical. One manager said, "I worry that we won't get it right this time and then I fear for the future of the NHS." A GP said, "The money needs to be used to change the system, not to reoxygenate the current system." The public appears to be skeptical about the difference the new resources and changes will make. "Thirty percent of the public believes more money will improve services, and 50 percent think the NHS will just waste it," says Nigel Crisp, executive director of the London Regional Office of the NHS. "The government gave us more new money than people expected. Now we have to make a difference or the public will walk away from support of the NHS." One of his colleagues added, "Ironically, our challenge is made greater by the new money. The NHS is at its best in times of stress. The new money becomes an excuse to maintain the status quo."

"THE NEW NHS: MODERN DEPENDABLE"

The Labour Government's plans for the NHS are outlined in its White Paper, *The New NHS: Modern Dependable*, published in 1997. It explains the plan to build a "modern and dependable health service fit for the twenty-first century. A National Health Service which offers people prompt high quality treatment and care when and where they need it. An NHS that does not just treat people when they are ill but works with others to improve health and reduce health inequalities" (chapter 1, section 1.1).

The government's goals for the new NHS are quite simple:

- To improve the health of the population as a whole
- To improve the health of the worst-off in society and to narrow the health gap
- To modernize the health and social care system

The plans for the NHS are part of a more general national emphasis on modernizing government. Modernization is based on several underlying themes: focusing on results (the White Paper on Health coined the now widely used phrase of Blair pragmatism, "what counts is what works"), rewarding success and not tolerating mediocrity, organizing services around the convenience of the people using them, partnership with the private and nonprofit sectors, harnessing information technology, revaluing public service, and making policy for the long term, including establishing linkages across all levels of government (national, regional, and local).

These are the six specific key goals outlined in the NHS White Paper on Health (chapter 2, section 2.4):

1. To renew the NHS as a genuinely **national** service, with fair access to consistently high quality, prompt and accessible services right across the country

2. To make the delivery of health care against these new national standards a matter of *local* responsibility. Local doctors and nurses who are in the best position to know what patients need will be in the driving seat in shaping services

3. To get the NHS to work in *partnership* . . . by breaking down organizational barriers and forging stronger links with local authorities [also known as "boroughs"—the local municipal governments]

4. To drive *efficiency* through a more rigorous approach to performance and by cutting bureaucracy

5. To shift the focus onto quality of care so that **excellence** is guaranteed to all patients, and quality becomes the driving force for decision-making at every level of the service

6. To rebuild **public confidence** in the NHS as a public service, accountable to patients, open to the public and shaped by their views.

The NHS modernization strategy focuses on providing accessible and convenient services for patients, ensuring uniformly high standards, integrating services around need, and tackling the causes of ill health and inequality. The scope of reform is very broad, touching every part of the NHS.

The most significant new initiatives fall into several general categories: setting clear national standards, creating strong local initiatives, strengthening external monitoring, improving access and convenience for patients, and modernizing information technology and systems.

Setting Clear National Standards

Quality and performance are major themes of the new reforms. "We have been so proud of social justice in the NHS, it has made us complacent about what people actually get," said one clinician. "We need strong national standards for quality and strong accountability."

Two of the major initiatives in this area are "National Service Frameworks" and the "National Institute for Clinical Excellence," or NICE.

NATIONAL SERVICE FRAMEWORKS. These are evidence-based national templates of care describing preferred organizational and delivery models. They encompass care at all levels, including clinical standards and configuration of services. The government has issued NSFs on coronary heart disease, mental health, and care of older people, and will issue a framework for diabetes in spring 2001.

NATIONAL INSTITUTE FOR CLINICAL EXCELLENCE. NICE is a new national body that has been created to promote cost- and clinical effectiveness of NHS services by giving guidance to the NHS. It will advise on best practice in the use of existing treatment options, appraise new treatments and technology, and advise the NHS how best to apply them. The goal is to have NICE's evidence-based guidelines used in the entire country, in an effort to help end geographical variations in care. NICE has issued guidelines in a number of areas, including responding quickly to give guidance to clinicians during last winter's flu epidemic on the appropriate use of flu shots.

The focus on national standards seems to have been well received in the NHS. According to one GP, "Many of us think this is a brilliant idea, but it is too early to tell if it will work. We desperately need accountability for quality in the system, but the challenge will be to create local service frameworks to deliver the national stuff, particularly when it requires integration across primary and secondary care, and with chronic care."

CLINICAL GOVERNANCE. This is a new framework through which all NHS providers will be held accountable for continuously improving the quality of their services and safeguarding high standards of care. NHS providers, including PCGs, are required to demonstrate that they have an effective clinical governance process in place that meets the following standards:

- Clear lines of responsibility and accountability for the overall quality of clinical care
- A comprehensive program of quality improvement systems (including clinical audit, supporting and applying evidence-based practice, implementing clinical standards and guidelines, and workforce planning and development)
- Education and training plans
- Clear policies aimed at managing risk
- Integrated procedures for all professional groups to identify and remedy poor performance

BEACONS PROGRAMME. This is a new national program for identifying and sharing good practice within the NHS. In its first round, the government identified nearly three hundred examples of best practice in the areas of primary care, cancer services, reducing waiting lists and times, mental health services, human resource management, and health improvement. The program distributed a catalog of model programs throughout the NHS. Each program agreed to be a resource for others in the NHS, including being available at certain times for site visits from other NHS programs, and to participate in "Beacon Fairs."

Creating Strong Local Initiatives: PCGs and PMS Pilots

Although the NHS reform plan sets national frameworks and guidelines, it relies on local providers and partnerships to deliver them. The major initiative in reforming local care delivery and quality is the establishment of PCGs, which are described in more detail in the next section of this chapter.

Another local initiative is Personal Medical Services (PMS) pilots. As noted in Chapter Eleven, GPs are not employees of the NHS, they are independent contractors who are paid by the NHS through a negotiated national contract. In 1997, the NHS established Personal Medical Services (PMS) pilots to allow greater flexibility in paying for primary care, in the hope of addressing recruitment and retention problems and improving the delivery of primary care services. GPs and other NHS providers such as nurses and community trusts can apply for pilot status, which permits them to provide primary care services under a local contract with the health authority instead of under the national GP contract. There are several hundred PMS pilots in England, covering approximately 8 percent of all GPs in the country. These pilots range from practice-based pilots, some with GPs and nurses working in partnership together to nurse-led pilots and pilots with salaried doctors employed by a community trust. Many pilots are focusing on a particular client group, such as elderly or mentally ill people, children, homeless people, or people with substance abuse problems.

The Castlefields Health Centre (CHC) in the town of Runcorn in the northwest of England (introduced in Chapter Eleven and described further in the "Local Postscript" at the end of this chapter) is one of the earliest PMS pilots. According to one physician at CHC,

> There have been lots of advantages of PMS. Some are financial: we have been able to have the GPs become salaried employees of the practice and use nurses in managerial roles. The GPS like being salaried and being able to focus solely on medicine. But the biggest attraction of PMS is the incentives it can provide to improve quality. Now we have meaningful clinical measures in our contract with the health authority, ones based on the prevalence of disease in *our* population, and performance targets that are longitudinal and that we can improve over time. The Red Book [the national schedule of fees and allowances] only pays extra for certain types of chronic care management, which are not necessarily the ones we want to focus on for our patients. We need to care much less about the form of the GP contract and much more about outcomes.

An executive at the local health authority also supported the PMS pilots:

> Independent contractor status can create perverse incentives for high patient lists and lack of investment in the practice. We have an expression, "gardening the list," that refers to a GP who keeps his patient list just below 3,500, which is the point at which they get no additional payment for more patients. Someone once said that 'at the first sign of change, GPs reach for their calculators.' There is too much of a focus among GPs on the Red Book. . . . From our perspective, we think PMS improves quality because we can set an improvement plan with the practice and then audit the practice based on that plan, instead of looking at individual service billings. But many GPs and the national doctors' council think PMS pilots are a plot to make them do more for less and take away their independent contractor status.

Strengthening External Monitoring

The new reforms include a range of new oversight mechanisms and processes, including the Commission for Health Improvement (CHI).

COMMISSION FOR HEALTH IMPROVEMENT. CHI is an independent statutory body established in November 1999 to "ensure that standards are being met throughout the NHS." Among its responsibilities are to review all local health care organizations in the NHS (NHS Trusts, PCTs, health authorities) at least every four years, focusing on the implementation of clinical governance, National Service Frameworks, and NICE guidelines. CHI also has the authority to intervene in any situation in which there is a "serious or persistent clinical problem," and to oversee and assist with external incident inquiries.

NATIONAL PERFORMANCE INDICATORS. The government is also developing a comprehensive set of national performance indicators intended to measure the performance of the NHS along six dimensions: health improvement (for example, changes in premature death), fair access (utilization by various socioeconomic groups), effective and efficient delivery of appropriate care (labor productivity, day surgery rates), patient experience (being measured by a new national survey of patients and users), and health outcomes of NHS (such as treating infectious diseases where immunizations are available).

Improving Access

Improving access is a matter of particular concern and focus for the government, and a number of new initiatives are designed to reduce waiting lists and times.

MODERNIZATION. The government has made significant new commitments to modernizing substandard hospital buildings and physician offices, investing £8 billion over three years. Investments have targeted emergency departments and primary care. The government has also raised more than £2 billion in private capital to redevelop twenty-five hospitals through the "Private Finance Initiative," to be repaid through public sector revenue funding.

NHS DIRECT. This is a new free NHS telephone help line, offering twenty-four-hour access to advice and information from a nurse about health problems and services, and if necessary, triage to emergency services.

PRIMARY CARE WALK-IN CENTERS. These centers provide minor treatment and health information to any member of the public on a walk-in basis. The goal is to have one center for every 240,000 people, or about seventy centers nationally. As of March 2000, there were thirty-eight centers, nine of them in London. The centers must be managed by an NHS body or a GP cooperative; have the support of the local PCG or PCT, the health authority, and the wider local health economy; and be consistent with the local Health Improvement Plan. They must be in a convenient location to enable easy access and have a "responsive style of service" (that is, be open early mornings, late evenings, and weekends).

Some critics worry that NHS Direct and the walk-in centers will weaken the gatekeeper function of GPs and undermine continuity of care. "These initiatives support a demand- and not a needs-based approach to care," said one GP. "They will cost a lot and just generate new care, not replace other services. And the money that's being spent on these programs is needed more for other critical services." But others dismiss these criticisms, arguing that the NHS needs to be much more responsive to the schedules and needs of working people. They also hope that these efforts will free up GPs to focus on patients with more serious problems. "There's unreasonable concern about the walk-ins," said one GP. "After all, there are only thirty-eight of them throughout Britain. Walk-ins are a great additional service, not a replacement for general practice. The early evidence is that people like these services." Another doctor agreed, "The walk-in centers are evoking undue hysteria from some GPs. They might actually help us if we work with them. There's this contradiction among GPs that we're overburdened with work but we can't let go." A health authority executive agreed, "These efforts have not helped GP paranoia about the role of GPs in the new NHS. They think it is a way to take away their patients. Our answer is that you should be pleased your workload is being diminished. But there will continue to be tension about whether we should be putting more resources into making care easier to obtain for people who don't really have much wrong, or to give better care to people with chronic conditions and a much greater burden of disease."

However, many observers noted that these initiatives will not improve the most significant access problem: waiting lists for consultant services. "The major change that needs to happen to decrease waiting lists is to change consultant payment," said one NHS executive. "The ability of consultants to have private practices is the biggest impediment to improving access and waiting times. Consultants make so much money on the private side." Approximately 18 percent of the English population has private insurance. The popularity of private insurance has been fueled in large part by concern about waiting lists, which have been growing. One-quarter of elective surgeries are private, paid either out-of-pocket or through private insurance. According to one recent story, 20 percent of business done in private hospitals is on a self-pay basis (Pridham, 2000). This story quotes prices for private surgeries ranging from £1,000 to £1,500 for hernia surgery to £9,500 to £12,500 for a heart bypass operation, all-inclusive of consultant fees and hospital stay.

A GP agreed that private practice saps consultant availability: "The waiting lists do not go down because specialists need the waiting lists to enable their private practices. Consultants hated fundholding because it put pressure on them to work harder for NHS. They now can have all the advantages of private practice with none of the risk." This GP gave as an example an ophthalmologist in his area who splits his time equally between the NHS and private practice and earns £25,000 from the NHS and £250,000 from his private patients. "And he is not atypical," noted the physician.

Other Initiatives

Here are quick summaries of some of the other initiatives currently under way:

INFORMATION FOR HEALTH. The NHS has committed to an extensive program as part of the health reform agenda. The government's strategy in this area, called "Information for Health," is a seven-year plan to "provide the right information wherever it is needed in the NHS, from the doctor's surgery to any hospital accident and emergency unit . . . and to ensure proper information is available to tackle the causes of ill health and to plan and monitor health care, and to make sure patient information remains confidential."

One component of this agenda is NHS Net, an "information superhighway" that will link all GPs to one another via the Internet by 2002. "Ninety-six percent of GPs have a computer and 20 percent of practices in England have paperless electronic medical records," according to a NHS executive, who continued,

> We decided that the Internet is the best medium for the transfer of
> clinical information across all parts of the NHS. We issued specs for a
> GP system but there are lots of vendors that can provide systems to

individual practices. The first year of this project failed miserably but now we are stepping up the effort, making more resources available for GP infrastructure. Perhaps we are just hanging ourselves from a higher tree. The GPs are very concerned about privacy of the information, although they have been happy for years to mail and fax patient information back and forth to one another.

HEALTH ACTION ZONES. HAZs are the government's vehicle for implementing a seven-year program to reduce health inequalities in England. When the initiative was announced in 1997, the government said the aim is to "target a special effort on a number of areas where we believe the health of local people can be improved by better integrated arrangements for treatment care." Twenty-six HAZs have been created, covering some of the most deprived areas of the country. The strategic objectives of the program are to identify and address the health needs of the local area, to develop partnerships, and to modernize services.

So far, the HAZs seem to have had little impact, in the opinion of most observers. "The results are disappointing," according to a senior executive of the NHS. "Some of them are producing good results but very little is happening in most. Most have approached the requirement that they do a needs assessment as a task and not a strategy. So now that they have the needs assessment, they don't know what to do with it." A GP activist added, "HAZs are designed to focus on health improvement, service improvement, and public health. They should be the playmaker, the Franz Beckenbauer of the entire system. But instead they are run by tired, recycled NHS managers. We have missed a real opportunity to engage new leadership and to engage the public. Public health is not an enthuser. It has become a report writer. We need passion to drive the public health improvement process." Another observer noted, "As a country, we are suffering from Zone-itis. We have education action zones, employment zones, better government zones, health action zones, all with no overlap. I fear HAZs were invented for political reasons without any prior thinking."

PCGs IN MORE DETAIL

Primary Care Groups are one of the major vehicles through which the government's national health agenda is to be realized. The concept of Primary Care Groups grew out of the range of commissioning models implemented by the Conservative government in the 1990s (fundholding, locality commissioning groups, total purchasing projects). In its White Paper on Health, the government stated that it was eliminating these elements of the "divisive internal market system of the 1990s . . . an approach which was intended to make the NHS more efficient but ended up fragmenting decision-making and distorting incentives to such an extent that unfairness and bureaucracy became its defining features."

PCGs have four main functions:

- To improve the health of, and address health inequalities in, their communities
- To develop primary care and community services across the Primary Care Group
- To advise on, or commission directly, a range of secondary hospital services for patients within their area that appropriately meet patient needs
- To better integrate primary and community services and work more closely with Social Services

As noted earlier, participation in PCGs by GPs and community nurses is mandatory. On April 1, 1999, 481 PCGs were created in England. As PCGs reconfigure or progress to Primary Care Trust (PCT) status, this figure will change on an annual basis. PCGs have a patient population ranging from 46,000 to 257,000, with an average of about 100,000. The organizations are governed by a board that is a committee of the parent health authority and must consist of

- Between four and seven GPs
- One or two community or practice nurses
- One Social Services representative
- One lay member
- One health authority representative (who may not be the authority's executive director)
- The chief executive of the PCG

The chair of the Board is selected by the Board from among its members.

Primary Care Groups may operate at one of four levels (although until April 1, 2000, all PCGs were at levels 1 or 2):

- *Level 1:* The PCG will, at a minimum, act in support of the health authority in commissioning care for its population, acting in an advisory capacity.
- *Level 2:* The PCG takes devolved responsibility for managing the budget for health care in its area, acting as part of the health authority.
- *Level 3:* The PCG becomes a free-standing body accountable to the health authority for commissioning services but not directly providing community services. It is able to employ a limited range of staff (with the expectation that these staff will replace functions now performed by health authority personnel).
- *Level 4:* The PCG becomes a free-standing body accountable to the health authority for commissioning care, and with added responsibility for the provision of community services for its population. The organization can run community hospitals and community health services, employ necessary staff, and own property.

PCGs that operate at level 3 or 4 are known as Primary Care Trusts (PCTs). The first wave of seventeen PCTs became operational on April 1, 2000. The NHS expects half of the PCGs to become PCTs by April 2001, and the goal is to move all PCGs to PCT status within three to five years. "The law says you cannot force a PCG to become a PCT," said an official from a health authority, "but the clear message from the NHS is you *will* become a PCT. The same thing happened with fundholding. Legally we could not force GPs but the NHS was more directive. The problem is going to be that most GPs are not desperate to be trusts. They think PCTs are a way to cap spending and make GPs salaried. They are suspicious of the government's motives."

Health authorities are the bodies charged with leading the development of PCGs (although PCTs will undertake many of the functions presently performed by the health authorities, including commissioning health services, investing in primary and community care, and improving the health of the local population). The Regional Offices of the NHS, which oversee the health authorities, have the management responsibility of fostering the development of PCGs, including overseeing the mechanisms used by health authorities to consult and establish PCGs. Health authorities and Regional Offices have undertaken a range of activities to help the development of PCGs, including identifying training needs and developing learning sets for PCG chairs and chief executives, and conducting training sessions for lay members of PCG Boards. The NHS Regional Offices have also been charged with assembling support teams made up of external facilitators from local universities, senior NHS managers, and clinicians to act as resources to health authorities when working with PCGs.

PCTs can only be established with the approval of the Secretary of State. The review process requires the preparation of an application followed by a "consultation process" to assess the degree of local support for the proposed PCT. Health authorities have responsibility for undertaking the consultation process, which lasts up to three months. It culminates in a report by the health authority to the relevant NHS Regional Office, presenting the health authority's view on the proposed PCT and its "state of readiness." The Regional Office then reviews the submission and makes its recommendation to the Minister of Health, who then passes it on to the Secretary of State.

PCGs AND PCTs IN NORTH CHESHIRE

North Cheshire Health is the NHS region that serves the three towns of Runcorn, Warrington, and Widnes in the northwest of England (near Manchester). The population of the area is 312,000 and is projected to grow only about 2 percent over the next twenty years. However, the proportion of residents aged sixty-five or older will increase significantly, from 14 percent in 1996 (slightly lower than the national average) to nearly 19 percent.

In fiscal year 1998–99, North Cheshire Health spent £207 million buying health care services for residents of the area. Table 12.1 shows the distribution of funding by type of service. In the 1999–2000 fiscal year, the budget for NCH climbed by approximately £4 million in real terms. Despite this significant increase in funding, the NHS in North Cheshire reports it is experiencing significant financial pressures, particularly as a result of increases in GP drug prescribing costs, which were £1 million over budget in the last fiscal year.

Category	Spending (£ 000)
Hospital and community services	161,887
General practitioner prescribing	27,570
General practitioner services	5,746
Dentistry	146
Ophthalmic services	1,459
Other	7,315
Management costs	2,500
Total	206,623

Table 12.1. North Cheshire Health 1998–99 Annual Spending.
Source: North Cheshire Health. Annual Report and Information Packet: 1998–99, Fact Sheet 07.

Provider System

Two acute hospital NHS trusts are located within the NCH area, Halton General and Warrington Hospital. In addition, many residents are treated at another hospital in a neighboring community. Community services for the area are provided mainly by two community trusts located in the area.

North Cheshire has forty-nine medical practices, of which twenty are one- or two-GP practices. (The area also has forty-eight general dental practices, fifty-seven pharmacies, and twenty-six optical practices.) The GPs and other primary care providers are organized into four PCGs: Runcorn, Warrington North West and Central, Warrington North East and South, and Widnes. Table 12.2 provides data on each of these PCGs, while Table 12.3 details their payments and budgets.

Most observers in the North Cheshire area predict significant consolidation in the provider system in the next few years. The Runcorn and Widnes PCGs are expected to merge, as are the two PCGs in Warrington. The boards of Halton and Warrington Hospitals have told the Secretary of State that they want to merge, and a consultation process is under way. The North Cheshire health authority will probably be consolidated with one or more health authorities in the North West region. According to one provider, "The end game is going to be one PCT for Runcorn and Widnes, one in Warrington, one acute trust, one mental health confederation, all part of one much larger health authority. But there is a lot of concern and politicking as the players try to position to be sure that they have a job at the end of the consolidation process."

PCG	Runcorn	Warrington North West and Central	Warrington North East and South	Widnes
PCG level	2	2	2	1
Practice population	64,057	99,062	94,752	60,283
Population of local area	64,965	96,468	93,312	57,776
Number of practices	7	16	12	11
Number of GPs	65	N/A	N/A	N/A
# of PCG Staff	7 FTEs	3 FTEs	3 FTEs	6 FTEs
Subgroups established by PCG	• Information Services • Commissioning • Primary care development • Coronary heart disease • Training and Development • Patient Involvement	• Information Management • Prescribing • Commissioning • Clinical Governance • HImP • Community Involvement • Strategy and Accountability	• Information Management and Technology • Prescribing • Commissioning • Clinical Governance • HImP • Finance • Organisational Development	• Information Management and Technology • Prescribing • Clinical Governance • HImP • Finance

Other working groups	• Practice managers • Nurses forum			• Practice managers group • Nursing Council
Health improvement program priorities	• Heart disease • Young peoples' health	• CHD and stroke • Mental health • Mental health of youth • Accidents	• CHD and stroke • Mental health • Mental health of youth • Accidents	• Respiratory disease • Smoking and sexual health in young people
Some sample projects	• Practice-based call and recall system for patients with CHD, based on protocol • Closer links with school health services • Providing financial advice services in practices • Baseline assessment of quality in practices • Survey of local people • Projects on nonsteroid anti-inflammatory drugs, drug returns, and repeat prescribing • Nursing strategy for PCG • Developing practice-focused services to be shared across practices	• Review of all patients with CHD • Development of mental health register • Development of community-based diabetes teams	• Same as Warrington North West and Central—working collaboratively	• New family doctor model for housing development • NP model for underserved neighborhood • Sure Start Initiative, to improve well-being of children under four

Table 12.2. PCGs in North Cheshire Health.

PCG	Runcorn	Warrington North West and Central	Warrington North East and South	Widnes
Primary Medical Services Cash-Limited:*				
Practice staff	574	1,091	1,076	811
Buildings	113	217	244	153
Computers	20	28	29	21
Allocated	57	65	51	59
Total	764	1,401	1,400	1,044
Non-Cash-Limited:	1,820	3,870	3,909	2,320
*Personal Medical Services under Pilots***	1,356	578	244	0
*PCG Budgets****				
Hospital and Community Services	28,626	45,000	35,000	0
Prescribing	5,946	9,500	8,500	6,150
General Medical Services	1,068	1,500	1,500	1,217
Other		8,700	6,000	
Management	183	300	300	232
Total	35,823	65,000	51,300	7,599
NHS Trust Responsibility****	33,000+			12,000+

Table 12.3.   PCG Payments and Budgets in Fiscal Year 1998–99 (£ 000s).
Note: *Cash-limited services are subject to line-item appropriation in the national NHS budget, distributed to regions and practices based on an allocation formula, and cannot be increased without further appropriation. Non-cash-limited items are subject to a budgeted amount but can be exceeded without specific federal action.
**There are four PMS pilot programs in North Cheshire, two in Runcorn and two in Warrington.
***Level 2 PCGs have unified budgets composed of hospital and community health services, prescribing, and cash-limited GMS. Level 1 PCGs do not have hospital and community service budgets.
****Each of the North Cheshire PCGs has agreed to take specific lead responsibility for negotiating contracts with certain hospital and community trusts for all of North Cheshire Health.

According to a member of the Runcorn PCG board, "A PCT is the direction of our travel. We hope to get there by 2002. We need to get the Runcorn and Widnes PCGs combined before then. But there are going to be immense social and cultural issues to overcome to make that happen." A NHS manager agreed: "There are differences in family structures, origin, level of social deprivation, and philosophies between the Widnes and Runcorn PCGs. They even like different sports: one is a rugby league town and in the other it's football. Widnes has mainly solo practice doctors, many of whom had never met each other until they became a PCG, even when they practiced in the same town for thirty years. In fact, the doctors in Widnes did not even want to become a PCG; they wanted to be a level 0. There was much less GP fundholding in Widnes. The GPs in the Runcorn PCG were almost all fundholders, and they have well-committed doctors and sharply defined practices. But the practices all want to do it their way and not the PCG way. . . . On the other hand, the Widnes PCG is doing very well and developing a sense of coherence and connection among the practices. They are also cheerfully aware of the low opinion in which they are held by the Runcorn PCG." Another observer at the health authority added, "The Runcorn GPs thinks the individual practice should be the building block of the entire system. But that can never happen. The PCG has to be above the practice level because the needs of the population are not discrete depending on what practice they go to."

How Do PCGs and PCTs Look from North Cheshire?

There seems to be much enthusiasm in North Cheshire and elsewhere about many of the changes that are under way in the primary care system. But this optimism is tempered somewhat by concerns over the enormous scope of the reforms, the rapid pace of change, and whether capacity is sufficient in many parts of the NHS to implement the reforms successfully. Said one NHS executive: "The agenda is too ambitious and we cannot do it all so quickly. The chief execs are looking pretty tired. There are too many expectations, standards, and hoops to jump through." One local NHS manager said, "On my good days, I think our glass is definitely at least half full. We have lots of good general practices, lots of extended primary care teams, lots of community-based specialists, lots of good general managers, and some experience with commissioning. But on my bad days, I think the whole thing is a bloody mess."

Even the most enthusiastic supporters of the reforms under way in primary care see a number of challenges ahead. Others are quite cynical about the prospects for improvement. The following sections summarize some of the most frequently voiced concerns and questions.

Are PCGs and PCTs an Improvement?

Observers disagree about whether to applaud or mourn the loss of fundholding and its replacement with PCGs and PCTs. Even senior officials of the NHS did not necessarily advocate for this change. According to a top NHS manager,

> Many of us thought fundholding was going rather well. It was allowing experimentation in primary care and was evolving toward a managed primary care system. Fundholding shook up primary care provision and made GPs more aware of resources. In fact, it improved primary care much more than secondary care. But the new government was quite centrist in its approach. It rejected the market and was keen on consistency, arguing that there was an inherent unfairness in the two-tier system created by fundholding. The government also needed the symbolism of changing. So we invented the primary-care-led NHS and PCGs. But I'm not sure it's really taken off as a concept. The goal was to use more teams and have more integration of care across the system. But the PCGs are not baring their teeth in the same way some of the fundholders did. Fundholding was much better fun—it was much more radical. Although it was really pinpricks in the system, its effects were more immediate. But PCTs potentially have even more power than fundholders ever could have, if they can get hold of community services and really develop truly integrated systems of care. The market is dead but the culture it created is not. Consultants are just waking up to the enormous power the GPs will have in the PCTs. Up until now they have thought the NHS managers had the power.

There is certainly grief in some quarters in North Cheshire over the elimination of GP fundholding. According to one GP from a former fundholding practice:

> Fundholding was much more exciting. We felt more in control, and we could take on the hospitals. Waiting lists were very personal for us

because we knew the patients, unlike the health authority. We could put pressure on consultants and be entrepreneurial. Now the PCG does everything by consensus, and we're not willing as a group to move volume. Under fundholding, we kept hospital costs and referrals down so it did not matter if drug costs rose, it all balanced out. But now there's no reason to be careful because the health authority holds the hospital budget so hospital costs don't matter to us. Why be critical, why wonder if we could manage a patient in the practice? The incentives to manage care were much closer and more real under fundholding.

Another former fundholder agreed: "The elimination of fundholding took resources away from our practice. We lost the funding that supported an acupuncturist and ENT clinic and other practice-based services. We cannot have practice-based services anymore because it's not equal, but equality is not the same as equity. Services should be based on need. We see the PCG as an organization that has taken away, and not given us back much of anything."

Others in North Cheshire do not mourn the loss of fundholding. "Fundholding was alienating and often counterproductive," according to an official at the health authority. "The fundholders bit lumps out of one another and often us. It had some bad effects on the system. It did get GPs to develop skills and expertise, and an interest in the hospital sector. But when they took all their services out of one of the hospital trusts, they still left all the fixed costs behind. This might have benefited their patients but it was not good for the system." A hospital official agreed, "Too often fundholding was about bossing people and getting back on them for past feuds. Few fundholders had any understanding of the entire system. They were very insular."

Can the NHS Culture Be Changed?

One of the most frequently voiced challenges to the reforms under way is that of changing what one GP termed "the whole genetic code of the NHS." "The political rhetoric is 'everyone up to the best.' But I suspect we will likely only move the distribution curve a bit to the right. This type of change is about learning and making change in complex systems. It does not occur because you write it down and provide more money," said one NHS executive. Another exec agreed: "We have sorted out the anatomy but not the physiology of the system. We took away the internal market but did not replace it by systems to support performance measurement and cultural change. The keys over time will be teamwork and integration of services, but we need to develop the levers to make this happen." But many local managers seem cynical about how to make this cultural change on the ground. A PCG manager said, "The national and regional offices keep telling us, in writing and in trainings, that we need to change the culture of the NHS, that we need to set up the PCGs and PCTs as true 'learning organizations.' But this just seems like crap rubbish from America to me. What does it mean?"

Do the PCGs and PCTs Have Adequate Managerial Capacity?

The almost universal answer to the question of managerial capacity seems to be no. "Based on what we read, it seems that managed care plans in the U.S. spend about 20 percent of their budgets on management," said one PCG staff person. "We spend very little in the NHS. We don't want to get to the U.S. level, but we are going to need to spend more. But instead, government has set very stringent cost rules, so overhead is being reduced." According to one PCG manager, "People buy the vision but the day-to-day challenge is very wearing. The ambition, scope, and pace are huge. The NHS has never been good at managing in a developmental way. And the problems are compounded because many of us know we will lose our jobs in the transition to PCTs because there will be consolidation among the PCGs. And it will be harder to recruit and keep good managers if the economy stays so hot. The NHS cannot compete with private sector pay." Another manager added, "When people take a job in primary care, it cannot be seen as the end of their careers, which it has been in the past. All the high-profile managers are always at the teaching hospitals. There are not enough people who want to run PCTs now." But a hospital executive thought this would change in the future: "I think PCTs will attract the premier league executives because the power and excitement will be there, not at the hospitals."

One source of new management talent for the PCGs and PCTs may be GPs. More and more GPs are spending time on managerial issues as they work in PCGs. "The good news is that many GPs are starting to get management training," said one NHS executive. "They didn't really think they needed it under fundholding because that was built on their own practices. There used to be terrible antagonism between managers and doctors but this is calming down. Doctors are more willing to get involved in management, and managers are more focused on patients and improving things that make practicing medicine hard." Another manager added, "The GPs used to just think the managers were bureaucrats and gray suits. Now the medical directors of the PCTs have gray trousers and are working up to the gray jackets."

But it's clear that many GPs have much to learn in terms of management. "Most GPs are not used to managing or being managed," observed a hospital manager. "GPs like autonomy. Consultants, on the other hand, are used to management and leadership." The weakness of the boards of the PCGs and PCTs causes particular concern. "The PCGs are spawning committees, having endless meetings, producing paper reports but not getting anything done because there is not good leadership. The health authorities are supposed to be doing the development, but most are not," said one observer. Another added, "The leadership and managerial issues increase considerably as PCGs evolve into PCTs. The roles and functions are different, and the leadership and management roles of clinicians and managers in primary care have to change. GPs must improve their ability to deliver care and to commission services. All this will take development and leadership both within the PCGs and the local health economies."

Lack of adequate information systems is viewed as a significant managerial challenge for the PCGs and PCTs. "There has been no significant extra money for information technology," according to one member of the Runcorn PCG. "We are trying to be consistent with IT across the PCG, but it's hard and is requiring a lot of administrative effort by the doctors. Any extra resources have generally gone to practices with the least technology. But should the priority of the PCG be to invest in the practices that are behind or the ones who are trying hardest?"

An executive at the North Cheshire health authority agreed that IT is a major issue: "It is critical, but the NHS strategy is too fancy and complex. It should be simpler and more concrete, like starting with saying that all GPs should have a computer. All the practices are at a different level in IT and there is no consistency. Every practice has a different level of funding for information technology, with no rationality. The resource allocation process was there and was followed and the result was none of the practices have the same level of IT investment. This is a big issue for the PCGs and PCT: How will they address IT?"

Will Health Authorities Support PCGs and PCTs—and How Will They Do It?

Under the reforms, the health authorities have a number of key roles:

- Assessing the health needs of the local population
- Providing strategic leadership for improving health and tackling health inequalities, and drawing up a plan called a Health Improvement Programme (or HImP) in partnership with all local interests
- Deciding on the range and location of health services for local residents, consistent with the HImP
- Determining local targets and standards to drive quality and efficiency in light of national priorities and guidance, and ensuring their delivery
- Supporting the development of PCGs and PCTs
- Allocating resources to PCGs and PCTs
- Holding PCGs and PCTs accountable, through effective performance management

Tension between the PCGs and the health authorities was a frequently mentioned problem, even by the regional and national executives of the NHS. According to one national manager, "The health authority needs to evolve into being a resource to the PCGs and PCTs and helping them manage. The health authorities have to move to performance management. But there is lots of tension between the PCGs and the health authorities right now. The regional NHS is spending lots of time sorting out rows between the PCGs and the health authorities because it has the ammunition to get the parties around the table and arbitrate." Another national executive added,

> The whole agenda is predicated on health authorities' helping the PCGs, but many health authorities are abandoning them. PCGs often get no information from the health authorities about what's going on. This has created an impression of secrecy. . . . Health authorities have failed miserably in the last seven or eight years to make many inroads into improving care—they have been a turnstile: focused on process, focused on units, focused on details like pricing in the internal market. Their biggest role could have been to challenge clinicians and quality

of care, but they rarely did. Now most of the health authorities either tell people to do things or they abdicate responsibility—they don't know how to work in any other way.

This last observation was confirmed by a conversation with the executive of the North Cheshire health authority. "I have done many jobs in the NHS but I have never shared power with anyone," he said. This executive expressed a great deal of frustration over what he perceives to be the unclear role of the health authority in the new NHS and the attitude of the local PCGs:

The role of the health authority is supposed to be to provide "strategic leadership." What does that mean? Am I supposed to sit in the crow's nest all day looking out? I think our role should be to help the mini-systems work well and deliver services well in an integrated manner, working across all local agencies, not just the health service. . . . A big problem now is that the central government is bypassing the health authorities and going directly to the GPs. It's stupid to have a dog and then bark yourself. . . . The Prime Minister and Health Minister think the health authorities are holding back on change because that's what they hear from GPs. So then we get letters telling us we have to support GPs more. But we are already spending 30–40 percent of our staff time on PCG development—but it's not recognized because it is never enough for the PCGs.

For example, while we focus a lot on waiting lists and I know my job is on the line if I have more than a certain number of people on the waiting list at the end of the fiscal year, we have never looked at which PCGs have patients on the list and for what type of services. The PCGs want this information to help them do their work, and we should help. But we just do not have the resources to do the level of analysis that they want. So they think we are being pigheaded and holding back. But we are having to make decisions about how to deploy resources. And we only have fifty-five people to do a lot of work.

The PCGs are a classic English administrative concept—no staff, no budgets, and no power. They are at an early stage of development spending more time bickering about fees for management services than clinical initiatives. But the GPs do not see the value in what the health authority does. We ran seminars to try to educate doctors about what we do but they did not come. They don't understand or value administration and bureaucracy. Most of the practices are small, simple operations and GPs are used to being the alpha male in their baboon packs. They are very hierarchical and used to dealing with low-level administrative staff and they think of the health authority staff in the same way. The health authority role is strategic—to be sure that all the different PCGs are not just doing their own things. We bring the broader perspective, to tell them that there needs to be sacrifice for the common good. GPs can't just focus on their own patients, they have a wider responsibility to the community.

Is the NHS Approach Too Centralized?

Clinicians and managers at all levels of the NHS are concerned that the management style of the new government is very centrist. "The government said we can't return to top-down management," said one doctor, "But we have." A top NHS executive agreed, "The new government is big on national standards and guidelines—a much more planned way, but not necessarily more participatory. It's quite a Stalinist approach really. The test will be whether the ministers will be willing to let go of the levers and let local initiatives and local partnerships really flourish. Only time will tell."

Will Resources Really Be Reallocated from the Hospitals to Community-Based Care?

Many GPs and PCG managers fear the government will be unwilling to allow resources to move out of the hospital trusts to primary and community-based services. "To improve primary care we must improve secondary care to make it more efficient and free up the resources and be able to reallocate them," said a GP. Many PCGs strongly suspect that providers will continue to get resources based on power and connections rather than need. Said one community-based provider, "The whole reform strategy is very centralized and very acute focused. There is still too much money flowing to hospitals and the consultants." A hospital executive in North Cheshire did not disagree:

> The acute trusts are the ones who need to sharpen up. We need much greater accountability. If you look around, you will see that hospitals have often been focused on the wrong thing. For example, we have the world's greatest collection of modern automatic doors at many hospitals but maybe the money would have been better spent on

providing more cataract surgery. . . . Consultants are effective with the public so they have lots of political power. But hospitals and consultants are so used to dominating the system that they don't react to change unless it happens immediately. So they don't realize the potential of PCTs.

But some community-based providers are afraid that PCTs will actually make the situation worse. One community trust manager said, "In fact, many of us are concerned that what will happen with PCTs is that the resources in the community trusts will be stripped to bail out the acute trusts. We are already feeling bereaved, strangled, and without adequate resources, but we think we would do better staying as stand-alone organizations. At least then we have an independent voice and more control."

Can (and Should) PCGs and PCTs Really Drive Health Reform?

Opinions are strong on both sides about the suitability of using PCGs and PCTs as one of the major mechanisms for health reform and resource allocation at the local level.

Proponents argue that the PCGs and PCTs will assume a key role in health system reform. "I see PCGs and PCTs not as commissioners but as engines for change," said one physician. "PCTs will have a community orientation and allow GPs to work more closely with colleagues in other parts of the system. For example, PCTs could really work with social services in new and exciting ways—they could become a central focus for all kinds of one-stop shopping. There's no stigma about going to the GP, like there is for lots of other social services. I think PCTs will treat the hospitals as facilities, just a commodity." A GP colleague agreed, "I think PCTs will evolve into multi-specialty groups, with greater integration between primary care and community services, perhaps becoming like the original HMOs."

In assessing the potential of the primary care group concept, many say it is critical to distinguish between PCGs and PCTs. According to one NHS executive, "My cynical view of PCGs is they were conceived as a way to make the transition to PCTs, which would have been too radical to propose as the initial reform. Any hopes that PCGs would actually be effective are fantasies. They have not been given the management support or the incentives to actually help them fly. But the

PCTs will become the fundamental health organizations, with big budgets, able to commission services and improve health."

But others are less sanguine about the potential of PCTs. "It's not clear if PCTs will really encourage GPs to work more collaboratively with one another and with others, or just become a turgid bureaucratic structure that stifles innovation and creates process," said a health authority official, adding,

> Most GPs did not go into medicine to have to worry about how to make decisions about spending limited amounts of money. I am not sure the PCTs will like being in the hot seat about how to allocate finite resources—they will find themselves being as attacked as HMOs in the States—as the people who just say no and refuse to pay for care that is too expensive. PCGs and PCTs have not yet been exposed to public action and advocacy when the public doesn't like the results of their actions. Actions that shut services at hospitals will generate a response. The PCGs and PCTs will need to develop the organizational strategy and strength to deal with the politics.

An executive at the NHS echoed a similar concern: "My fear is that we have will have created hundreds of individual empires, each working on their own issues and concerns with no sense to the whole, despite the national framework."

Whether PCGs and PCTs can ever become an effective force for improving public health seems to be an open question. "GPs are very insular about things—they face toward their patients, not the system as a whole," said a health authority official. "Personal medical services and public health are not the same. GPs are not experts in public health. GPs are not good at meeting public health and population health needs—they are experts at anatomy and physiology and individual ill health. They don't have the skills or outlook to think about public health—they run small businesses." A senior NHS executive shared a related concern: "It's not clear to me that PCTs are big enough to be able to take a really strategic view of health, let alone do much about it. There are lots of hard questions to answer, like what should happen with community services and how PCTs should relate to social services. Even though the PCTs are bigger than the PCGs, most are still too small for health planning. Plus the accountability is not clear—what will the relationship be between the PCTs and the health authority? Fundholding was destabilizing because practices shifted care without regard for the impact on institutions or for the entire populations, but at least they were very small. PCTs will be big enough to really destabilize the system but it might not be in the best interests of public health."

As in most policy discussions, there are also cautiously optimistic moderates, including this senior executive at the NHS:

My guess is that PCGs and PCTs will be more effective in some areas than in others. They should help reduce variations in clinical practice and help with quality in primary care. They can also help with the development of new models of primary care, the development of disease management programs, encouraging more collaboration, better use of nurses and other models of interdisciplinary practice, shared services across practices, like physiotherapy and audiology, and improved prescribing. PCGs and PCTs will help GPs take a more population-based approach rather than focusing on their own local patch. They can also be a means to share GP expertise, like subspecialization in asthma, drug abuse, et cetera. They could develop new models like contracting with community pharmacists for disease management. But I don't think they will have much overall effect in the public health area—they are too small and they lack the skills and training. GPs are not used to looking at health in a wider sense.

Despite these concerns, the development of PCGs and PCTs seems certain to continue apace. In the words of one academic who is a long-time observer of the NHS: "We need to be careful not to load up PCTs with totally unrealistic expectations. But no matter what happens, we need to try again, fail again—but fail better. This will not be the last time we modernize the NHS. No one will fix all of this now. Muddling through is a great and unglamorous British tradition." A GP colleague was equally practical: "We need to have passion about where we are going. We can't get caught up in the structure and the technical details. The NHS culture has been one of enabling and dependency, and clinicians and managers have to view each other as resources and not rely on the NHS for answers. This is all a mess but an exciting one if you can keep the vision in place."

—w— Epilogue: Making
the Elephant Dance

Dr. David Colin-Thome
National Director for Primary Care, National Health Service
General Practitioner, Castlefields Health Centre

Just after the case in this chapter was written, the government made two significant announcements. On average, it would increase the funding of the NHS by at least 6 percent for the next four years, double the rate of normal increase. And it set out its aspirations, plans, and targets to improve the NHS over the next ten years in a document called the "NHS Plan," which had as co-signatories the main doctors', nurses', and trade union organizations together with government ministers.

The government wished to ensure the continuation of the principle of fairness and equality, on which the NHS was founded, but accepted that the system was underfunded and in urgent need of reform, not least in focusing the service on the user and not the provider of services, and in achieving improved quality that was uniformly available throughout the country. To this end the government set up many formal committees so as to influence the development of the NHS. These are mainly called either Modernisation Boards or Task Forces and are composed of clinicians, managers, and the public.

The NHS Plan was greeted with great acclaim, not least by doctors, but the enthusiasm for the changes gradually began to dissipate. One of the reasons for the frustration, particularly of doctors, was the

428

slowness with which the increased resources reached them, thus preventing the increasing autonomy of action and improvement of services that seemed to be on offer. Another cause of frustration, particularly for doctors, is the perceived undue emphasis on improved access for patients and the number of targets being set for the NHS.

To sharpen up the management of the Health Service and to involve clinicians, especially those from primary care, in the management of the Health Service, the government in March 2001 embarked on a radical restructure of the NHS by deciding to abolish health authorities by 2002 and Regional Offices by 2003. This development has been named "Shifting the Balance of Power." The principal aspects of the restructuring are as follows:

• PCTs will become the lead NHS organizations in assessing need, planning and securing all health services. To improve health they will engage local communities and lead the NHS contribution to working with local government and other partners. It is expected that every PCG will have become a budget-holding PCT by October 2002. Most of these were in place by April 2002. By 2004 and possibly 2003, after transitional arrangements, the PCTs will have at their disposal 100 percent of local NHS money, amounting to some 75 percent of total NHS resources. The other 25 percent is held at central level for costs such as new capital expenditure, GPs' pay, and the administration of the Health Service.

• NHS trusts will continue to provide services, working within service agreements with the PCTs. All high-performing trusts will earn greater freedoms and autonomy in recognition of their achievements. Such NHS trusts will be existing hospitals, PCTs, and ambulance services and, once well established, the stand-alone mental health trusts that will be set up in conurbations.

• As of April 2002, just under thirty strategic health authorities have replaced the existing ninety-five health authorities. They will step back from service planning and commissioning to lead the strategic development of the local Health Service and performance manage PCTs and NHS trusts on the basis of local accountability agreements.

• The Department of Health will change the way in which it relates to the NHS, focusing on supporting the delivery of the NHS Plan. The eight NHS Executive Regional Offices will be abolished by 2003 and four new regional directors of health and social care will oversee the development of the NHS and provide the link between NHS organizations and the central department.

• Directors of public health will be on the boards of all PCTs and there will be directors of public health attached to Government Offices, of which there are nine. These Government Offices have a much wider view over the public sector beyond the Health Service. Previously directors of public health were at health authority and Regional Office levels. PCTs will have clinicians on the main board and a majority of clinicians on the Executive Board, which will be in charge of everyday planning and management.

In June 2001 the general election gave the Labour government a majority of 167, the largest overall majority ever given to a second-term administration. Despite this vote of confidence by the British public, all members of the Labour administration during the election campaign were put under enormous pressure about the poor running of the Health Service. This pressure has culminated in a determination to deliver the NHS Plan and to set, year on year, very specific targets. These are the key immediate targets:

• For the conditions with the greatest clinical priority—cancer and heart disease and services for the elderly and those with a mental illness, covering the areas of prevention, treatment, and rehabilitation—the ambition is "to give our country levels of cancer and cardiac care that are no longer behind the rest, but up with the best in Europe."

• For primary care—the point of contact of most patients with the NHS—the priority is to increase the number of GPs as well as nurses and other primary care professionals, to get extra investment to the front line in primary care and in measures that will give patients easier access to primary care services, including a major rebuilding program for primary care premises. (GPs and their staff currently undertake approximately 300 million consultations a year.)

• For emergency care—invest more in ambulance services, build on the investment in accident and emergency departments, and expand the NHS Direct twenty-four-hour phone service staffed by nurses.

• For waiting time, which is the biggest concern about the NHS today, make significant reductions. Waiting times need to be improved in primary care, for ambulance services, in outpatient clinics, and for inpatient treatment and accident and emergency care as well.

To help meet these targets, numerous organizations and processes have been introduced. Although all are relevant, they will need to be managed to create a coherent service understandable to patient, public, and NHS staff alike. Here are some examples of the new initiatives:

National Service Frameworks. These frameworks have been published in the four clinical priority areas discussed. They are drawn up by clinical experts and the service is then expected to meet the targets set. Extra monies have been found for many of these areas, and national clinical directors (known as czars) have been identified for the four initial clinical areas with further national clinical directors for primary care services and children's services subsequently appointed.

Part of the plan is to increase the numbers of all types of clinical professionals over the next few years by rapidly expanding training at both undergraduate and postgraduate levels. Other frameworks are planned over the next few years for diabetes, renal service, children's services, and services for patients with long-term clinical problems such as neurological conditions.

The Modernisation Agency. This is now a considerable support agency that incorporates a leadership center and employs many staff for the support of clinical professionals in redesigning services and care processes to make them more effective and efficient. The methodologies are evidence-based, and many of them draw on the work of Dr. Donald Berwick and his Institute for Healthcare Improvement, based in Boston, Massachusetts.

A proposed NHS University, similar in function to other corporate universities.

· The Plan notes that primary care is to continue its lead role in the NHS, building on previous initiatives such as fundholding but now made more systematic through the development of PCTs. Primary care, until the last ten years, was excluded from the strategic development of the National Health Service.

Patient and public involvement is to be incorporated, again systematically, into the National Health Service at both operational and strategic levels, and, furthermore, local health systems are to be scrutinized by local government—thus addressing, to some extent, the democratic deficit of the Health Service.

Quality and accountability are to be tackled in several ways. All clinical staff will be appraised yearly and revalidated using summative methodology every five years. The independent Commission for Health Improvement will review local health systems regularly and a Patient's Safety Agency will receive and review any adverse incidents affecting patients. All clinical professionals are involved in reviewing quality through the local clinical governance arrangements set up some four years ago. Much of this quality agenda developed over many years but has been given added force by recent revelations of wrongdoing. (A GP named Dr. Shipman was found to have been systematically murdering his patients. In addition, several well-documented instances of poor-quality services have been reported, in particular regarding the care of children undergoing surgery in the Bristol Hospital. The latter culminated in an independent enquiry that made various recommendations about accountability and quality, which the government is to respond to in the near future and is likely to accept in toto.)

Targets are set to ensure that the NHS Plan is delivered and, in the short term, for the key priority areas described here. Organizations that meet these targets are given more autonomy in spending further resources and have access to extra monies through a performance fund. Underperforming organizations would also access the performance fund but can only spend these extra resources with the help and support of local management review and working with the Modernisation Agency.

The description of some of the organizations will give a flavor of the many initiatives introduced into the NHS to ensure increasing quality, accountability, and a consistent approach throughout the country. Doctors in particular, even GPs to whom much more influence has been given, are feeling very poorly motivated at present, in part due to the rising pressure of workload but also, I suggest, because of the demand of higher patient aspirations and a need for more accountability. In this they are similar to doctors in other parts of the world who similarly describe disaffection.

Doctors and their leaders will need to grasp and accept changing patient aspirations, the demand for better and more consistent quality, and a more overt accountability; these pressures are inevitable and, to many of us, desirable if we are to have a truly responsive health service. To many the changes and new organizations may seem too numerous and too centralist, but if we have a National Health Service the "Headquarters" have a right and responsibility to set a national framework and structures to describe what is needed. Local staff need to be engaged in the "how" and by delivering the "how" will increasingly influence the "what." That will be the challenge and, if grasped, the opportunity for all—but in particular for the clinical professionals. The future may give less perceived power but more accountable influence.

To many, more money and a higher percentage of GDP devoted to the Health Service would solve the problems of the NHS, and indeed the need for increasing resources has been accepted. Improvement will also need to come from a change of culture, including of management. Such a change is predictably less universally accepted. As professor Ilona Kickbusch of Yale University has observed, health systems tend to concentrate mainly on finance and access to care when they should also concentrate on the redesigning of health care systems and the wider concept of the betterment of health (1999). Health care systems, however richly funded, are relatively peripheral to health gain; what we need, as health professionals, is to ensure that the money we receive for health care is spent to maximum effectiveness so that monies are available for government and others to concentrate on and address the wider social determinants of health that do damage to so many of our population.

The U.K. government is devoting a large amount of its resources outside the NHS in areas such as lessening child poverty, improving the education system for all, and building up a decaying national infrastructure as health needs take a higher priority than health care systems alone. Despite some increasing private provision, the health system in the United Kingdom for the foreseeable future will be funded almost entirely from taxation as it is part of the wider concept of "solidarity," it being an integral part of a system to address social and economic justice as much as improving technical aspects of clinical care. The NHS as a concept still retains massive popularity in the United Kingdom even though there is a widespread acceptance that quality and responsiveness need to improve.

LOCAL POSTSCRIPT

The Castlefields Health Centre continues to innovate and challenge clinical practice. It has been, since 1997, a personal medical services (PMS) pilot, taking part in an initiative that now covers 20 percent of all GPs in England. The government wishes this figure to be at least a third of all GPs as PMS fulfills government philosophy by encouraging local autonomy in return for very specific quality markers. The new national GP contract currently being negotiated may well follow a similar path.

Under personal medical services, the practice receives a budget for all the team. The Castlefields Practice, by working closely with our nursing colleagues and offering systematic care to our patients, has produced over three years a 47 percent fall in death rate in patients suffering with existing heart disease. This figure has now been achieved by the PCG and has been set as a national marker. Separately through working with nurses in the lead, we have identified savings of more than £2.5 million in patients who are elderly or patients suffering from mental disease. This has been achieved by cutting dramatically admission rates and lengths of stay in hospital.

Halton and Warrington Hospitals have merged to form a single acute hospital trust delivering care on two sites. Runcorn PCG in 2002 will merge with Widnes PCG and become a PCT, incorporating the local Community Services Trust—which will then cease to exist.

Halton Health Authority and the Northwest Regional Office will go out of existence (in 2002 and 2003, respectively) following national restructuring and will be replaced by a strategic health authority covering a larger area than the health authority but less than the previous Regional Office.

References

Department of Health. *The New NHS: Modern Dependable* (White Paper). London: National Health Service, 1997.

Kickbusch, I. "Community Health Initiatives." Presentation to conference titled "Health Care: A Global Perspective V," Wroclaw, Poland, Aug. 5, 1999.

Langlands, A., and Dixon, J. "The Promise of Innovation: Can Elephants Dance?—The NHS and beyond." *NHS Executive.* Unpublished paper dated Mar. 30, 1999.

Pridham, H. "Jumping the Theatre Queue." *LondonTimes*, Mar. 25, 2000, p. 43.

—✶— Index

AARP, 242, 257, 299
Abbott Northwestern Hospital, 320, 321
Access to care: cost-sharing and, 34;
    and decentralization, 95; fair, 401;
    goal of, 1; improving, 406–408;
    overstating issue of, 354; patient
    satisfaction survey on, *157–158*;
    purchasing specifications on,
    287–288
Access to drugs. *See* Pharmaceuticals,
    access to
Accountability: for asthma
    management, increasing, among
    providers, 215–217; of business
    units, 62–67; of businesses, issue
    of, 325; of cities, 136–137;
    of health plans, 310, 311; at the
    local and practitioner level, 381,
    426, 429, 432, 433
Accreditation requirement, 345.
    See also National Committee
    for Quality Assurance
    (NCQA)
ACE inhibitors, use of, 51, 52, 218
Action plans, network managers
    developing, 74–76
Active employees, plans for, 57–60
Acute care, 130; purchasing
    specifications on, *282–284*
Acute myocardial infarction (AMI),
    49–50, 76, *77*, 350
Additional Medical Insurance
    (AMI), 46–47
Additional payments, 381, 382
Adjusted average per capita cost
    (AAPCC), 254–255, 264

Administration: benefits, outsourcing,
    62, 66; changes in, confusion over,
    62; fees for, 70, 73; of fundholding,
    379; and funding levels, 5, 6;
    increasing resources for, concern
    with, 43; for private physician
    group practice, 148; of sickness
    funds, 183–184
Admission rates: cutting, 434; by
    disease category, *41*; by year, 128
Adult day health center, 255
Adverse risk selection, 194
Advertising and marketing, 142, 144,
    184, 194, 267; direct-to-consumer,
    32, 224
Advertising campaign, counter-
    tobacco, 319
Agency for Health Care Policy and
    Research (AHCPR), 207, 319
Agency for Healthcare Research and
    Quality, 333
Aging population, 2, 87, 168, 205, 298,
    347–348, 349, 412. *See also* Elderly
    population
Aging Services Access Points (ASAPs),
    250–251, 254, 257, 258, 262, 263,
    264, 267, *272*, 296
"Aging Society," 27, 47
Agreement on Trade-Related Aspects
    of Intellectual Property Rights,
    Including Trade in Counterfeit
    Goods (TRIPS agreement), 105
AHCPR-funded project, 207, 319
Ahrens, R., 303
Allina Foundation, 321
Allina Health System, 306, 320, 321, 322